Neurosurgical Aspects of Pregnancy

AANS Publications Committee
Christopher M. Loftus, MD, Editor

Neurosurgical Topics

The American Association of
Neurological Surgeons

Library of Congress Catalog
ISBN: 1-879284-36-7

Neurosurgical Topics ISBN: 0-9624246-6-8

Printed in U.S.A.

The American Association of Neurological Surgeons
22 South Washington Street
Park Ridge, Illinois 60068-4287

This publication is published under the auspices of the Publications Committee of the American Association of Neurological Surgeons (AANS). However, this should not be construed as indicating endorsement or approval of the views presented by the AANS, or by its committees, commissions, affiliates, or staff.

Daniel L. Barrow, MD, Chairman
AANS Publications Committee

Gay Palazzo, AANS Staff Editor

AANS1.75M1195

Neurosurgical Topics Series

Forthcoming Books

1996

Subarachnoid Hemorrhage: Pathophysiology and Treatment
Edited by Joshua B. Bederson, MD

Syringomyelia and the Chiari Malformations
Edited by John A. Anson, MD, Edward C. Benzel, MD, and Issam A. Awad, MD

Surgery of the Visual Pathways
Edited by Linda L. Sternau, MD

Neural Tube Defects
Edited by J. Gordon McComb, MD

Dedication

to my daughter

Mary Catherine Loftus

whose gestation and birth
formed the inspiration for this project

CONTENTS

List of Contributors

Harold P. Adams, Jr., MD
Division of Cerebrovascular Disorders
Department of Neurology
University of Iowa
Iowa City, Iowa

Hans E. Bakken, MD
Division of Neurosurgery
Department of Surgery
University of Iowa College of Medicine
Iowa City, Iowa

H. Hunt Batjer, MD
Professor and Chief
Division of Neurological Surgery
Northwestern University Medical School
Chicago, Illinois

Steven J. Beer, MD
Division of Neurosurgery
Department of Surgery
University of Iowa Hospitals and Clinics
Iowa City, Iowa

John Bodensteiner, MD
Professor, Department of Neurology
West Virginia University
Morgantown, West Virginia

Patricia H. Davis, MD
Division of Cerebrovascular Disorders
Department of Neurology
University of Iowa
Iowa City, Iowa

Jerry Day, MD
Department of Surgery
Division of Neurosurgery
Milton S. Hershey Medical Center
Hershey, Pennsylvania

Mark Gibson, MD
Professor and Chairman
Department of Obstetrics and Gynecology
West Virginia University
Morgantown, West Virginia

Mark G. Hamilton, MDCM, FRCS(C)
Department of Clinical Neurosciences
University of Calgary
Foothills Hospital and
Alberta Children's Hospital
Calgary, Alberta, Canada

William C. Hanigan, MD,PHD
Clinical Professor of Neurological Surgery
and Pediatrics
Department of Neurosurgery
University of Illinois
College of Medicine at Peoria
Peoria, Illinois

Robert Hoeldtke, MD
Professor, Department of Medicine
West Virginia University
Morgantown, West Virginia

Russell D. Hull, MB,BS,MSC,FCCP
Department of Medicine
University of Calgary
Foothills Hospital
Calgary, Alberta, Canada

Michael R. Jacoby, MD
Division of Cerebrovascular Disorders
Department of Neurology
University of Iowa
Iowa City, Iowa

Howard H. Kaufman, MD
Professor and Chairman
Department of Neurosurgery
West Virginia University
Morgantown, West Virginia

John P. Laurent, MD
Chief, Section of Pediatric Neurosurgery
Baylor College of Medicine
Texas Children's Hospital
Houston, Texas

Christopher M. Loftus, MD
Professor of Neurological Surgery
Department of Surgery
University of Iowa Hospitals and Clinics
Iowa City, Iowa

Michael D. Medlock, MD
Assistant Professor of Neurosurgery
and Pediatrics
Georgetown University
Washington, DC

Leon Moores, MD
Department of Neurological Surgery
Walter Reed Army Medical Center
Washington, DC

Michael G. Muhonen, MD
Division of Neurosurgery
Department of Surgery
University of Iowa
Iowa City, Iowa

John D. Olson, MD, PHD
Professor, Vice Chairman for Clinical Affairs
Department of Pathology
University of Iowa
Iowa City, Iowa

Richard K. Osenbach, MD
Assistant Professor of Surgery
F. Edward Hebert School of Medicine
Uniformed Services
University of Health Sciences
Bethesda, Maryland
Attending Neurosurgeon
Walter Reed Army Medical Center
Washington, DC

Nelson M. Oyesiku, MD, PHD
Assistant Professor
Department of Neurosurgery
Emory University School of Medicine
Atlanta, Georgia

Donald H. Penning, MD, MSC,FRCP
Department of Anesthesiology
University of Iowa Hospital
Iowa City, Iowa

Graham F. Pineo, MD, FRCP(C)
Department of Medicine
University of Calgary
Foothills Hospital
Calgary, Alberta, Canada

John G. Piper, MD
Division of Neurological Surgery
The University of Iowa College of Medicine
Iowa City, Iowa

Setti S. Rengachary, MD
Professor, Department of Neurosurgery
University of Minnesota
Minneapolis, Minnesota

Timothy C. Ryken, MD
Assistant Professor of Neurological Surgery
State University of New York
Upstate Medical Center
Syracuse, New York

Michael Salcman, MD, FACS
Clinical Professor of Neurosurgery
George Washington University
Washington, DC

Paul D. Sawin, MD
Division of Neurosurgery
University of Iowa Hospitals and Clinics
Iowa City, Iowa

Joel D. Siegal, MD
Department of Neurosurgery
University of Minnesota
Minneapolis, Minnesota

Dale M. Swift, MD
Assistant Clinical Professor of Neurosurgery
University of Texas
Southwestern Medical Center
Children's Medical Center
Dallas, Texas

Karen A. Valentine, MD, PHD, FRCP(C)
Department of Medicine
University of Calgary
Foothills Hospital
Calgary, Alberta, Canada

Wendy Ziai, MD
Department of Clinical Neurosciences
University of Calgary
Foothills Hospital
Calgary, Alberta, Canada

AANS Publications Committee

The American Association of Neurological Surgeons is accredited by the Accreditation Council for Continuing Medical Education (CME) to sponsor continuing medical education for physicians.

The American Association of Neurological Surgeons designates the continuing medical education activity as 15 credit hours in Category I of the Physician's Recognition Award of the American Medical Association.

PREFACE

This volume of the *Neurosurgical Topics Series* is dedicated to neurosurgical topics related to pregnancy. This is a broad subject which crosses several disciplines. It became apparent to the editor that although a significant amount of information was available on the neurosurgical care of pregnant patients, the problem was sufficiently rare that this information was not organized in any specific place. When faced with a difficult clinical problem requiring a better understanding of the physiology of pregnancy, the natural history of neurosurgical disorders (especially cerebrovascular disorders) in pregnant patients, and/or the propriety of and options available for surgical intervention in pregnant women, the references were rather diffuse and difficult to pull together. A decision was made in concert with the Publications Committee of the American Association of Neurological Surgeons and its Chairman, Dr. Daniel Barrow, to prepare a text on neurosurgery in pregnancy.

The book breaks naturally into three major divisions. The first section addresses nonsurgical topics that affect decision-making in pregnant patients. These include chapters on physiology and thrombosis, radiation protection, anesthesia, and drug toxicity. This information is often very difficult for neurosurgeons to access elsewhere. The second section deals with specific neurosurgical disorders that are either unique to or substantially different in pregnant patients. A sincere effort has been made to address the relevant surgical considerations related to each of these disorders. The third major section includes those topics which did not fit readily in the previous two, including positioning issues, intrauterine diagnosis, intrauterine neurosurgery, and finally ethical concerns. While the chapter on intrauterine neurosurgery may not be applicable to practicing neurosurgeons it was included because of the fascinating nature of this developing field and the long-term implications of this research. The concluding chapter on ethical issues and brain death considerations in pregnant patients will certainly have applicability to any neurosurgical practice.

This book was intended to serve two purposes. We hope that it will provide a reference source, bringing together the entire constellation of problems referable to pregnancy. Likewise, we hope that the second section in which specific neurosurgical disorders are dealt with on an individual basis will prove helpful in surgical planning and in surgical management of pregnant patients for the individual neurosurgeon. I have been pleased with the individual efforts of the various chapter authors and appreciate their willingness to contribute to this work. I would likewise like to express my gratitude to my colleagues on the Publications Committee for their constructive commentary and to Gay Palazzo and her staff at the AANS Publications Office for successfully producing the volume. Finally, I would like to express my gratitude to my secretary at The University of Iowa Hospitals, Kathy Escher, for her efforts in preparing these manuscripts for publication.

Christopher M. Loftus MD, FACS
Iowa City, Iowa

CHAPTER 1

FETAL TOXICITY OF COMMON NEUROSURGICAL DRUGS

JOHN G. PIPER, MD

A variety of neurosurgical disorders may arise in the pregnant patient.[38,42,55,65,85,93,99,110,112,117,124,129,160] All of these conditions share fundamental principles of medical management in the pre- and postoperative periods which are imperative for successful outcomes. Some common medications can cause serious fetal toxicity, so the treating neurosurgeon requires an understanding of appropriate drug therapy in the pregnant neurosurgical patient. This need is strengthened by the fact that commonly used neurosurgical drugs are not widely prescribed by other physicians caring for pregnant patients. It may fall upon the neurosurgeon most to make informed decisions regarding proper medication selection.

The principles that guide drug prescription during pregnancy are based on the concept of the fetomaternal unit.[82] The well-being of the fetus is dependent on maintenance of maternal health. Active untreated disease of the mother will have adverse affects on both maternal and fetal well-being. In the words of Gideon Koren, "the well being of the mother should dictate her need for drug therapy."[82] No serious medical condition in the mother should go untreated. Fortunately, numerous therapeutic options are available for the treatment of most clinical conditions, so the physician should seek an appropriate treatment which offers the best maternal outcome while minimizing risks to the developing fetus. This chapter will review commonly used drugs in neurosurgery (Table 1) and discuss their respective risks of fetal toxicity to provide the necessary information for an informed decision regarding treatment.

DEVELOPMENTAL TOXICOLOGY

Developmental toxicology is the study of the relationship between chemical or environmen-

TABLE 1

COMMONLY USED DRUGS IN NEUROSURGERY

Anticonvulsants
Phenytoin
Phenobarbital and primidone
Carbamazepine
Other anticonvulsants
Bromocriptine
Anticoagulants
Warfarin
Heparin
Corticosteroids
Diuretic medications
Mannitol
Other diuretics
Nimodipine

tal agents and the development of congenital anomalies.[138] Congenital malformations are identified in 3% to 5% of all live births, and in 1% to 2%, these malformations are severe.[138] In up to two-thirds of the cases, no known cause for a malformation can be identified.[138] Between 25% and 30% of the malformations are related to chromosomal abnormalities, 3% to radiation, infection, or maternal disease, and between 2% and 6% to drugs and environmental chemicals. During the time of gestation, 60% to 75% of pregnant patients will receive between three and 10 medications. While accurate figures are not available, illicit drug use has been suspected in >10% of all pregnancies. Because medications are one area that can be controlled, the realm of developmental toxicology takes on great clinical importance.

The main focus of developmental toxicology is on structural malformations associated with exposure to various agents (Table 2). The term "teratology" is derived from the Greek word "teras," meaning malformation.[138] In practical use, teratology applies not only to malformations but also to other manifestations including growth retardation, impaired function, and fetal and neonatal death.[138] Equally important areas of concern are transient toxic, metabolic, or physiological side effects of medications used during pregnancy.[138] Examples include adrenal cortex suppression from maternal use of glucocorticoids and coagulation defects in neonates whose mothers are treated with various anticonvulsant medications. As a general rule, the fetus appears to be much more susceptible than the mother to the adverse side effects of medications.

Numerous factors determine teratogenic susceptibility of the developing fetus to various medications (Table 2). Of prime importance is species susceptibility.[10,16,138] Chemicals which are known teratogens in the human population may produce very few malformations in animal studies. Conversely, many agents used safely in the pregnant patient have been shown to cause birth defects in animals, often with supratherapeutic doses. While animal research can serve as a screening tool and reveal insight into teratogenic mechanisms, results of these experiments cannot be extrapolated directly to human beings.

TABLE 2

Developmental Toxicology

Teratogenic effects
Congenital malformations
Growth retardation
Functional impairment
Metabolic or physiological impairment
Fetal wastage or neonatal death
Issues involved in teratogenicity
Species susceptibility
Timing of exposure
Drug administration
Dosage
Duration of exposure
Pharmacokinetic alterations in pregnancy
Placental transfer and metabolism

Another important aspect in developmental toxicology is the timing of drug exposure.[83,121,138] In order for teratogenic effects to occur, fetal exposure to a chemical agent must occur at a susceptible stage in development. The highest susceptibility occurs typically during the period of organogenesis in the first trimester. An excellent example of this phenomenon is the high incidence of birth defects in mothers taking warfarin during the first trimester compared to a much lower rate when this drug is taken during the second and third trimesters.[83]

Developmental toxicology also examines potential dose-dependent relationships between drugs and birth defects. It would be anticipated that higher doses should correlate with a higher incidence of teratogenicity. For example, most anticonvulsants show a dose-dependent teratogenic relationship. Teratogenicity is not always dose-dependent, however, as demonstrated by the teratogenic effects of phenytoin, which may not be dose-dependent.[48] The duration of exposure to a given drug and the dosing interval may also play an important role.[45,93,138]

Other factors influencing teratogenicity include changes in maternal pharmacokinetics and the role of the placenta during pregnancy. The volume of distribution of nearly all drugs is increased during pregnancy.[93] The placenta also has metabolic and placental transfer functions.[46,74,82,101,155,175] The placenta contains nu-

TABLE 3

FOOD AND DRUG ADMINISTRATION CATEGORIES OF DRUG RISK IN PREGNANCY*

Category	Risk in Pregnancy	Human and/or Animal Data
A	None known	Controlled human studies fail to show fetal risk
B	Unlikely	Either: A) animal studies fail to show risk but no controlled human studies, or B) fetal risk in animal studies but controlled human studies fail to show risk
C	Unknown	No controlled human studies and either: A) fetal risk in animal studies, or B) no animal studies available
D	Definite but *may* be acceptable	Controlled human studies show fetal risk, but medication *may* be necessary in certain circumstances
X	Definite and unacceptable	Animal and/or controlled human studies show fetal risk, and medication is absolutely contraindicated

*Adapted from Federal Register.[47]

merous bioactivating enzymes, such as the cytochrome P450 mono-oxygenase system, which participate in biotransformation of medications taken by the mother.[74,101] Placental transfer is also regulated by drug characteristics (molecular weight, ionization, and lipid solubility) and by placental properties (rates of maternal and fetal placental blood flow, placental metabolism, and placental age).[82,101,155]

Given the complex factors involved in developmental toxicology, it is not surprising that much remains to be discovered regarding the safe medical management of the pregnant woman. Approximately 3,000 chemicals have been tested for teratogenicity, with 600 agents shown to produce developmental toxicity in experimental animals. Only 35 of these agents have clearly been shown to cause birth defects in human beings.[94] Because of concern over the remaining agents, drugs are often designated by their manufacturer to be contraindicated during pregnancy or that their safety has not been established. To maximize safety, the Food and Drug Administration (FDA) has developed a classification system to assist the physician in drug selection during pregnancy (Table 3).[23,47,94,176] This classification system divides drugs into risk categories A, B, C, D, and X and provides physicians with a rapid source of information regarding the relative safety of medications from both animal and human studies.

COMMONLY USED MEDICATIONS IN THE NEUROSURGICAL PATIENT

Anticonvulsants

The most common issue of drug prescription during pregnancy that neurosurgeons will encounter is the treatment of maternal seizure disorders. Children of epileptic mothers have been shown to have an increased risk of congenital anomalies, even after attempts to control extraneous factors such as parity and maternal age.[13,42,75,95,167,178] At best, 14% of such children have congenital anomalies compared with 5.6% of the general population.[48] Other studies substantiate a two- to three-fold increase in the risk of congenital anomalies.[13,70,78,107,153,156] In addition to congenital anomalies, other complications can arise in the pregnant patient who is taking anticonvulsants, and a normal outcome following pregnancy is anticipated in only 80% of cases.[107,177,178]

Some have suggested that the high incidence of birth defects is related to the underlying seizure disorder or other factors.[41,44,52,80,81,107,141,157] While these may be contributory, it appears that anticonvulsant use contributes significantly to birth defects.[13,41,48,62,70,78,85,123] This view is supported by studies in which seizure frequency failed to correlate with higher rates of birth defects.[48] Furthermore, the teratogenic effects are compounded when multiple anticonvulsant medications are employed.[48] Despite the documented risks of anticonvulsants, it is clear that risks to both the mother and fetus are much greater if an active seizure disorder goes untreated.[85,162]

Some generalizations can be made regarding adverse effects of anticonvulsants. These medications are strongly associated with the development of cleft lip and cleft palate, limb abnormalities, and cardiac malformations.[2,5,42,44,70,78,85,113,141] Increased rates of prematurity, intrauterine growth retardation, and perinatal/neonatal mortality have all been observed.[18] The risk of spontaneous abortion, stillbirth, microcephaly, and mental retardation may also be increased.[4] The infants of mothers on anticonvulsants have an increased risk of epilepsy (3%), and the mothers may also experience increased seizure activity during gestation, although the latter remains controversial.[177] Patients with epileptic seizures during pregnancy are at an increased risk for toxemia.[177] Finally, infants of mothers taking anticonvulsants have a higher rate of fetal hemorrhage (10%), and the incidence of maternal vaginal bleeding is increased as well (10%).[177] Given the variety of potential complications, the epileptic mother should be considered to have a high-risk pregnancy.[18]

The etiology of anticonvulsant fetal toxicity remains obscure. Some have suggested that underlying genetic factors or anticonvulsant metabolites may play an important role, especially with phenytoin.[23,49,70,78,157] Recent reports have also noted an association between folic acid deficiency from anticonvulsants and birth defects.[5,13,85,179] In particular, folic acid deficiency is strongly associated with the use of phenytoin and phenobarbital.[13,85] Support for this theory includes the observation that other medications which lower folic acid levels are associated with birth defects.[170] While this is only one of many possible underlying factors in the teratogenicity of anticonvulsants, it is a correctable problem.

Phenytoin

Phenytoin is one of the most widely used anticonvulsants in the management of neurosurgical patients. It readily crosses the placental barrier, with fetal blood levels approximately one-half that of the mother.[105,113] Phenytoin appears to concentrate in the fetal liver, kidneys, adrenal glands, and heart.[105] In addition, maternal phenytoin consumption has been associated with induction of the fetal hepatic cytochrome P-450 system.[105]

Both animal and human studies have shown a strong correlation between phenytoin use during pregnancy and development of congenital anomalies.[13,49,50,62,78] This phenomenon may not be dose-dependent.[23,48] Because of known teratogenicity and the potential concurrent need during gestation, this medication is classified in FDA category D.[23] While the etiological factors involved in the teratogenicity of this medication remain obscure, recent studies have demonstrated that phenytoin's teratogenic effects may arise from underlying genetic factors, epoxide metabolites, and/or folic acid deficiency.[13,49,70,78,85,113] Patients taking this medication during gestation should receive folic acid supplementation.[13]

Birth defects caused by phenytoin may vary widely.[49,50,62,78,85] Most characteristic is the fetal hydantoin syndrome, which is identified in 5% to 40% of infants whose mothers have taken this medication during gestation.[13,60,78] Characteristic features include craniofacial anomalies such as a broad nasal bridge, upturned nose, hypertelorism, ptosis, epicanthic folds, and low-set ears (Figure 1A and B).[60,61,78,85,113] Cleft lip and cleft palate appear to be correlated strongly with the use of Dilantin.[13,44,45,48,60,78,85] Fontanelles may be enlarged or craniosynostosis may occur, with the fused sutures forming prominent bony ridges.[60,61,78] Limb involvement is quite common and includes hypoplasia of the distal phalanges and nails (Figure 1C and D).[60,61,78,79,85] The thumb often appears morphologically indistinguishable from other fingers.[60,61] Atypical palmar creases are also commonly encountered. Growth and development may be altered, and mild to moderate mental retardation is common.[60,61,78,85]

Additional findings include widely spaced nipples as well as rib and sternal malformations.[61] Spine abnormalities associated with a low hairline and nuchal webbing have been reported.[60,61,78] Other major congenital anom-

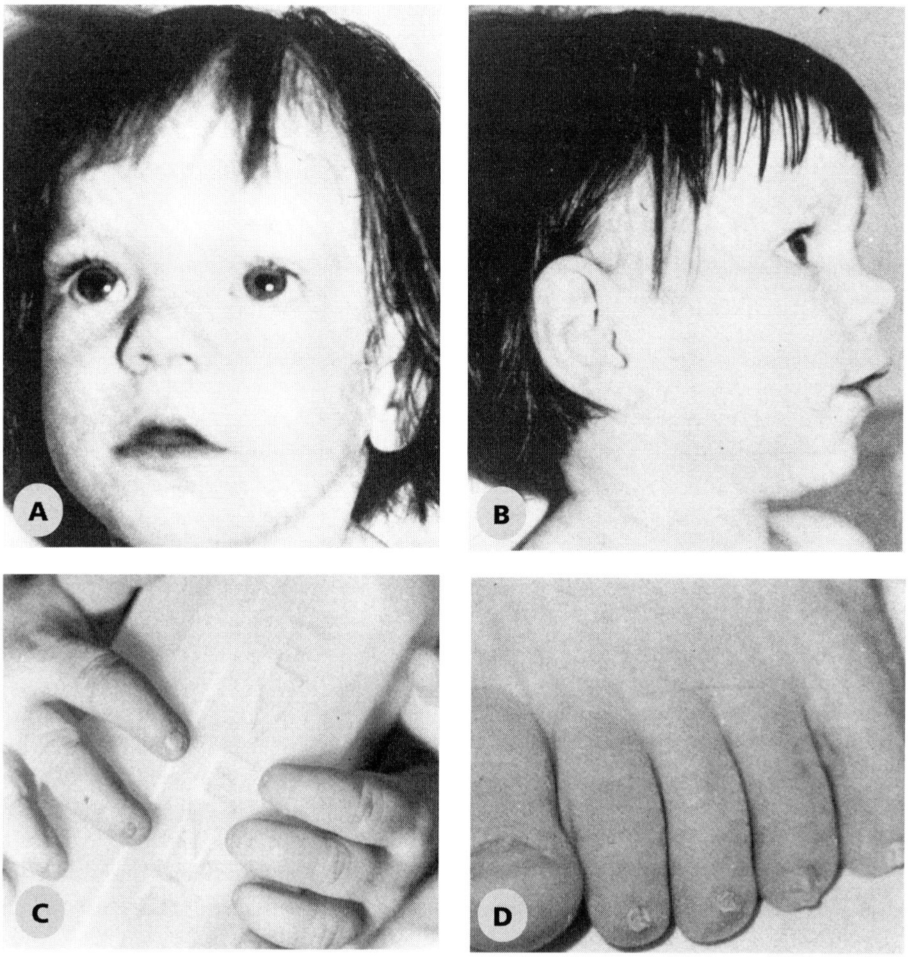

Figure 1: A and B) A fetal hydantoin syndrome patient exhibiting the characteristic facies with hypertelorism, epicanthic folds, and a shallow nasal bridge. **C and D)** Limb involvement is also common, often taking the form of hypoplasia of the distal phalanges and nails of the upper (C) and lower (D) extremities. (Courtesy of James Hanson, M.D., The University of Iowa, Iowa City, Iowa.)

alies include cardiovascular and genitourinary malformations.[60,61] Diaphragmatic hernias have also been reported.[60] Phenytoin may also be a transplacental carcinogen associated with neuroblastoma and other tumors.[23] The risk of such malformations appears to be two- to three-fold greater in infants whose mothers took phenytoin.[60,61]

Phenobarbital and Primidone

Barbiturates and other related anticonvulsant drugs readily cross the placenta and concentrate within fetal tissues, particularly the liver and brain.[25,105] They are capable of inducing fetal hepatic mono-oxygenase activity and cause folic acid deficiency during pregnancy.[5,13,85,105] Furthermore, barbiturate medications may alter sex steroid levels and produce metabolic alterations such as lowering serum calcium levels by alterations in vitamin D metabolism.[30,48,105,137] The use of phenobarbital and related medications during pregnancy has been strongly associated with congenital malformations, prompting designation as FDA category D drugs.[23,110,139] The teratogenic effects of these medications are dose-dependent.[13,48]

Common congenital anomalies reported following the use of phenobarbital and related medications during pregnancy include numerous craniofacial anomalies.[23,110,139] A shortened nose with a low nasal bridge is often associated with hypertelorism, epicanthic folds, and ptosis.[110,139] Cleft lip and palate, relative prognathism, a widened mouth, and hypoplastic pharynx are also commonly reported.[139] Retarded skeletal development and limb abnormalities have been described, and psychomotor delay may also occur.[23,110,139]

Carbamazepine

Carbamazepine (FDA category C) is a tricyclic anticonvulsant which is commonly used in pregnancy.[23] Like the previously mentioned medications, it readily crosses the placenta and reaches fetal serum levels that are 50% to 80% of maternal levels.[42,105] Carbamazepine is almost evenly distributed in fetal tissues but has exhibited slightly higher levels within the liver and kidneys.[105] Carbamazepine levels are relatively low within the brain early in gestation but accumulate in later pregnancy and during infancy.[105] Like other anticonvulsants, carbamazepine is suspected of inducing hepatic mono-oxygenase activity, although this has not been demonstrated conclusively.[105] Carbamazepine has been associated with congenital defects in both animal and human studies.[45,73] While the etiological factors involved remain unclear, an epoxide metabolic intermediate may be involved in this medication's teratogenicity and that of phenytoin.[73,75,92]

Apart from common side effects of this medication (bone marrow suppression with aplastic anemia, agranulocytosis, thrombocytopenia, or leukopenia), several congenital anomalies have been specifically associated with carbamazepine's use during pregnancy.[95] Most common appear to be fingernail hypoplasia, which is identified in 26% of patients, and developmental delay, which occurs in 20%.[73] Craniofacial anomalies are identified in 11% and include microcephaly, narrow bifrontal diameter, upslanting palpebral fissures, and a short nose with long filtrum.[73] Cardiac defects have also been described.[73] The risk of spina bifida is increased 10-fold in patients taking carbamazepine.[85,131] This yields a 1% risk of spina bifida, which should prompt the use of prenatal diagnostic measures if the mother so desires.[85]

Other Anticonvulsant Medications

Ethosuximide (FDA category C) is a frequently used drug in the treatment of petit mal seizure disorders.[23,42] This medication has been widely used during pregnancy, and studies have revealed placental transfer with approximately equal maternal and fetal blood levels.[42,105,113] While clinical experience with this medication remains limited, ethosuximide does appear to have a low incidence of teratogenicity in human and animal studies.[13,21] This drug is often considered the anticonvulsant of choice for management of petit mal seizures in pregnancy.[42]

Benzodiazepines (diazepam and lorazepam, FDA category D; clonazepam, FDA category C) are occasionally employed in the management of epileptic patients, particularly acutely.[23] These medications readily cross the placenta and have a low rate of teratogenicity in animal studies.[13,21] Some studies in humans have demonstrated a weak relationship between this medication class and craniofacial anomalies such as cleft lip and palate.[13,21] When given close to the time of delivery, these medications can also cause withdrawal symptoms in the infant or the floppy infant syndrome.[21] All of the adverse effects appear to be dose-related.[21] These medications have been used in the treatment of status epilepticus during pregnancy.

Valproic acid (FDA category D) readily crosses the placental barrier, and while the fetal serum level is variable, it often exceeds that found in the maternal circulation.[23,105,106] The teratogenicity of this anticonvulsant has been clearly shown in animals.[24,35,45,83] In human studies, this anticonvulsant has been associated with fetal distress in almost one-half of reported cases and with low Apgar scores in 28%.[164] Major and minor congenital anomalies, collectively known as the fetal valproate syndrome, are also common.[7,128,161]

Features of fetal valproate syndrome include brachycephaly, a small nose with flat nasal bridge, hypertelorism, and shallow orbits (Figure 2).[161,164] The mouth has a thin upper vermil-

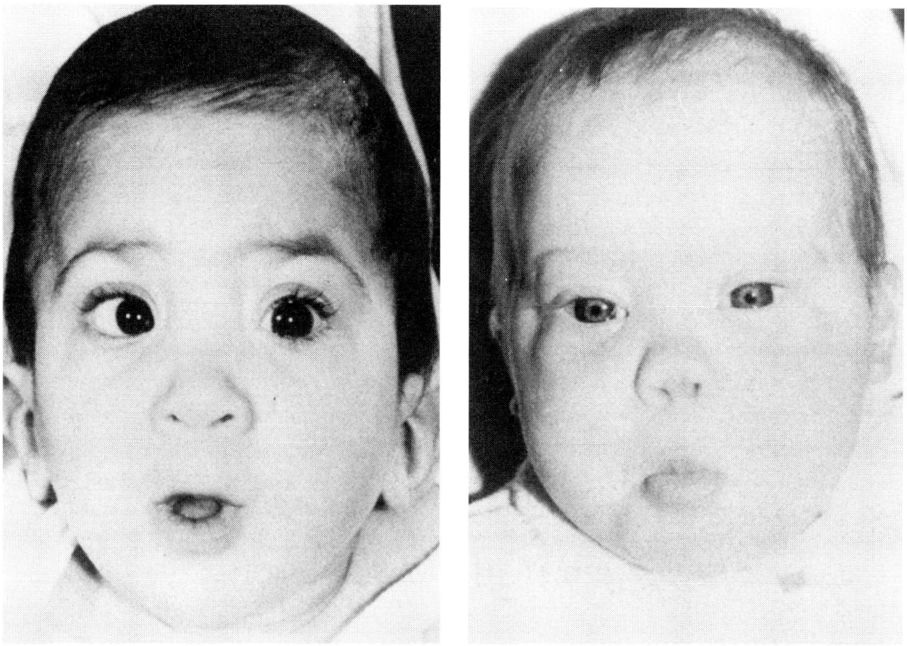

Figure 2: Fetal valproate syndrome is characterized by a typical facies which includes an upturned nose, elongated filtrum, hypertelorism, and epicanthic folds. The mouth is characteristically small with a thin upper vermilion border. Additional anomalies include low-set ears and brachycephaly. (From *Am J Med Genet 19:*473-481, 1984. Reprinted by permission of John Wiley & Sons, Inc.)

lion border and long upper lip, with micrognathia and microstomia also possible.[164] The ears are typically low-set with posterior rotation.[161,164] Inspection of the trunk reveals a broad chest with widely spaced nipples. The fingers and toes are often elongated and thin with hyperconvexity of the nails. Fetal valproate syndrome is frequently associated with growth retardation.[161] Other major congenital anomalies affecting the cardiovascular and genitourinary systems have also been reported.[7,83,128,164] Of specific concern is a higher incidence of neural tube defects, which are found in 1% to 2% of babies of patients taking this medication.[7,19,35,42, 71,83,85,127,161,173] Because of the high incidence of myelodysplasia, prenatal diagnosis should be offered to the mother. The risks associated with this anticonvulsant are dose-dependent and are increased with single daily dose administration because of the high peak serum levels.[71] Serum concentrations of valproic acid should be monitored closely if use of this anticonvulsant cannot be avoided.[71,173]

The anticonvulsant *trimethadione* (FDA category D) is often used in the treatment of petit mal seizures.[23,54,113] A distinct congenital syndrome, the fetal trimethadione syndrome has been reported in infants of mothers taking this medication.[35,42,54,69,78,113] Short stature is common, as is developmental and speech delay.[23,34,56,78,83] Characteristic facial features include V-shaped eyebrows and epicanthic folds (Figure 3).[35,56,78,83] The ears are low-set, and the helix is frequently folded anteriorly.[56,69] Palatal and dental anomalies are also common.[56,83,113] Inguinal hernias and hypospadias have been reported, and examination of the extremities frequently reveals digital anomalies and simian creases.[35,54,69] Additional major congenital anomalies have also been reported, including trigonocephaly, microcephaly, and major cardiovascular malformations.[35,54,56,69,78]

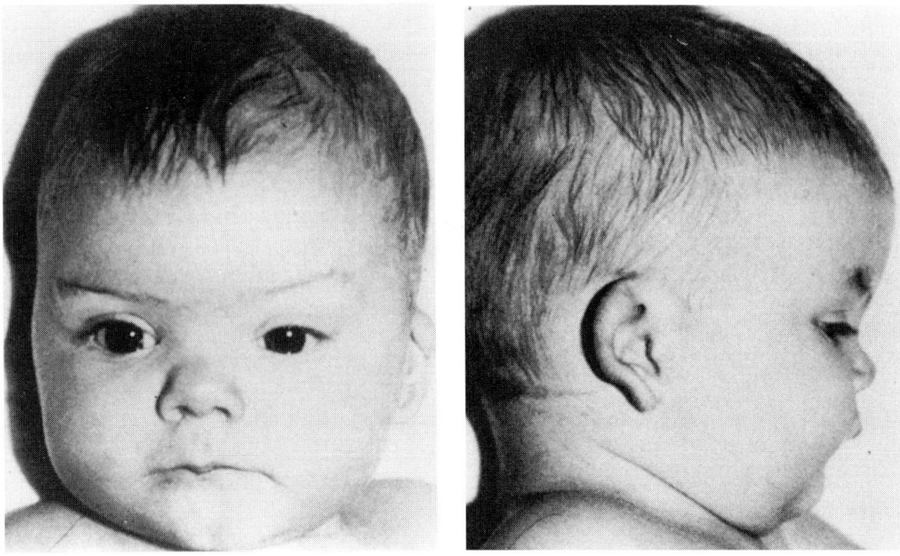

Figure 3: Fetal trimethadione exposure may result in a characteristic facies exhibiting V-shaped eyebrows, a shallow nasal bridge, and epicanthic folds. Also, the helix of the ear is often folded anteriorly. (Courtesy of James Hanson, M.D., The University of Iowa, Iowa City, Iowa.)

Treatment Recommendations During Pregnancy

It is clear that all anticonvulsant medications are potentially teratogenic.[48,104,146,147,156] This risk needs to be conveyed to the pregnant woman when anticonvulsants are started.[83,85,113,151] Furthermore, patients in the childbearing years who are already on anticonvulsant medications should be made aware of these risks so that they can make informed decisions regarding pregnancy.[35,88,113,151] They should be informed that the chances of having a normal child are 80% to 90% despite anticonvulsant therapy.[35,64,151]

The most common seizure disorders treated by neurosurgeons during pregnancy are of a generalized nature. Although both have been successfully employed, carbamazepine (FDA category C) in general may be preferable over phenytoin (FDA category D) during pregnancy.[23,35,95,102,133,149,150,165] It should be recalled that carbamazepine is associated with a higher risk of neural tube defects, so prenatal diagnosis should be offered to the patient on this medication.[35] The other anticonvulsants are best reserved as second-line therapy unless the patient's seizure disorder is known not to respond to carbamazepine.

Some fundamental principles apply to the prescription of anticonvulsant medications during gestation. If a patient has been seizure-free for a period of several years, withdrawing the anticonvulsant(s) may be attempted in order to minimize fetal and maternal risk.[35,151] The patient should be slowly tapered from medication with close follow-up so that anticonvulsants can be restarted if seizure activity recurs. If the patient's epilepsy is active, discontinuation of medication is not advised since the risks of prolonged seizure to both the mother and child outweigh the risks of the anticonvulsant medication.

The risks of congenital anomalies and side effects appear to increase with the number of anticonvulsant medications used.[35,48,71,85,104] One anticonvulsant should be employed whenever possible, and anticonvulsant levels followed closely.[85,104] If the patient develops seizure activity on one medication, a careful review of the patient's compliance and anticonvulsant level should be undertaken prior to increasing the dose or adding additional medications.[35] Also, the drug levels of most anticonvulsant medications can be expected to decrease during gestation, so dose adjustments are likely to be required throughout gestation.[36,87,90,177] While it is controversial whether seizure frequency actually increases during pregnancy, studies which show such an association often link inadequate anticonvulsant levels with increases in seizure activity.[85,87,104,177,178] If a different medication is to be tried, adequate therapeutic levels should be achieved with the new drug prior to discontinuation of the previously utilized anticonvulsant. Only when refractoriness to multiple single agents has been demonstrated should multiagent therapy be instituted.[35,71]

As previously mentioned, numerous anticonvulsants have been associated with folic acid deficiency, which may be an important factor in teratogenesis.[30,37,42,85,179] Folic acid supplementation should be employed concurrently if anticonvulsants are instituted during pregnancy.[42,85,179] For epileptic patients who are contemplating pregnancy, this medication should be started prior to conception when possible. The earlier that supplementation can be instituted, the more likely that severe congenital anomalies can be avoided since these tend to occur early in gestation during the period of organogenesis.

In addition to teratogenic effects, there are other possible side effects seen with anticonvulsant medications during pregnancy. A well-described phenomenon is the anticoagulant effect of these medications leading to hemorrhagic disease of the newborn.[25,35,85,103,123,154,159] These drugs cause depression of fetal vitamin K-dependent coagulation factors (factors II, VII, IX, and X) and prolongation of coagulation parameters.[25,35,85,103,154,159] Hemorrhage typically occurs within 24 hours of delivery, but intrapartum hemorrhage may occur.[85,154,159] Pathological findings include gastrointestinal, intra-abdominal, intrathoracic, and/or intracranial hemorrhage.[85,154,159] Medications most strongly associated with bleeding include phenytoin and barbiturate derivatives (phenobarbital and primidone), which produce bleeding in up to 7% of pregnancies.[25,35,85,103]

TABLE 4
TRANSMISSION RATES OF COMMON ANTICONVULSANT MEDICATIONS IN BREAST MILK

Medication	Kaneko et al[76]	Janz et al[71]
Valproic acid	not applicable	2%
Phenytoin	18.1%	30%
Phenobarbital	45.9%	40%
Carbamazepine	39.4%	45%
Primidone	80.9%	60%
Ethosuximide	78.8%	90%

Treatment includes maternal vitamin K_1 administration during the last 2 to 4 weeks of pregnancy and during labor.[35,39,85,103,154] Coagulation parameters should be checked at birth in every infant whose mother had received anticonvulsant therapy to identify coagulation defects, with specific factor assays performed as needed.[39,103,159] The risk of bleeding is high if vitamin K-dependent factors are less than 5% to 20% of the adult standard.[154,159] Infants should also be given 1 mg vitamin K_1 routinely, although this may not in all cases prevent hemorrhage.[35,103,154] If hemorrhage occurs, 10 ml/kg of fresh frozen plasma should be administered.[159] Some have also recommended prophylactic fresh frozen plasma if the vitamin K-dependent coagulation factors are severely depressed.[35,85,103,159] With prolonged labor, the risk of hemorrhage may be increased and cesarean section should be considered early.[159] Of final note, the mother's coagulation studies are almost always normal and should not be relied upon to predict the status of her infant.

Breast-Feeding and Anticonvulsant Treatment

Concern regarding anticonvulsant medications continues after delivery in mothers who are breast feeding their infants. Maternal milk transmission rates vary widely but are highest with primidone and ethosuximide (Table 4).[23,71,76,126] In general, breast feeding is only relatively contraindicated for mothers on anticonvulsants.[71,76,106] Factors to consider when making a decision regarding advisability of breast feeding include the type and dose of the anticonvulsant medication, the volume of milk used, the medication's transmission rate, and the infant's metabolic capacity.[71,76,126] Since anticonvulsant medications often produce sedative effects, the infant's mental status can be followed to determine if breast feeding is exposing the infant to significant levels of these medications.[14,71,126] Sedation, particularly common with benzodiazepines, phenobarbital, and primidone, is also seen with phenytoin.[23,71] The infant's serum drug levels should be monitored when these anticonvulsants are in maternal use. Because of sedation, breast feeding is contraindicated while nursing mothers are on most benzodiazepines.[14,23,118,126] There is insufficient data to make recommendations on breast feeding for mothers on trimethadione.[23]

Bromocriptine

Bromocriptine has revolutionized the medical management of patients with prolactin-secreting pituitary adenomas.[15,38,112,135,163] Bromocriptine exerts its effect by decreasing mitotic activity and inhibiting estrogen-induced proliferation of lactotrophs, causing a decrement in the serum prolactin level and tumor size.[38,41,112,163] When used indefinitely, it may be the only treatment required for small tumors.[17,135] Female infertility is a common symptom in the amenorrhea/galactorrhea syndrome produced by hyperprolactinomas.[15,17,38,41,42,58,112,113,135] The use of bromocriptine often reverses infertility, creating concern over the use of this medication during pregnancy and the effects of pregnancy on pituitary tumors.[38,41,58,113]

Despite initial concerns, numerous reports of patients harboring pituitary adenomas have shown that pregnancy can be safely undertaken with close follow-up.[17,38,58,113,130] Due to concerns of teratogenicity, it is common practice for physicians to discontinue bromocriptine use during pregnancy to avoid any potential effects on fetal development.[41] While bromocriptine readily crosses the placenta and has been shown to have effects on the fetal pituitary gland, numerous animal and human studies have failed to show significant teratogenic effects on the developing fetus.[17,38,41,113] Bromocriptine is therefore classified as a category C medication on the FDA scale.[23]

If a patient taking bromocriptine desires to become pregnant, initial evaluation should focus on the existence of suprasellar extension.[41] If there is no supracerebellar extension, bromocriptine can be safely discontinued and pregnancy undertaken.[41,58] Close neurological follow-up should be provided, particularly noting headache, visual field changes, or elevation of prolactin levels.[15,41] Should any of these arise, treatment with bromocriptine is reinstituted in an attempt to control the tumor size.[15,17,38,41] If the pregnancy has progressed well into the third trimester, consideration can be given to induction of labor.[15,41] If treatment fails and induction of labor is not possible, treatment with steroids and surgery is recommended.[15] Concern also continues into the postpartum period, when breast feeding is contraindicated while the mother is on bromocriptine.[23] This drug also suppresses lactation, further necessitating bottle feeding.[41,42,77]

Anticoagulation Therapy

The use of anticoagulation during neurosurgical procedures such as carotid endarterectomy is well established.[42] These medications are also utilized in medical management of conditions such as stroke, venous sinus thrombosis, and deep venous thrombosis.[3,13,22,42,65] The mainstays of anticoagulation therapy are heparin for rapid initiation and short-term treatment and coumarin derivatives (warfarin) for maintenance therapy. While well-monitored anticoagulation is safe and effective in the general population, it carries substantial fetal and some maternal risk when given during pregnancy.[13,59,84,153,168] Fortunately, the need for anticoagulation during childbearing years is low, but should the need arise, a brief review of anticoagulant management is needed.

The neurological and neurosurgical literature is sparse regarding the use of anticoagulants during pregnancy, due to the low incidence of neurological disorders which require anticoagulant therapy in females of childbear-

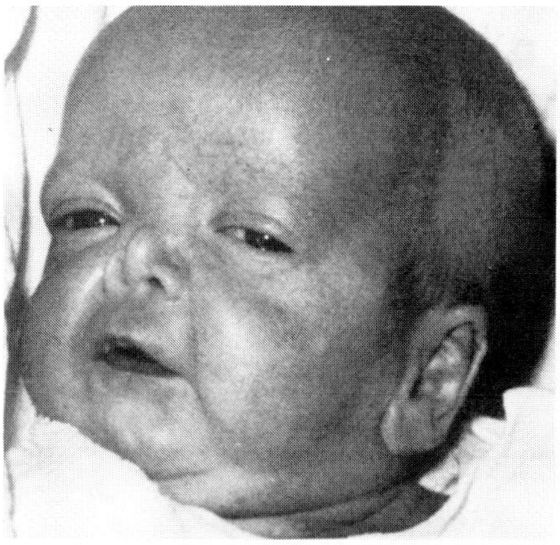

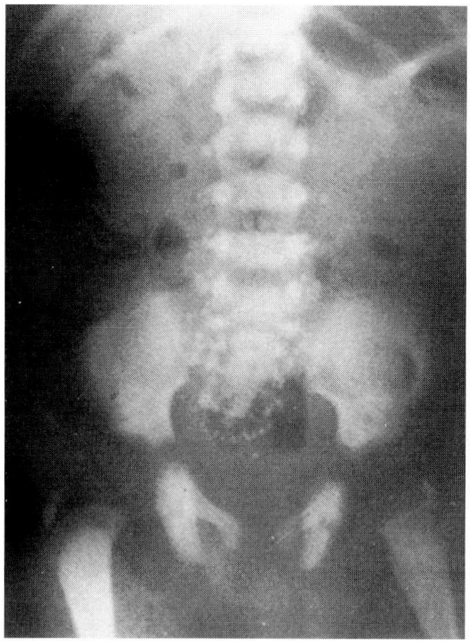

Figure 4: The fetal warfarin syndrome is manifest by nasal hypoplasia, a shallow nasal bridge, and pronounced grooves near the alae nasi *(left).* Stippled calcification of the skeleton is also common *(right).* (From *Am J Dis Child 129:*360-362, 1975, American Medical Association.)

ing age.[42] Fortunately, there is a large body of literature addressing the management of prosthetic heart valves during pregnancy which can serve as a guide for rational anticoagulant use for neurosurgical disorders.[28,59,65-67,109,122,134,136,168] While anticoagulation during pregnancy can never be rendered totally safe, steps can be taken to minimize maternal and fetal risks if anticoagulant therapy is unavoidable.

Coumarin Derivatives

Warfarin is the prototypical coumarin anticoagulant which interferes with synthesis of vitamin K-dependent coagulation factors (factors II, VII, IX, and X).[3,22,65,113] This medication readily crosses the placental barrier and is a known teratogen, but may have some clinical use in pregnancy and is therefore classified in FDA category D (category X by the manufacturer).[3,22,23,65,84] The risk of congenital anomalies in the infants of mothers treated with coumarin derivatives is approximately 5%, with some series reporting an incidence up to 30%.[3,59,67,109]

The most common effect of coumarin derivatives on the fetus is the fetal warfarin syndrome (warfarin embryopathy).[13,51,59,83,120,125,153,171] This syndrome arises from drug exposure by the mother during the first trimester and specifically during weeks 6 to 9 of gestation.[3,22,59,67,109,134] Characteristic facial features include nasal hypoplasia, narrowing of the nares, and choanal stenosis with resultant respiratory distress (Figure 4 *left*).[13,22,51,59,120,125,144,153] The epiphyses show characteristic stippled calcifications which are especially common in the axial skeleton, proximal femur, and calcaneus (Figure 4 *right*).[13,22,51,59,120,125,144,153] There is also a high incidence of scoliosis.[59] These aspects of the fetal warfarin syndrome have a similar phenotypic appearance to the genetic disorders chondrodysplasia punctata and Conradi-Hunermann syndrome.[11,13,22,51,59,119,143,153,171] Additional findings of the fetal warfarin syndrome include low birth weight in 40%, hypoplasia of the digits or extremities in 50%, and developmental retardation in 31% of affected cases.[59,120]

Coumarin exposure during the second and third trimesters of pregnancy can lead to central nervous system and ocular abnormalities, but these are far less common than warfarin embryopathy.[22,59,67,109,144,145] Specific abnormalities include optic atrophy, microphthalmia, hydrocephalus, agenesis of the corpus callosum, Dandy-Walker syndrome, midline cerebellar atrophy, and encephaloceles.[59,109] Mental retardation is also commonly reported. Other findings include spasticity in 31% and seizure disorders or neonatal death in up to 23% of cases; deafness, scoliosis, and growth retardation have also been reported in 7.7% of patients with second or third trimester exposure to this medication.[59]

In addition to congenital anomalies, numerous other risks are associated with anticoagulant use during pregnancy. Prematurity, stillbirth, and fetal hemorrhages are all commonly encountered.[12,20,30,31,65] Spontaneous abortions have also been reported in up to 50% of cases when the medication is given during the first trimester.[31,136] Maternal bleeding may also occur.[31]

As previously mentioned, warfarin produces the anticoagulated state by inhibition of post-translational carboxylation of vitamin K-dependent coagulation factors. It has been hypothesized that similar effects exerted during fetal development may contribute to the high incidence of birth defects, although the precise etiology remains obscure. In addition, the strong phenotypic similarities between chondrodysplasia punctata and Conradi-Hunermann syndrome alluded to previously may provide further insight into genetic aspects contributing to the teratogenicity of this medication.

Heparin

Heparin is a mucopolysaccharide which inhibits fibrin formation by increasing antithrombin III activity.[3,22] Unlike warfarin, heparin does not cross the placental barrier.[3,22,109,113] In concordance with this observation, no specific congenital syndromes have been conclusively associated with the use of heparin during pregnancy.[109,113] There are, however, other risks associated with heparin use during pregnancy which have prompted its assignment to FDA category C.[23,109,113]

Heparin carries the same clinical risks during pregnancy that are observed in the general patient population, including thrombocytopenia related to antiplatelet antibodies.[3,26,109] Osteoporosis is common with long-term heparin use and is related to reduction of maternal 1,25-dihydroxyvitamin D.[1,3,12,40,109] Additional side effects can include anaphylaxis, fat necrosis, and alopecia.[3] For these reasons, close follow-up is needed in all patients on heparin therapy.

More specific to pregnancy are the high rates of maternal and fetal complications with heparin use. While this may be in part related to the underlying disease process, the medication almost certainly plays a major role. The absence of placental transfer of heparin prevents fetal hemorrhage, but the risk of maternal hemorrhage is 10%, with deaths occurring in 2% of these mothers.[3,22,67] Outcome with respect to the fetus is little better than that achieved with warfarin.[59] Stillbirth is reported in 1/8 of cases, and prematurity occurs in 1/5 of cases.[59] In fact, the risk of maternal hemorrhage at delivery may actually be higher with heparin compared to warfarin, but this risk is offset by reduction in the fetal risk and the fact that maternal anticoagulation can be more rapidly controlled.[3,22] More recently, the results of heparin use in pregnancy have improved, possibly due to more vigilant monitoring of the anticoagulated state.[23]

Treatment Recommendations

The safest approach is to avoid anticoagulant use during pregnancy, but if maternal anticoagulation is required for all or part of pregnancy, several important factors can minimize the risk of these medications. After an extensive review of the literature, Hall et al[59] concluded that there was no clear evidence to favor the use of one anticoagulant over another. Other clinicians feel strongly that the timing of medication delivery may be quite significant.[22,23,59,67] In several large series of pregnant patients with a prosthetic cardiac valve, the use of heparin during the first trimester has resulted in good outcome to avoid the fetal warfarin syndrome.[30,65,67,83,109,134,144,152] In the second and third trimesters, warfarin was substituted for convenience given the low incidence of congenital anomalies associated with this medication after the first trimester.[42,65,67,152] Anticoagulation with heparin was reinstituted at approximately 36-38 weeks of gestation to allow more rapid control of coagulation parameters during delivery.[20,22,30,67,109,122,134,144,152] Institution of heparin 1 month prior to the anticipated delivery date is also prudent given the high incidence of prematurity in anticoagulated patients. Of final note, because of changes in the maternal coagulation status near parturition, higher doses of heparin may be required to maintain anticoagulation.[67]

Because of the high risks associated with anticoagulants in both medication classes, the neurosurgical patient who requires anticoagulation should be fully advised of the potential adverse effects.[134] Also, women of childbearing age should be encouraged to avoid pregnancy until anticoagulation can be discontinued.[134] If inadvertent pregnancy occurs or if the patient chooses to become pregnant despite the known risks of these medications, she should be advised that a normal outcome can be anticipated in approximately two-thirds of cases.[22,109] When desired by the patient, referral should be made for discussion of options concerning prenatal diagnosis and/or therapeutic abortion. Finally, there are no absolute contraindications to breast feeding full-term infants if the mother requires anticoagulation, but it is wise to give vitamin K_1 to infants of mothers on warfarin.[14,89,97]

Corticosteroids

Glucocorticoids are widely used in the field of neurosurgery. These drugs are of clear benefit for treatment of peritumoral cerebral edema.[38,42,112,129,142] In addition, glucocorticoids are employed in the treatment of spinal cord injury and arthritic conditions involving the spine.[99] A number of neurological disorders such as multiple sclerosis, myasthenia gravis, and vasculitis may also respond to glucocorticoid therapy.[42,46,117,124,132] Given the serious nature of these disease states, it is often felt that institution or continuation of glucocorticoid therapy is required during pregnancy.[21,38,42,117] Studies examining the safety of glucocorticoids in pregnancy are often difficult to interpret given problems separating drug toxicity from effects of the underlying maternal disease state, but these medications certainly have some adverse side effects.[34,43,114,148]

The general side effects of long-term corticosteroid therapy are reported in up to 67% of cases; this can have an adverse impact on pregnant patients as well as the general population.[60,63,117] Possible complications include adrenal cortex suppression and loss of the stress response.[60,63,117,148] Adequate stress doses of glucocorticoids should be given to the pregnant patient who is on chronic steroid therapy near parturition. Other general side effects include cushingoid appearance, cataracts, osteoporosis, aseptic necrosis of the hip, hypertension, hypokalemia, and peptic ulcer disease.[60,63,117,148] Numerous drug interactions have also been reported and are especially common with nonsteroidal anti-inflammatory medications, aspirin, anticoagulants, anticonvulsants, and diuretics.[60,63,117]

Some adverse effects of glucocorticoid medications are more specific to pregnancy. Glucocorticoids have been demonstrated to be teratogens in various animal models, particularly mice and rats.[34,43,114,148] Alterations in cerebral function have been demonstrated in a rat model of gestational steroid use.[34,43,148,172] No definitive evidence exists for teratogenic effects in humans except for a slight increase in the incidence of cleft lip and/or palate.[6,12,43,46,86,140] Some investigators have suggested that glucocorticoid therapy may be associated with a diverse spectrum of major and minor congenital anomalies, but it remains unclear if such associations truly exist.[46,114,176] There is no relationship between spontaneous abortion and the use of glucocorticoids, and in fact these medications may actually serve to prevent this complication.[114,148] There is a small risk of adrenocortical insufficiency in children of mothers on steroid therapy, which is more likely to occur if steroid use is chronic.[12,111,148] These children should be observed closely for signs of adrenal suppression.[12,111] Finally, there appears to be a slightly increased risk of infectious complications following prolonged rupture of the membranes in mothers on glucocorticoids.[34,148]

Recommendations regarding steroid use during pregnancy have focused on several issues. The doses should be maintained at the lowest level possible to achieve therapeutic benefit. While studies have shown glucocorticoid therapy to be safe during gestation, these studies have been performed with low doses, typically less than the equivalent of 10 mg of prednisone (FDA category B) per day.[12,23,176] Furthermore, certain steroid preparations (e.g., prednisone) are considered much safer due to placental metabolism. This property is not characteristic of other glucocorticoids such as dexamethasone.[30] Placental metabolism provides an added level of safety to consider when weighing the risks and benefits of various corticosteroid preparations. For these reasons, prednisone is often considered first-line therapy as long as it is capable of controlling the patient's symptoms. Dexamethasone (FDA category C) has also been used during gestation with few side effects; however, the greatest experience with this medication is during later trimesters.[23,29,43,113] In the critically ill neurosurgical patient in whom induction of labor is considered, dexamethasone also has the added benefit of promoting fetal lung maturity within 24-48 hours.[29,33,34,43,57,91,108,116,140,158] This drug may also promote labor in prolonged pregnancy.[72] To date, studies of glucocorticoid use in spinal cord injury have utilized methylprednisolone. Unfortunately, little data is available on the use of this medication during pregnancy, and no specific recommendations can be made beyond giving appropriate therapy to the injured mother.[114]

Breast feeding of infants by a mother who is receiving glucocorticoids also presents a dilemma.[98,115,126] Overall, very small amounts of glucocorticoids are transferred within breast milk.[115,126,148] It can be concluded that if the mother is receiving less than 20-40 mg of prednisone per day, breast feeding can be considered safe.[115,126] Insufficient data on breast feeding is available for dexamethasone and many other corticosteroids.[23]

Diuretic Therapy

Neurosurgical patients with intracranial mass lesions (tumors, abscesses, hematomas, etc.) are frequently treated with diuretics to help control intracranial hypertension.[38,42,112] The most commonly employed agent is mannitol, a hexahydric alcohol which functions as an osmotic diuretic by being excreted by direct glomerular filtration without prior metabolism. Mannitol crosses the placenta, is excreted in fetal urine, and subsequently accumulates in the amniotic fluid.[9] Animal studies performed in the rabbit have shown that serum osmolality can be increased by 25% in the mother, with serious fetal side effects such as dehydration, contraction of the blood volume, cyanosis, loss of amniotic fluid, and bradycardia. Human studies examining effects of mannitol during pregnancy are limited.[9] Administration of 20% mannitol to pregnant mothers has been shown to produce an increase in serum osmolality of approximately 10%.[42] This was matched by a similar increase in fetal serum osmolality. Unfortunately, no mention of fetal outcome was made in this study.[42] Others have reported the use of mannitol during pregnancy without apparent ill effect.[42] Given the potential side effects, mannitol is considered an FDA category C medication.[23] While utilization of mannitol in pregnancy should be limited, this medication should not be withheld in the case of serious or life-threatening intracranial hypertension.[23,42]

In addition to osmotic diuretics, other diuretic therapies have been employed safely during pregnancy.[27,30,46,68] The largest experience is with thiazide diuretics (FDA category C), which are of little use in the management of intracranial hypertension. The effects of the loop diuretic furosemide during pregnancy are less well defined. Jacobs reported five cases where furosemide use during pregnancy caused no increase in the incidence of congenital anomalies, and a similar opinion was shared by Barrillon and co-workers.[8,68] On the other hand, furosemide has been linked with diminished placental reserve and metabolic abnormalities such as elevated serum uric acid levels and hyponatremia.[8,27,174] Furosemide has also been shown to have a paradoxical effect in pregnancy by actually increasing the volume of distribution.[53] Furosemide is classified as an FDA category C drug, and its use should be limited to serious or life-threatening situations when the benefits are felt to outweigh potential risks.[23]

Nimodipine

Aneurysmal subarachnoid hemorrhage is occasionally encountered during pregnancy. Cerebral vasospasm associated with aneurysmal subarachnoid hemorrhage is a common cause of ischemic deficits with resultant morbidity and mortality.[55] Potential complications of vasospasm are lessened by the physiological increase in intravascular volume which accompanies pregnancy, but vasospasm remains a serious problem.[55] The use of nimodipine, a cerebral-specific calcium channel blocker, has been shown to improve outcome from vasospasm related to subarachnoid hemorrhage in patients with good neurological function (Hunt and Hess grades I to III).[96,100]

Very few studies are available which address the risks of this medication during pregnancy. Animal studies in the rabbit have shown an increased incidence of congenital malformations and intrauterine growth retardation.[96,100] Embryotoxicity has also been demonstrated in rats, with increased skeletal variation, growth retardation, and stillbirth, but no malformations were noted.[96,100] There are no adequate human studies which examine the risks of this medication during pregnancy.[96,100] Other calcium channel blockers have been successfully used in pregnancy but have been shown to exert a tocolytic effect.[32,160,166,169] Animal studies of these agents have also been associated with fetal acidosis and hypoxemia.[32]

Given a paucity of pregnancy data and a known beneficial role for good-grade subarachnoid hemorrhage patients, nimodipine has been classified as an FDA category C agent.[23] It should be offered to all patients in Hunt and Hess grades I to III following subarachnoid hemorrhage if the benefits are felt to outweigh potential risks to the fetus.[160] Fortunately, a good clinical grade allows consultation with the mother herself regarding the possible adverse effects. Finally, nimodipine is highly concentrated within breast milk in animal studies; however, no human studies are available[96,100] and breast feeding is not recommended while this medication is being used.[96,100]

CONCLUSIONS

The successful treatment of neurosurgical disorders during pregnancy requires a thorough understanding of the principles guiding appropriate drug prescription. The fetal toxicity of commonly used neurosurgical drugs is often substantial, but maternal well-being may necessitate such intervention. The risks of treatment can be minimized by a thorough understanding of the various medication options. Issues regarding drug prescription during pregnancy most often surround the treatment of seizure disorders. While all anticonvulsants appear to be teratogenic, the risks may be less than an untreated seizure disorder. Adverse drug effects can be minimized by careful drug selection, adherence to monotherapy when possible, close monitoring of drug levels, and folic acid supplementation. Additional medications prescribed in the management of the pregnant neurosurgical patient include bromocriptine, corticosteroids, diuretics, and calcium channel blockers. All of these medications have well-defined or potential side effects which could adversely affect the fetus. Drug prescription must take into account the risks of untreated maternal disease on the well-being of the mother and fetus versus the fetal toxicity of a prescribed medication. Finally, concern regarding drug prescription does not end with delivery of the child, since breast feeding may continue to expose the newborn infant to adverse effects of maternal medications. Decisions regarding the safety of breast feeding rely heavily on the type of medication given, its dosage level, and the infant's health.

REFERENCES

1. Aarskog D, Aksnes L, Markestad T, et al: Heparin-induced inhibition of 1,25-dihydroxyvitamin D formation. **Am J Obstet Gynecol 148:**1141-1142, 1984
2. Anderson RC: Cardiac defects in children of mothers receiving anticonvulsant therapy during pregnancy. **J Pediatr 89:**318-319, 1976
3. Angel JL, Knuppel RA, Hoffman M, et al: Anticoagulant use in pregnancy, in Petrie RH (ed): **Perinatal Pharmacology.** Oradell, NJ: Medical Economics Books, 1989, pp 95-108
4. Annegers JF, Baumgartner KB, Hauser WA, et al: Epilepsy, antiepileptic drugs, and the risk of spontaneous abortion. **Epilepsia 29:**451-458, 1988
5. Annegers JF, Elveback LR, Hauser WA, et al: Do anticonvulsants have a teratogenic effect? **Arch Neurol 31:**364-373, 1974
6. Baden M, Bauer CR, Colle E, et al: A controlled trial of hydrocortisone therapy in infants with respiratory distress syndrome. **Pediatrics 50:**526-534, 1972
7. Bailey CJ, Pool RW, Poskitt EME, et al: Valproic acid and fetal abnormality. **Br Med J 286:**190, 1983
8. Barrillon A, Grand A, Gerbaux A: Thérapeutique cardiologique et grossesse. **Ann Med Interne 125:**437-445, 1974
9. Basso A, Fernandez A, Althabe O, et al: Passage of mannitol from mother to amniotic fluid and fetus.

Obstet Gynecol **49**:628-631, 1977
10. Beck F: Model systems in teratology. **Br Med Bull 32**:53-58, 1976
11. Becker MH, Genieser NB, Finegold M, et al: Chondrodysplasia punctata. Is maternal warfarin therapy a factor? **Am J Dis Child 129**:356-359, 1975
12. Beeley L: Adverse effects of drugs in later pregnancy. **Clin Obstet Gynaecol 8**:275-290, 1981
13. Beeley L: Adverse effects of drugs in the first trimester of pregnancy. **Clin Obstet Gynaecol 8**: 261-274, 1981
14. Beeley L: Drugs and breast feeding. **Clin Obstet Gynaecol 8**:291-295, 1981
15. Bergh T, Nillius SJ, Wide L: Clinical course and outcome of pregnancies in amenorrhoeic women with hyperprolactinaemia and pituitary tumours. **Br Med J 1**:875-880, 1978
16. Berry CL, Barlow S: Some remaining problems in the reproductive toxicity testing of drugs. **Br Med Bull 32**:34-38, 1976
17. Bigazzi M, Ronga R, Lancranjan I, et al: A pregnancy in an acromegalic woman during bromocriptine treatment: effects on growth hormone and prolactin in the maternal, fetal, and amniotic compartments. **J Clin Endocrinol Metab 48**:9-12, 1979
18. Bjerkedal T, Bahna SL: The course and outcome of pregnancy in a woman with epilepsy. **Acta Obstet Gynecol Scand 52**:245-248, 1973
19. Bjerkedal T, Czeizel A, Goujard J, et al: Valproic acid and spina bifida. **Lancet 2**:1096, 1982 (Letter)
20. Bloomfield DK: Fetal deaths and malformations associated with the use of coumarin derivatives in pregnancy. A critical review. **Am J Obstet Gynecol 107**:883-888, 1970
21. Bologa M, Koren G, McGuigan M, et al: Drugs and chemicals most commonly used by pregnant women, in Koren G (ed): **Maternal-Fetal Toxicology. A Clinician's Guide.** New York, NY: Marcel Dekker, 1990, 29-51
22. Bonnar J: Venous thromboembolism and pregnancy. **Clin Obstet Gynaecol 8**:455-473, 1981
23. Briggs GG, Freeman RK, Yaffe SJ: **Drugs in Pregnancy and Lactation. A Reference Guide to Fetal and Neonatal Risk, 4th ed.** Baltimore, MD: Williams & Wilkins, 1994
24. Brown NA, Kao J, Fabro S: Teratogenic potential of valproic acid. **Lancet 1**:660-661, 1980 (Letter)
25. Bryant Jackson CL, Quirk JG: The use of barbiturates in obstetrics, in Petrie RH (ed): **Perinatal Pharmacology.** Oradell, NJ: Medical Economics Books, 1989, pp 235-243
26. Calhoun BC, Hesser JW: Heparin-associated antibody with pregnancy: discussion of two cases. **Am J Obstet Gynecol 156**:964-966, 1987
27. Carswell W, Semple PF: The effect of furosemide on uric acid levels in maternal blood, fetal blood and amniotic fluid. **J Obstet Gynaecol Br Commonw 81**:472-474, 1974
28. Casanegra P, Avilés G, Maturana G, et al: Cardiovascular management of pregnant women with a heart valve prosthesis. **Am J Cardiol 36**:802-806, 1975
29. Caspi E, Schreyer P, Weinraub Z, et al: Changes in amniotic fluid lecithin-sphingomyelin ratio following maternal dexamethasone administration. **Am J Obstet Gynecol 122**:327-331, 1975
30. Catz CS, Abuelo D: Drugs and pregnancy. **Drug Ther 4**:79-91, 1974
31. Chong MKB, Harvey D, de Swiet M: Follow-up study of children whose mothers were treated with warfarin during pregnancy. **Br J Obstet Gynaecol 91**:1070-1073, 1984
32. Clark SL: Actions of cardiac drugs during pregnancy, in Petrie RH (ed): **Perinatal Pharmacology.** Oradell, NJ: Medical Economics Books, 1989, pp 133-140
33. Collaborative Group on Antenatal Steroid Therapy: Effect of antenatal dexamethasone administration on the prevention of respiratory distress syndrome. **Am J Obstet Gynecol 141**:276-286, 1981
34. Crowley P: Corticosteroids in pregnancy: the benefits outweigh the costs. **J Obstet Gynaecol 1**:147-150, 1981
35. Dalessio DJ: Seizure disorders and pregnancy. **N Engl J Med 312**:559-563, 1985
36. Dam M, Christiansen J, Munck O, et al: Antiepileptic drugs: metabolism in pregnancy. **Clin Pharmacokinet 4**:53-62, 1979
37. Dansky LV, Andermann E, Rosenblatt D, et al: Anticonvulsants, folate levels, and pregnancy outcome: a prospective study. **Ann Neurol 21**:176-182, 1987
38. DeAngelis LM: Central nervous system neoplasms in pregnancy. **Adv Neurol 64**:139-152, 1994
39. Deblay MF, Vert P, Andre M, et al: Transplacental vitamin K prevents haemorrhagic disease of infant of epileptic mother. **Lancet 1**:1247, 1982 (Letter)
40. de Swiet M, Dorrington Ward P, Fidler J, et al: Prolonged heparin therapy in pregnancy causes bone demineralization. **Br J Obstet Gynaecol 90**: 1129-1134, 1983
41. De Wit W, Coelingh Bennink HJT, Gerards LJ: Prophylactic bromocriptine treatment during pregnancy in women with macroprolactinomas: report of 13 pregnancies. **Br J Obstet Gynaecol 91**:1059-1069, 1984
42. Donaldson JO. **Neurology of Pregnancy, 2nd ed.** Philadelphia, PA: WB Saunders, 1989
43. Doran TA, Swyer P, MacMurray B, et al: Results of a double-blind controlled study on the use of betamethasone in the prevention of respiratory distress syndrome. **Am J Obstet Gynecol 136**:313-320, 1980
44. Dronamraju KR: Epilepsy and cleft lip and palate. **Lancet 2**:876-877, 1970
45. Eluma FO, Sucheston ME, Hayes TG, et al: Teratogenic effects of dosage levels and time of administration of carbamazepine, sodium valproate, and diphenylhydantoin on craniofacial development in the CD-1 mouse fetus. **J Craniofac Genet Dev Biol 4**:191-210, 1984
46. Eriksson M, Catz CS, Yaffe SJ: Drugs and pregnancy. **Clin Obstet Gynecol 16**:199-224, 1973
47. Federal Register **44**:37,434-37,467, 1980
48. Fedrick J: Epilepsy and pregnancy: a report from the Oxford record linkage study. **Br Med J 2**:442-448, 1973
49. Finnell RH, Chernoff GF: Genetic background: the elusive component in the fetal hydantoin syndrome. **Am J Med Genet 19**:459-462, 1984 (Editorial comment)
50. Finnell RH, Chernoff GF: Variable patterns of malformation in the mouse fetal hydantoin syndrome. **Am J Med Genet 19**:463-471, 1984
51. Fourie DT, Hay IT: Warfarin as a possible teratogen.

S Afr Med J 49:2081-2083, 1975
52. Friis ML: Epilepsy among parents of children with facial clefts. **Epilepsia 20**:69-76, 1979
53. Gant NF, Madden JD, Siiteri PK, et al: The metabolic clearance rate of dehydroisoandrosterone sulfate. IV. Acute effects of induced hypertension, hypotension, and naturesis in normal and hypertensive pregnancies. **Am J Obstet Gynecol 124**:143-148, 1976
54. German J, Kowal A, Ehlers KH: Trimethadione and human teratogenesis. **Teratology 3**:349-362, 1970
55. Giannotta SL, Daniels J, Golde SH, et al: Ruptured intracranial aneurysms during pregnancy. A report of four cases. **J Reprod Med 31**:139-147, 1986
56. Goldman AS, Yaffe SJ: Fetal trimethadione syndrome. **Teratology 17**:103-106, 1978
57. Gonzalez Ruiz AR, Sibai BM: Glucocorticoids for lung maturation in preeclampsia, in Petrie RH (ed): **Perinatal Pharmacology**. Oradell, NJ: Medical Economics Books, 1989, pp 289-296
58. Griffith RW, Turkalj I, Braun P: Outcome of pregnancy in mothers given bromocriptine. **Br J Clin Pharmacol 5**:227-231, 1978
59. Hall JG, Pauli RM, Wilson KM: Maternal and fetal sequelae of anticoagulation during pregnancy. **Am J Med 68**:122-140, 1980
60. Hanson JW: Teratogen update: fetal hydantoin effects. **Teratology 33**:349-353, 1986
61. Hanson JW, Smith DW: The fetal hydantoin syndrome. **J Pediatr 87**:285-290, 1975
62. Hanson JW, Smith DW: Fetal hydantoin syndrome. **Lancet 1**:692, 1976 (Letter)
63. Haynes RC Jr: Adrenocorticotropic hormone, adrenocortical steroids and their synthetic analogs: inhibitors of the synthesis and actions of adrenocortical hormones, in Gilman AG, Rall TW, Nies AS, et al (eds): **The Pharmacological Basis of Therapeutics, 8th ed.** New York, NY: Pergamon Press, 1990, pp 1431-1462
64. Hill RM: Anticonvulsant medication. **Am J Dis Child 133**:449-450, 1979 (Letter)
65. Hirsh J, Cade JF, Gallus AS: Anticoagulants in pregnancy: a review of indications and complications. **Am Heart J 83**:301-305, 1972
66. Hurwitz A, Milwidsky A, Medina A, et al: Failure of continuous intravenous heparinization to prevent stroke in a pregnant woman with a prosthetic valve and atrial fibrillation. A case report. **J Reprod Med 30**:618-620, 1985
67. Iturbe-Alessio I, Del Carmen Fonseca M, Mutchinik O, et al: Risks of anticoagulant therapy in pregnant women with artificial heart valves. **N Engl J Med 315**:1390-1393, 1986
68. Jacobs D: Maternal drug ingestion and congenital malformations. **S Afr Med J 49**:2073-2080, 1975
69. Jäger-Roman E, Deichl A, Jakob S, et al: Fetal growth, major malformations, and minor anomalies in infants born to women receiving valproic acid. **J Pediatr 108**:997-1004, 1986
70. Janz D: The teratogenic risk of antiepileptic drugs. **Epilepsia 16**:159-169, 1975
71. Janz D, Beck-Mannagetta G, Andermann E, et al (Commission on Genetics, Pregnancy, and the Child, International League Against Epilepsy): Guidelines for the care of epileptic women of childbearing age. **Epilepsia 30**:409-410, 1989
72. Jenssen H, Wright PB: The effect of dexamethasone therapy in prolonged pregnancy. **Acta Obstet Gynecol Scand 56**:467-473, 1977
73. Jones KL, Lacro RV, Johnson KA, et al: Pattern of malformations in the children of women treated with carbamazepine during pregnancy. **New Engl J Med 320**:1661-1666, 1989
74. Juchau MR, Rettie AE: The metabolic role of the placenta, in Fabro S, Scialli AR (eds): **Drug and Chemical Action in Pregnancy. Pharmacologic and Toxicologic Principles.** New York, NY: Marcel Dekker, 1986, pp 153-169
75. Kaneko S, Otani K, Fukushima Y, et al: Teratogenicity of antiepileptic drugs: analysis of possible risk factors. **Epilepsia 29**:459-467, 1988
76. Kaneko S, Sato T, Suzuki K: The levels of anticonvulsants in breast milk. **Br J Clin Pharmacol 7**:624-627, 1979
77. Katz M, Kroll D, Pak I, et al: Puerperal hypertension, stroke, and seizures after suppression of lactation with bromocriptine. **Obstet Gynecol 66**:822-824, 1985
78. Kelly TE: Teratogenicity of anticonvulsant drugs. I. Review of the literature. **Am J Med Genet 19**: 413-434, 1984
79. Kelly TE: Teratogenicity of anticonvulsant drugs. III. Radiographic hand analysis of children exposed *in utero* to diphenylhydantoin. **Am J Med Genet 19**:445-450, 1984
80. Kelly TE, Edwards P, Rein M, et al: Teratogenicity of anticonvulsant drugs. II. A prospective study. **Am J Med Genet 19**:435-443, 1984
81. Kelly TE, Rein M, Edwards P: Teratogenicity of anticonvulsant drugs. IV. The association of clefting and epilepsy. **Am J Med Genet 19**:451-458, 1984
82. Koren G: Changes in drug disposition in pregnancy and their clinical implications, in Koren G (ed): **Maternal-Fetal Toxicology. A Clinician's Guide.** New York, NY: Marcel Dekker, 1990, pp 3-13
83. Koren G: Teratogenic drugs and chemicals in humans, in Koren G (ed): **Maternal-Fetal Toxicology. A Clinician's Guide.** New York, NY: Marcel Dekker, 1990, pp 15-27
84. Kronick J, Phelps NE, McCallion DJ, et al: Effects of sodium warfarin administered during pregnancy in mice. **Am J Obstet Gynecol 118**:819-823, 1974
85. Krumholz A: Epilepsy in pregnancy, in Goldstein PJ, Stern BJ (eds): **Neurological Disorders of Pregnancy, 2nd ed.** Mount Kisco, NY: Futura, 1992, pp 25-50
86. Kullander S, Källén B: A prospective study of drugs and pregnancy. 3. Hormones. **Acta Obstet Gynecol Scand 55**:221-224, 1976
87. Landon MJ, Kirkley M: Metabolism of diphenylhydantoin (phenytoin) during pregnancy. **Br J Obstet Gynaecol 86**:125-132, 1979
88. Leeder JS, Spielberg SP: Teratogenicity and litigation, in Koren G (ed): **Maternal-Fetal Toxicology. A Clinician's Guide.** New York, NY: Marcel Dekker, 1990, pp 415-425
89. L'e Orme M, Lewis PJ, de Swiet M, et al: May mothers given warfarin breast-feed their infants? **Br Med J 1**:1564-1565, 1977
90. Levy RH, Yerby MS: Effects of pregnancy on antiepileptic drug utilization. **Epilepsia 26 (Suppl 1)**: S52-S57, 1985
91. Liggins GC, Howie RN: A controlled trial of antepartum glucocorticoid treatment for prevention of the

respiratory distress syndrome in premature infants. **Pediatrics 50:**515-525, 1972

92. Martz F, Failinger C III, Blake DA: Phenytoin teratogenesis correlation between embryopathic effect and covalent binding of putative arene oxide metabolite in gestational tissue. **J Pharmacol Exp Ther 203:** 231-239, 1977
93. Mattison DR: Physiologic variations in pharmacokinetics during pregnancy, in Fabro S, Scialli AR (eds): **Drug and Chemical Action in Pregnancy. Pharmacologic and Toxicologic Principles.** New York, NY: Marcel Dekker, 1986, pp 37-102
94. Mattison DR, Kozlowski K, Quirk JG, et al: Effects of drugs and chemicals on the fetus, in Petrie RH (ed): **Perinatal Pharmacology**. Oradell, NJ: Medical Economics Books, 1989, pp 13-41
95. Mattson RH, Cramer JA, Collins JF, et al: Comparison of carbamazepine, phenobarbital, phenytoin, and primidone in partial and secondarily generalized tonic-clonic seizures. **N Engl J Med 313:**145-151, 1985
96. McEvoy GK, Litvak K, Welsh OH Jr, et al: **AHFS Drug Information 94**. American Society of Hospital Pharmacists, 1994, pp 1182-1187
97. McKenna R, Cole ER, Vasan U: Is warfarin sodium contraindicated in the lactating mother? **J Pediatr 103:**325-327, 1983
98. McKenzie SA, Selley JA, Agnew JE: Secretion of prednisolone into breast milk. **Arch Dis Child 50:**894-896, 1975
99. Meyerhoff J: Neurological manifestations of rheumatic diseases in pregnancy, in Goldstein PJ, Stern BJ (eds): **Neurological Disorders of Pregnancy, 2nd ed.** Mount Kisco, NY: Futura, 1992, pp 293-311
100. Miles, Inc: **Nimotop Packing Insert.** Elkhart, Indiana, July 1993
101. Miller RK: Placental transfer and function: the interface for drugs and chemicals in the conceptus, in Fabro S, Scialli AR (eds): **Drug and Chemical Action in Pregnancy. Pharmacologic and Toxicologic Principles.** New York, NY: Marcel Dekker, 1986, pp 123-152
102. Moosa SM, El Zayat SG: Phenytoin infusion in severe pre-eclampsia. **Lancet 2:**1147-1148, 1987 (Letter)
103. Mountain KR, Hirsh J, Gallus AS: Neonatal coagulation defect due to anticonvulsant drug treatment in pregnancy. **Lancet 1:**265-268, 1970
104. Nakane Y, Okuma T, Takahashi R, et al: Multi-institutional study on the teratogenicity and fetal toxicity of antiepileptic drugs: a report of a collaborative study group in Japan. **Epilepsia 21:**663-680, 1980
105. Nau H, Kuhnz W, Egger H-J, et al: Anticonvulsants during pregnancy and lactation. Transplacental, maternal and neonatal pharmacokinetics. **Clin Pharmacokinet 7:**508-543, 1982
106. Nau H, Rating D, Koch S, et al: Valproic acid and its metabolites: placental transfer, neonatal pharmacokinetics, transfer via mother's milk and clinical status in neonates of epileptic mothers. **J Pharmacol Exp Ther 219:**768-777, 1981
107. Nelson KB, Ellenberg JH: Maternal seizure disorder, outcome of pregnancy, and neurologic abnormalities in the children. **Neurology 32:**1247-1254, 1982
108. Nochimson DJ, Petrie RH: Glucocorticoid therapy for the induction of pulmonary maturity in severely hypertensive gravid women. **Am J Obstet Gynecol 133:**449-451, 1979
109. Oakley C: Valve prostheses and pregnancy. **Br Heart J 58:**303-305, 1987
110. O'Brien CF, Kurlan R: Movement disorders in pregnancy, in Goldstein PJ, Stern BJ (eds): **Neurological Disorders of Pregnancy, 2nd ed.** Mount Kisco, NY: Futura, 1992, pp 181-201
111. Ohrlander S, Gennser G, Nilsson KO, et al: ACTH test to neonates after administration of corticosteroids during gestation. **Obstet Gynecol 49:** 691-694, 1977
112. Olivi A, Brem RF, McPherson R, et al: Brain tumors in pregnancy, in Goldstein PJ, Stern BJ (eds): **Neurological Disorders of Pregnancy, 2nd ed.** Mount Kisco, NY: Futura, 1992, pp 85-105
113. Onnis A, Grella P: **The Biochemical Effects of Drugs in Pregnancy**. New York, NY: Halsted Press, 1984, Vol 1, pp 119-172
114. Onnis A, Grella P: **The Biochemical Effects of Drugs in Pregnancy**. New York, NY: Halsted Press, 1984, Vol 2, pp 72-89
115. Öst L, Wettrell G, Björkhem I, et al: Prednisolone excretion in human milk. **J Pediatr 106:**1008-1011, 1985
116. Papageorgiou AN, Desgranges MF, Masson M, et al: The antenatal use of betamethasone in the prevention of respiratory distress syndrome: a controlled double-blind study. **Pediatrics 63:**73-79, 1979
117. Pascuzzi RM, Coslett HB, Johns TR: Long-term corticosteroid treatment of myasthenia gravis: report of 116 patients. **Ann Neurol 15:**291-298, 1984
118. Patrick MJ, Tilstone WJ, Reavey P: Diazepam and breast-feeding. **Lancet 1:**542-543, 1972 (Letter)
119. Pauli RM, Madden JD, Kranzler KJ, et al: Warfarin therapy initiated during pregnancy and phenotypic chondrodysplasia punctata. **J Pediatr 88:**506-508, 1976
120. Pettifor JM, Benson R: Congenital malformations associated with the administration of oral anticoagulants during pregnancy. **J Pediatr 86:**459-462, 1975
121. Poswillo D: Mechanisms and pathogenesis of malformation. **Br Med Bull 32:**59-64, 1976
122. Pridmore BR, Murray KH, McAllen PM: The management of anticoagulant therapy during and after pregnancy. **Br J Obstet Gynaecol 82:**740-744, 1975
123. Rall TW, Schleifer LS: Drugs effective in the therapy of the epilepsies, in Gilman AG, Rall TW, Nies AS, et al (eds): **The Pharmacological Basis of Therapeutics, 8th ed.** New York, NY: Pergamon Press, 1990, pp 436-462
124. Repke JT: Myasthenia gravis in pregnancy, in Goldstein PJ, Stern BJ (eds): **Neurological Disorders of Pregnancy, 2nd ed.** Mount Kisco, NY: Futura, 1992, pp 269-291
125. Richman EM, Lahman JE: Fetal anomalies associated with warfarin therapy initiated shortly prior to conception. **J Pediatr 88:**509-510, 1976 (Letter)
126. Rieder MJ: Drugs and breastfeeding, in Koren G (ed): **Maternal-Fetal Toxicology. A Clinician's Guide.** New York, NY: Marcel Dekker, 1990, pp 63-85
127. Robert E: Valproic acid in pregnancy—association with spina bifida: a preliminary report. **Clin Pediatr 22:**336, 1983
128. Robert E, Rosa F: Valproate and birth defects. **Lancet 2:**1142, 1983 (Letter)
129. Roelvink NCA, Kamphorst W, van Alphen HAM, et

al: Pregnancy-related primary brain and spinal tumors. **Arch Neurol 44**:209-215, 1987
130. Rogers JD, Fahn S: Movement disorders and pregnancy. **Adv Neurol 64**:163-178, 1994
131. Rosa FW: Spina bifida in infants of women treated with carbamazepine during pregnancy. **N Engl J Med 324**:674-677, 1991
132. Rudick RA, Birk KA: Multiple sclerosis and pregnancy, in Goldstein PJ, Stern BJ (eds): **Neurological Disorders of Pregnancy, 2nd ed.** Mount Kisco, NY: Futura, 1992, pp 165-180
133. Ryan G, Lange IR, Naugler MA: Clinical experience with phenytoin prophylaxis in severe preeclampsia. **Am J Obstet Gynecol 161**:1297-1304, 1989
134. Salazar E, Zajarias A, Gutierrez N, et al: The problem of cardiac valve prostheses, anticoagulants, and pregnancy. **Circulation 70 (Suppl I)**:I-169-I-177, 1984
135. Samaan NA, Schultz PN, Leavens TA, et al: Pregnancy after treatment in patients with prolactinoma operation versus bromocriptine. **Am J Obstet Gynecol 155**:1300-1305, 1986
136. Sareli P, England MJ, Berk MR, et al: Maternal and fetal sequelae of anticoagulation during pregnancy in patients with mechanical heart valve prostheses. **Am J Cardiol 63**:1462-1465, 1989
137. Schachter SC: Endocrine aspects of epilepsy in women. **Adv Neurol 64**:35-44, 1994
138. Schardein JL: **Chemically Induced Birth Defects.** New York, NY: Marcel Dekker, 1985
139. Seip M: Growth retardation, dysmorphic facies and minor malformations following massive exposure to phenobarbitone *in utero*. **Acta Paediatr Scand 65**:617-621, 1976
140. Semchyshyn S, Zuspan FP, Cordero L: Cardiovascular response and complications of glucocorticoid therapy in hypertensive pregnancies. **Am J Obstet Gynecol 145**:530-533, 1983
141. Shapiro S, Slone D, Hartz SC, et al: Anticonvulsants and parental epilepsy in the development of birth defects. **Lancet 1**:272-275, 1976
142. Shapiro WR, Posner JB: Corticosteroid hormones. Effects in an experimental brain tumor. **Arch Neurol 30**:217-221, 1974
143. Shaul WL, Emery H, Hall JG: Chondrodysplasia punctata and maternal warfarin use during pregnancy. **Am J Dis Child 129**:360-362, 1975
144. Shaul WL, Hall JG: Multiple congenital anomalies associated with oral anticoagulants. **Am J Obstet Gynecol 127**:191-198, 1977
145. Sherman S, Hall BD: Warfarin and fetal abnormality. **Lancet 1**:692, 1976
146. Sibai BM: Magnesium sulfate is the ideal anticonvulsant in preeclampsia-eclampsia. **Am J Obstet Gynecol 162**:1141-1145, 1990
147. Sibai BM: Eclampsia, in Goldstein PJ, Stern BJ (eds): **Neurological Disorders of Pregnancy, 2nd ed.** Mount Kisco, NY: Futura, 1992, pp 1-24
148. Sidhu RK, Hawkins DF: Prescribing in pregnancy. Corticosteroids. **Clin Obstet Gynaecol 8**:383-404, 1981
149. Slater RM, Wilcox FL, Smith WD, et al: Phenytoin infusion in severe pre-eclampsia. **Lancet 1**: 1417-1421, 1987
150. Slater RM, Wilcox FL, Smith WD, et al: Phenytoin in pre-eclampsia. **Lancet 2**:1224-1225, 1989 (Letter)
151. Smith DW: Teratogenicity of anticonvulsive medications. **Am J Dis Child 131**:1337-1339, 1977 (Comment)
152. Smith J, Koren G: Drugs of choice in pregnancy, in Koren G (ed): **Maternal-Fetal Toxicology. A Clinician's Guide**. New York, NY: Marcel Dekker, 1990, pp 53-61
153. Smithells RW: Environmental teratogens of man. **Br Med Bull 32**:27-33, 1976
154. Solomon GE, Hilgartner MW, Kutt H: Coagulation defects caused by diphenylhydantoin. **Neurology 22**:1165-1171, 1972
155. Sonawane BR, Yaffe SJ: Physiologic disposition of drugs in the fetus and newborn, in Fabro S, Scialli AR (eds): **Drug and Chemical Action in Pregnancy. Pharmacologic and Toxicologic Principles**. New York, NY: Marcel Dekker, 1986, pp 103-121
156. Sullivan FM, McElhatton PR: A comparison of the teratogenic activity of the antiepileptic drugs carbamazepine, clonazepam, ethosuximide, phenobarbital, phenytoin, and primidone in mice. **Toxicol Appl Pharmacol 40**:365-378, 1977
157. Speidel BD, Meadow SR: Maternal epilepsy and abnormalities of the fetus and newborn. **Lancet 2**:839-843, 1972
158. Spellacy WN, Buhi WC, Riggall FC, et al: Human amniotic fluid lecithin/sphingomyelin ratio changes with estrogen or glucocorticoid treatment. **Am J Obstet Gynecol 115**:216-218, 1973
159. Srinivasan G, Seeler RA, Tiruvury A, et al: Maternal anticonvulsant therapy and hemorrhagic disease of the newborn. **Obstet Gynecol 59**:250-252, 1982
160. Stern BJ: Cerebrovascular disease and pregnancy, in Goldstein PJ, Stern BJ (eds): **Neurological Disorders of Pregnancy, 2nd ed.** Mount Kisco, NY: Futura, 1992, pp 51-84
161. Tein I, MacGregor DL: Possible valproate teratogenicity. **Arch Neurol 42**:291-293, 1985
162. Teramo K, Hiilesmaa V, Bardy A, et al: Fetal heart rate during a maternal grand mal epileptic seizure. **J Perinat Med 7**:3-6, 1979
163. Thorner MO, Martin WH, Rogol AD, et al: Rapid regression of pituitary prolactinomas during bromocriptine treatment. **J Clin Endocrinol Metab 51**:438-445, 1980
164. Tropper P: The pharmacology of antiseizure agents during pregnancy, in Petrie RH (ed): **Perinatal Pharmacology**. Oradell, NJ: Medical Economics Books, 1989, pp 85-93
165. Tuffnell D, O'Donovan P, Lilford RJ, et al: Phenytoin in pre-eclampsia. **Lancet 2**:273-274, 1989 (Letter)
166. Ulmsten U, Andersson KE, Wingerup L: Treatment of premature labor with the calcium antagonist nifedipine. **Arch Gynecol 229**:1-5, 1980
167. Venning GR: Identification of adverse reactions to new drugs. I. What have been the important adverse reactions since thalidomide? **Br Med J 286**:199-202, 1983
168. Vitali E, Donatelli F, Quaini E, et al: Pregnancy in patients with mechanical prosthetic heart valves. Our experience regarding 98 pregnancies in 57 patients. **J Cardiovasc Surg 27**:221-227, 1986
169. Walters BNJ, Redman CWG: Treatment of severe pregnancy-associated hypertension with the calcium antagonist nifedipine. **Br J Obstet Gynaecol 91**: 330-336, 1984
170. Warkany J: Aminopterin and methotrexate folic acid

deficiency. **Teratology 17**:353-358, 1978
171. Warkany J: A warfarin embryopathy? **Am J Dis Child 129**:287-288, 1975 (Comment)
172. Weichsel ME Jr: The therapeutic use of glucocorticoid hormones in the perinatal period: potential neurological hazards. **Ann Neurol 2**:364-366, 1977
173. Weinbaum PJ, Cassidy SB, Vintzileos AM, et al: Prenatal detection of a neural tube defect after fetal exposure to valproic acid. **Obstet Gynecol 67 (Suppl)**:31S-33S, 1986
174. Witter FR, King TM, Blake DA: Adverse effects of cardiovascular drug therapy on the fetus and neonate. **Obstet Gynecol 58 (Suppl)**:100S-105S, 1981
175. Wood SM, Hytten FE: The fate of drugs in pregnancy. **Clin Obstet Gynaecol 8**:255-259, 1981
176. Yeast JD: Immunosuppressive agent use in pregnant patients with transplantation, in Petrie RH (ed): **Perinatal Pharmacology**. Oradell, NJ: Medical Economics Books, 1989, pp 201-207
177. Yerby MS: Problems and management of the pregnant woman with epilepsy. **Epilepsia 28 (Suppl 3)**: S29-S36, 1987
178. Yerby MS, Devinsky O: Epilepsy and pregnancy. **Adv Neurol 64**:45-63, 1994
179. Zhu M, Zhou S: Reduction of the teratogenic effects of phenytoin by folic acid and a mixture of folic acid, vitamins, and amino acids: a preliminary trial. **Epilepsia 30**:246-251, 1989

CHAPTER 2

NEURORADIOLOGICAL DIAGNOSIS DURING PREGNANCY: RISKS AND GUIDELINES

RICHARD K. OSENBACH, MD, AND LEON MOORES, MD

Neuroradiological imaging procedures play a central role in the diagnosis and management of neurosurgical disease. These procedures include plain film radiography, computed tomography (CT), cerebral angiography, ultrasonography, and more recently magnetic resonance imaging (MRI). During pregnancy, neurological problems may occasionally arise which pose a threat to the health of the mother, the fetus, or both. Alternatively, a woman may harbor a pre-existing neurological condition which requires ongoing evaluation and treatment during pregnancy. Such situations often dictate the requirement for some type of neuroradiological imaging procedure in order to delineate the problem and formulate a plan for appropriate management. It goes without saying that any type and degree of radiation exposure during pregnancy is extremely anxiety-provoking. Indeed, the use of almost any diagnostic imaging during pregnancy invariably raises concerns regarding potential teratogenic risk to the developing fetus. It is understood that no radiological procedure should be performed during pregnancy without medical necessity. However, it should also be clear that the medical welfare of the mother should never be jeopardized by withholding diagnostic procedures deemed essential simply because of the fear of potentially detrimental effects on the fetus. However, when imaging procedures are required, appropriate precautions and measures should be employed whenever feasible to ensure that the exposure to the fetus is minimal.

The purpose of this chapter is to discuss the use of some of the more common imaging modalities in the pregnant patient. Issues of occupational exposure to radiologists and technologists who are pregnant will also be discussed briefly. The effects of radiation on the fetus will also be reviewed briefly. Hopefully, this will help allay the undue fear of many physicians and patients who overestimate the risk of radiation.

BASIC ASPECTS OF RADIATION PHYSICS AND EXPOSURE

The major concern regarding radiation exposure to the fetus during pregnancy is related to exposure to high-energy ionizing radiation. Radiation is characterized according to the type of emission and associated energy. The two major forms of ionizing radiation are electromagnetic waves (x-rays and gamma rays) and particle radiation (alpha and beta).[14]

High-energy radiation has the ability to pass through tissues. As it does so, energy is transferred to atoms, which results in the removal of electrons and the generation of ion pairs; hence the term ionizing radiation. This transfer of energy and deposition in tissue results in molecular damage by disruption of chemical bonds in DNA, proteins, and lipids. Usually, this results in cell death or at least significant cellular dysfunction. Ionizing radiation can also interact with cellular water to produce free radicals, which in turn can alter chemical bonds.[6]

The potential for tissue damage from ionizing radiation is largely related to two factors, the amount of energy transferred to the tissue and the degree of tissue penetration. Electromagnetic waves and particles possess different energies and tissue penetration capabilities. Ionizing electromagnetic waves such as x-rays and gamma rays are short-wavelength, high-frequency emissions which have a relatively high energy. They are able to transfer energy and produce ionization while deeply penetrating tissues. In contrast to x-rays and gamma rays, high-energy particles are capable of producing a greater amount of ionization but exhibit relatively poor tissue penetration. This difference has important clinical implications. For example, because radionuclides are particle emitters, they are relatively safe to the fetus when outside the mother. However, when introduced into the mother and concentrated near the fetus (e.g., concentration of technetium-99 in the bladder) they may present significant risk of radiation exposure. Fortunately, radionuclide studies are not generally considered a critical part of the neuroimaging armamentarium in neurosurgery and would not be expected to have a large impact on fetal radiation exposure in this population.

In order to intelligently estimate the risk of radiation exposure, it is necessary to have a basic understanding of the methods by which radiation dosage is measured. The unit by which radiation is measured is dependent on the type of radiation, its energy, the medium through which it travels, and the qualities of the tissue absorbing a given radiation dose.[14] The basic unit of radiation exposure is the roentgen (R). However, the roentgen applies only to x-rays or gamma rays ionizing air. The "absorbed dose" is the term used to describe the effect of radiation on tissue and is defined as the quantity of energy absorbed per unit mass of tissue. The unit of measure for absorbed dose is the "rad" (radiation absorbed dose), which is equal to 0.01 joule/kg. As it turns out, 1 rad of absorbed dose in tissue is approximately equivalent to 1 roentgen of exposure. More recently, the International System of Units has gained wide acceptance and usage. In this system, the unit term for absorbed dose is termed the "gray" (Gy); 1 Gy is equivalent to 100 rad or 1 rad = 1 cGy.

Any type of ionizing radiation can be quantified in terms of rad or gray. However, a special unit has been defined which takes into account the specific type of radiation and its energy as well as the qualities of the absorbing tissue. This has been defined as the "dose-equivalent unit" or "rem" (roengten-equivalent-man) or the "sievert" (Sv) in the International System. The rem is equivalent to the rad multiplied by a qualitative factor. In the case of ionizing radiation, the qualitative factor is 1; therefore, 1 rem is equal to 1 rad.[11]

Effects of Radiation on the Embryo and Fetus

Radiation can have three major effects on the developing conceptus. It can be lethal, result in malformations, or result in growth retardation. Which effect occurs will depend on a number of factors including the radiation dose, dose rate (acute vs. chronic exposure), and stage of development.[1,2,6] In assessing the risks of exposure, it is important to recognize that the majority of data are derived from animal studies which have been extrapolated to humans.[6] There is little, if any, reliable human data from which valid conclusions can be drawn. Indeed, information on irradiation of human concepti is limited to two major sources: therapeutic irradiation during the early part of the century, and studies of atomic bomb survivors in Japan.

Fetal development can be divided into three major stages: 1) preimplantation, 2) organogenesis, and 3) fetal stage. The major effect of exposure to ionizing radiation prior to or immediately following implantation (fertilization up to 15 days) is embryonic death. During this time, the embryo is extremely sensitive to the lethal effects of radiation but relatively resistant to the teratogenic and growth retarding effects. If the number of cells which are damaged is low enough such that the embryo survives, the remaining undifferentiated cells will usually undergo enhanced proliferation to compensate for the cellular loss and to allow implantation and embryonic survival. In other words, the preimplantation effect of radiation on the embryo during a period when all the cells remain undifferentiated is an "all-or-none" phenomenon; the embryo either dies or survives and develops normally. Although no reliable human data exist, animal data suggest that the critical dose or median lethal dose (LD_{50}) for embryonic death is in the range of 1 Gy (100 rad).[1,2]

During the major period of organogenesis (Days 15 to 50 following conception), the embryo is highly sensitive to the teratogenic effects of radiation. Irradiation at this time can also lead to growth retardation, although postnatal catch-up is possible. The developing nervous system is especially vulnerable to the effects of radiation. In fact, the human nervous system is the only organ system in which radiation doses less than 250 to 500 mGy (25-50 rad) have been associated with developmental malformations.[1,2] This association was noted primarily in patients exposed in utero at Hiroshima. This sensitivity is primarily during the period of organogenesis although it persists to some extent into the later stages of fetal development. The major human developmental anomalies induced by radiation exposure include microcephaly, mental retardation, and eye malformations; neural tube and skeletal defects are also described. Following completion of organogenesis, irradiation results primarily in cellular depletion and growth retardation; moreover, as gestation progresses there is less ability for postnatal compensation.

Risks of Diagnostic Imaging

A number of authors have examined the potential for developmental malformations related to diagnostic x-rays performed during pregnancy.[3,5,15,17] Tabuchi et al[15] studied 117 children whose mothers received diagnostic x-rays during the first trimester of pregnancy. Developmental anomalies were noted in four (3.4%) of these children. Granroth[5] retrospectively studied 1,420 children both with and without central nervous system defects (710 children in each group). Although there were a few cases of congenital malformations and prenatal diagnostic x-ray exposure, there was no statistical correlation between the diagnostic radiation exposure and the malformations. Finally, Villemsun[17] studied 3,157 women who were exposed to diagnostic radiographs during pregnancy. Abdominal radiographs were performed in 829 (26%) of these women, 44 during the first trimester and 785 during the second or third trimester. Although dosimetry data were not available, there was no evidence of a statistically significant increase in the incidence of malformations in the offspring of these women.

There are clearly situations when diagnostic imaging must be performed during pregnancy. There is a natural tendency to have an inherent fear of being exposed to radiation, no matter how insignificant the exposure may be. Therefore, it is essential that women be accurately counseled regarding the risk of radiation exposure compared to the natural background rates of spontaneous abortion, genetic diseases, and developmental anomalies. In other words, the risks of radiation exposure must be placed in the context of the general risks of human reproduction. Between 30% and 50% of all known human conceptions abort spontaneously. The incidence of major congenital malformations *at birth* is approximately 3% to 4%. However, this incidence rises to approximately 10% once all malformations and genetic diseases become manifest.[1,2,6]

Although the true minimum threshold dose for the induction of congenital malformations is not known in humans, experimental studies would indicate that it is significantly greater than the radiation dosages used in diagnostic radiology, which are in the range of 20 to 5000 mrad (0.02-5.0 cGy). Therefore, it would make sense that the risk of major congenital malformations, mutations, and growth retardation from the doses utilized in diagnostic radiology would be extremely small. Indeed, Brent[1,2] has maintained that no such effects have occurred with doses of <5 rad.

The imaging studies employed most commonly in the diagnosis of neurosurgical disease are outlined in Table 1. Although radionuclide

TABLE 1

COMMONLY USED DIAGNOSTIC IMAGING STUDIES IN NEUROSURGERY

Plain radiographs
Skull
Cervical spine
Thoracic spine
Lumbar spine
Conventional tomography
Computed tomography
Head
Spine
Magnetic resonance imaging
Head
Spine
Cerebral angiography

TABLE 2

ESTIMATED MAXIMUM DOSE TO FETUS FROM SELECTED IMAGING PROCEDURES

Procedure	Dose in mSv (rem)*
Plain x-rays	
Skull	<0.5 (0.05)
Cervical spine	<0.5 (0.05)
Thoracic spine	<1.0 (0.10)
Lumbar spine	<1.5 (0.15)
Head CT (1-cm slice thickness)	<0.5 (0.05)
Cerebral angiogram	<1.0 (0.10)

* 1 rem = 10 mSv.

studies are occasionally employed in selected instances, they do not play a major role in the primary diagnostic evaluation of the majority of neurosurgical problems. The radiation dose to which the conceptus will be exposed depends on a number of factors including the specific technology employed (plain radiographs, CT, etc.), the technical aspects of a particular study (e.g., exposure factors, filtration, collimation), the size of the patient, the location of the conceptus within the pelvis, the number of films performed, and the duration of fluoroscopy if utilized.[3,4,9,20] For examinations which do not directly involve imaging of the abdomen or pelvis, the only radiation exposure to the conceptus will be through scatter. Obviously, those studies which are of greatest concern involve direct examination of the abdomen and pelvis. Table 2 lists estimates of the maximum dose received by the conceptus for a number of imaging procedures.[14,20] These values assume that the pelvis is shielded by a lead apron and/or is outside the direct path of the x-ray beam. These doses do not necessarily reflect the actual dose; indeed, the actual doses are typically much less than those listed in the table. It has been recommended that the equivalent dose to the conceptus not exceed 0.5 rem (5 mSv) for the entire gestational period.[10] As one can see from the data in Table 2, the conceptus dose for the majority of neuroimaging studies will be well below the recommended guidelines. However, this does not mean that these radiological studies should be ordered with impunity. In spite of the apparent safety, it is still incumbent upon the clinician to dutifully consider the potential risks of the study versus the benefits to the patient. However, it is fairly evident that an unfounded fear of fetal injury should never cause one to withhold a study which might significantly impact on the care of the patient.

OCCUPATIONAL EXPOSURE DURING PREGNANCY

In recent years, there has been an assimilation of growing numbers of women into the fields of neurosurgery, radiology, and radiological technology. Consequently, the issue of occupational radiation exposure and protection has become an important consideration in daily job performance. This issue is of tremendous professional and economic concern, not to mention the health of their progeny. The influence that this issue has on an individual will be affected by concerns of the individual prospective mother, her family, and peers. In order to make informed decisions, any woman with significant occupational exposure to ionizing radiation should have an understanding of the magnitude of the radiation dose to the conceptus that is likely to result from her particular specialty and the precautions which she should employ to guarantee that the conceptus dose is as low as possible.

The National Council on Radiation Protection and Measurements (NCRP) has developed a number of guidelines for pregnant women with occupational exposure to ionizing radiation.[10] The NCRP has recommended that the equivalent dose to the conceptus should not exceed 5 mSv (0.5 rem) during the entire period of gestation. Additionally, once pregnancy is confirmed, the dose should be less than 0.5 mSv in any given month. More recently, the International Commission on Radiological Protection (ICRP) has stated that once pregnancy is declared, the total equivalent dose should not exceed 1 mSv.[7] Based on this figure, the NCRP is considering modifying its recommendations. Finally, the "ALARA" (*A*s *L*ow *A*s *R*easonably *A*chievable) principle should be employed at all times. The latter requires high levels of quality assurance regarding equipment performance and regular evaluations of techniques and procedures.

Much of the concern regarding occupational exposure, particularly for radiologists and technologists, centers on procedures which employ fluoroscopy. In the subspecialty of neuroradiology, cerebral angiography and myelography are two classic examples of studies which are dependent on the use of fluoroscopy. Studies have shown that the dose to the conceptus of a pregnant angiographer will be well within the guidelines set forth by the NCRP and ICRP as long as high acceptable standards of radiation protection are consistently practiced.[4,9,18,19] These practices include wearing a 0.5-mm equivalent lead apron during filming. A special maternity lead apron has been designed which not only accommodates the maternal physique but also contains a 1.0-mm layer of shielding material throughout the entire width of the apron, which extends from the xiphoid process to approximately 3 inches below the symphysis pubis.[22] This effectively creates a belt around the fetus. Doubling the amount of lead in the apron decreases the body exposure by a factor of five. In addition to shielding, the fluoroscopist should maintain the greatest distance from the patient that is technically feasible during the examination and step behind a radiation barrier during serial filming. By following these standard practices, the equivalent dose to the conceptus should be significantly less than 0.01 mSv, well within the guidelines of the NCRP and ICRP. To put this figure in some perspective, one only need examine the levels of background radiation in various regions. For example, a pregnant woman living in Denver accumulates a 0.01-mSV (1 mrem) equivalent dose of background radiation every 3 days, which, extrapolated for the entire pregnancy, comes to just about 1 mSv. Santen et al[13] have published data concerning cerebral angiography and conceptus dose. These authors estimated that the average conceptus dose *per examination* was less than 0.001 mSv. This figure is based on an average of 17 minutes of fluoroscopy time and 60 films per examination. Assuming an average of 200 work days during gestation, Santen's figures would allow an angiographer to perform five examinations per day without exceeding the ICRP-recommended maximum dose of 1 mSv. The level of exposure from this is so small that the actual risk to the conceptus is essentially, if not actually, zero. Using data generated by the NCRP, Wagner and Hayman[19] estimated the risk of malformation based on the magnitude of conceptus dose above background levels of exposure and compared this to the natural incidence of malformation, which they assumed to be on the order of 4% (a 96% chance of birthing a child *without* a malformation). For a conceptus dose of 0.5 mSv above background (approximately corresponding to the conceptus exposure for women in radiology), the probability of having a child without a congenital anomaly is 95.999%.

Obviously, radiation protection cannot be carried out effectively without employing accurate dosimetry practices. This is accomplished by the use of film badges, which should be worn by all individuals with occupational exposure. Perhaps for all women of childbearing potential, but especially for fluoroscopists involved in high-exposure interventional procedures, it may be appropriate to utilize dual-film badging. One badge is used to monitor the dose to unprotected areas of the body while the second badge is worn beneath the protective lead apron and is indicative of the "under-apron" dose. With such practices, should the woman become pregnant, the prior under-apron dose can be used to retrospectively document the dose during the interim period when pregnancy was not suspected as well as prospectively predict the future dose to the conceptus.

Whether women should alter their practice or career planning based on this data is likely to be an individual decision. Clearly, the greatest risk of exposure is during the first trimester when the woman may be unaware or unable to confirm she is pregnant. Therefore, if an individual decides that the risk is sufficient to justify curtailing certain procedures, the primary concern should be to minimize the risks during the first trimester. Ultimately, each individual must decide for herself whether the conservative estimates of radiation risk are acceptable. If a woman does decide that the level of risk is acceptable, then she should be encouraged to pursue her profession and limit her exposure to the lowest practical levels by employing good standards of radiation protection.

Magnetic Resonance Imaging During Pregnancy

In recent years, MRI has become the imaging procedure of choice for a wide spectrum of intracranial as well as intraspinal pathology. MRI is clearly superior to other modalities for the evaluation of a number of pathological conditions. Indeed, MRI has almost become a "routine" study in the evaluation of nearly all patients with suspected neurological conditions.

MRI is thought to be safe. Thus far, there have been no reports of detrimental effects on chromosome structure, DNA synthesis, or rates of mutation.[8,21] However, because MRI is a relatively new imaging modality there are no studies to determine whether MRI has any long-term detrimental effects. Specifically, no data exist as to whether MRI can result in any adverse physiological or behavioral consequences. Johnson et al[8] studied 15 patients who underwent MRI examinations during Weeks 10 to 20 of gestation and observed no detrimental effects on the fetus in these women.

Despite the presumption that MRI has no adverse effects on fetal development, prudence would dictate that MRI be avoided if possible during the first trimester of pregnancy, especially during the first month, which is the period of neurological development. The British National Radiological Protection Board has adopted the policy that MRI be avoided during the first trimester.[12] During the second or third trimesters, MRI is permitted with approval of local medical ethics boards. In 1982, the Food and Drug Administration (FDA) required labeling of MRI units with regard to the safety of fetal imaging.[16] The FDAs position was that "the safety of MRI when used to image fetus has not been established." Although not specifically addressing the potential risks of MRI for pregnant patients, the FDA did not prohibit the use of MRI in pregnant patients. In 1987, a National Institutes of Health consensus panel advised that while no specific evidence exists to indicate that MRI adversely affects human development, "MRI as with all interventions in pregnancy should be used during the first trimester only when there are clear medical indications and when it offers a definite advantage over other tests."[11]

Pregnant women should be studied with MRI only after informed consent has been obtained. As a responsible clinician in such situations, one must constantly assess the risk/benefit ratio for the patient. If a complication of pregnancy poses a threat to the health of the mother, the *potential* risk to the conceptus must be carefully weighed against the risks of incorrect diagnosis or failure to detect a potentially health-threatening and potentially curable medical condition.

Conclusions

It goes without saying that the issue of fetal exposure to radiation and its potential harmful effects is highly emotional and sensitive. While the risks of radiation should not be trivialized, they should not be exaggerated to the point where sound medical judgment is compromised. There are circumstances in which the benefits of radiological imaging far outweigh any potential risk to the unborn child. The risks of radiation-induced defects are trivial compared with the exigent needs of the patient and failure to perform a medically indicated procedure cannot be justified. Hopefully, education of the medical community as well as the public will help allay some of the unfounded fear which has long been associated with radiation.

References

1. Brent RL: Radiation teratogenesis. **Teratology 21:** 281-298, 1980
2. Brent RL: The effects of embryonic and fetal exposure to x-ray, microwaves, and ultrasound. **Clin Perinatol 13:**615-648, 1986
3. Edwards FM: Risks of medical imaging, in Putnam CE, Ravin CE (eds): **Textbook of Diagnostic Imaging.** Philadelphia, PA: WB Saunders, 1988, p 91
4. Fry MRJ: Radiation protection, in Siegel BA, Stephens DH, Theros EG (eds): **Radiation Bioeffects and Management Test and Syllabus.** Baltimore, MD: John D Lucas Printing, 1991, pp 152-159
5. Granroth G: Defects of the central nervous system in Finland. IV. Association with diagnostic x-ray examinations. **Am J Obstet Gynecol 133:**191-194, 1979
6. Hall EJ: **Radiobiology for the Radiologist, 4th ed.** Philadelphia, PA: JB Lippincott, 1994, pp 363-378
7. International Commission on Radiological Protection: **1990 Recommendations of the International Commission on Radiological Protection.** New York, NY: Pergamon Press, ICRP Publication No. 60, 1991
8. Johnson IR, Symonds EM, Kean DM, et al: Imaging of the pregnant human uterus with nuclear magnetic resonance. **Am J Obstet Gynecol 148:**1136-1139, 1984
9. Mettler FA, Wagner LK: X-ray exposure to technologists during fluoroscopy, in Siegel BA, Stephens DH, Theros EG (eds): **Radiation Bioeffects and Management Test and Syllabus.** Baltimore, MD: John D Lucas Printing, 1991, pp 182-191
10. National Council on Radiation Protection and Measurements: **Recommendations on Limits for Exposure to Ionizing Radiation. NCRP Report No. 91.** Bethesda, MD: National Council on Radiation Protection, 1987
11. National Institutes of Health Consensus Conference: Magnetic resonance imaging. **JAMA 259:**2132-3128, 1988
12. National Radiological Protection Board: Revised guidelines on acceptable limits of exposure during nuclear magnetic resonance clinical imaging. **Br J Radiol 56:**974-977, 1983
13. Santen BC, Kan K, Velthuyse HJM, et al: Exposure of radiologists to scattered radiation during angiography. **Radiology 115:**447-450 , 1975
14. Sprawls P Jr: **Physical Principles of Medical Imaging, 2nd ed.** Gaithersburg, MD: Aspen Publishers, 1993
15. Tabuchi A, Nakagawa S, Hirai T, et al: Fetal hazards due to x-ray diagnosis during pregnancy. **Hiroshima J Med Sci 16:**49-66, 1967
16. United States Food and Drug Administration: **Guidelines for Evaluating Exposure Risk for Clinical NMR Systems.** Rockville, MD: Food and Drug Administration, Bureau of Radiological Health, 1982
17. Villemsun AL: **Environmental Factors in Congenital Malformations.** Copenhagen: FADL's Forlag, 1970, pp 130-142
18. Wagner LK, Fabrikant JI: Occupational exposure to radiologists, in Siegel BA, Stephens DH, Theros EG (eds): **Radiation Bioeffects and Management Test and Syllabus.** Baltimore, MD: John D Lucas Printing, 1991, pp 168-181
19. Wagner LK, Hayman LA: Pregnancy and women radiologists. **Radiology 145:**559-562, 1982
20. Wagner LK, Mettler FA: Diagnostic X-ray and radionuclide studies during pregnancy, in Siegel BA, Stephens DH, Theros EG (eds): **Radiation Bioeffects and Management Test and Syllabus.** Baltimore, MD: John D Lucas Printing, 1991, pp 254-271
21. Weinreb JC, Yuh WTC: Obstetrics, in Stark DD, Bradley WG Jr (eds): **Magnetic Resonance Imaging.** Toronto: CV Mosby, 1992, pp 1987-1988
22. Witrak BJ, Sprawls P: Maternity lead apron. **Radiology 150:**597, 1984

The opinions and assertions contained herein represent the views of the authors and do not necessarily reflect those of the United States Army Medical Department or the Department of Defense.

CHAPTER 3

FETAL EFFECTS OF ANESTHESIA

DONALD H. PENNING, MD, MSC, FRCP

The majority of neurosurgical procedures require some form of anesthesia. Many can be done under monitored anesthesia care or local anesthetic infiltration. For the purposes of this chapter, I will confine my comments to the fetal effects of general, epidural, or spinal anesthesia. Much information has been omitted about the effects of anesthesia on the pregnant patient if it did not pertain to neurosurgical patients; for example, the effects of epidural or spinal anesthesia on the course of labor and delivery per se. Persons interested in these and other topics should consult one of a number of recent and comprehensive texts on this subject.[10,43]

Very little specific information exists about the anesthetic care of the parturient for neurosurgical procedures. Some of the advice contained here is subjective and is based on a synthesis of sound anesthetic principles for neurosurgery combined with those applied to obstetrics. The risk of fetal morbidity and mortality that can be attributed to anesthesia alone during neurosurgery is not known. Indeed, that risk is not even known when considering all surgical procedures combined. It is impossible to separate the effects of anesthesia from the effects of the surgery and the underlying disease process. The best that we can hope to achieve, short of doing away with the need for anesthesia altogether, is to discover which anesthetic technique(s) is (are) associated with the lowest fetal and maternal morbidity and mortality rates for each type of patient and procedure. Several studies and reviews are devoted to the topic of anesthesia for nonobstetric surgery during pregnancy.[11,14,28]

FACTORS INFLUENCING FETAL RESPONSES TO ANESTHESIA

Physiological Changes of Pregnancy

The changes that accompany human pregnancy can complicate the administration of anesthesia to the pregnant patient. In general, anything that is bad for the parturient is also bad for the fetus and thus should be avoided. There are a number of reviews on the anesthetic implications of the physiological changes of pregnancy.[9,12,42] This discussion is limited to the most pertinent changes.

Respiratory System

Weight gain and soft-tissue swelling may make tracheal intubation difficult. This problem is exaggerated in pre-eclampsia. Functional residual capacity is decreased by 20% and oxygen consumption increased by 20%. Taken together, these changes contribute to the rapid hemoglobin desaturation that occurs at induction of general anesthesia. This serves to emphasize the need for adequate pre-oxygenation and rapid intubation in these patients.

Cardiovascular System

There is an increased cardiac output beginning early in pregnancy (8 weeks) and rising to approximately 40% above normal in the second trimester. It remains at that level until term, when it rises again during the painful contractions of labor and is maximum (80% increased) immediately postpartum. A so-called physiological anemia of pregnancy (hematocrit = 35%) occurs, despite the increased red cell mass, due to the relatively greater increase in plasma volume. There is normally a decrease (20%) in arterial blood pressure accompanied by decreased peripheral vascular resistance. Aortocaval obstruction can occur due to the compressive effects of the gravid uterus. The aorta may be partially occluded and the inferior vena cava (IVC) may become totally compressed. These results can be partially overcome by placing the parturient in the lateral position or by placing a wedge under the left hip of the mother, thus displacing the uterus from the IVC. While up to 15% of parturients are symptomatic in the supine position (anything from slight lightheadedness to overt shock), other patients may feel normal and yet have significantly compromised uterine perfusion.

Central Nervous System

The minimum alveolar concentration (MAC) is defined as the alveolar concentration of an anesthetic agent that produces immobility to a noxious stimulus in 50% of subjects.[19] In pregnancy, the MAC is reduced up to 40%, an effect thought to be mediated by progesterone. Less clear is the mechanism of the apparent increased neural sensitivity to local anesthetics. This may partially explain the reduced dose of local anesthetic required to produce epidural or spinal anesthesia. Another reason may be the engorged epidural veins reducing the size of the epidural and subarachnoid space.

Gastrointestinal System

A number of factors combine to place the parturient at increased risk for pulmonary aspiration of gastric contents. The stomach is displaced upward and toward the thorax by the gravid uterus. This effect is pronounced in the supine and especially in the lithotomy position. There is increased production of gastrin. Increased concentrations of progesterone and estrogen lead to decreased esophageal sphincter tone and an inhibition of gastrointestinal motility. For these reasons, and despite their fasting status, all parturients must be regarded as having a "full stomach." These changes are estimated to have onset around the 19th week of pregnancy and persist until at least 48 hours postpartum.[42]

Genitourinary System

There is an approximately 60% increase in renal blood flow and glomerular filtration rate during pregnancy. This leads to a serum blood urea nitrogen (BUN) and creatinine level that is roughly one-half that of the nonpregnant patient. A normal or even slightly elevated BUN or creatinine may suggest renal impairment. In that situation care should be exercised in administering renally excreted drugs. The increased glomerular filtration rate and decreased renal threshold for glucose can lead to slight glucosuria.

Hepatic System

The liver maintains normal synthetic function during pregnancy. There is a slight dilutional hypoalbuminemia due to the increased plasma volume. There is a hypercoagulable state due to increased circulating levels of fibrinogen and factors VII, VIII, X, and XII.

Regulation of Uterine Blood Flow

The uterus receives its blood supply by paired uterine arteries arising from the anterior division of the internal iliac artery. There is also a small contribution from the ovarian arteries which arise from the aorta. The nonpregnant uterus receives less than 5% of the cardiac output and 50-100 ml/min of blood. In pregnancy this increases to 12% of cardiac output and 700 ml/min at term. Approximately 90% of this blood is distributed to the intervillus space.[15]

The anesthesiologist can influence a number of the determinates of uteroplacental blood flow. The following is a classification of the causes of decreased uterine blood flow:[15] Placental perfusion can be decreased by *decreasing* mean uterine artery pressure, *increasing* uterine venous pressure, or *increasing* uterine vascular resistance. Clinically, uterine artery pressure can be lowered secondary to partial aortic compression by the gravid uterus in the supine position. Other causes include maternal hypovolemia or hemorrhage,[36] hypotension due to maternal sympathetic blockade by spinal or epidural anesthesia, or by drug-induced hypotension. Deliberately induced hypotension, which may be desirable in some neurosurgical procedures, will be discussed in a separate section.

Increased uterine venous pressure will decrease uterine perfusion pressure (uterine arterial minus venous pressure). Uterine venous pressure will be increased due to IVC obstruction by the gravid uterus in the supine position. Uterine contractions and drug-induced uterine hypertonicity will raise venous pressure, as will generalized maternal hypertonicity such as during seizures or the Valsalva maneuver.

Uterine vascular resistance can be increased by endogenous (catecholamines, vasopressin) or exogenous vasoconstricting substances. Occasionally (such as with paracervical block), high concentrations of local anesthetics may reach the myometrium or uterine arteries. This can cause uterine hypertonicity or uterine artery vasospasm, respectively. During a normal pregnancy, there is a decreased responsiveness of the maternal vasculature to vasoconstricting substances, namely epinephrine, norepinephrine, phenylephrine, and angiotensin II. It is thought that increasing levels of angiotensin II may be responsible for the normal increase in uterine blood flow, due to a lesser decrease in the response of systemic than uterine vessels. To be confusing, alpha-agonists in sheep cause greater vasoconstriction in uterine vessels than systemic vessels! Even in sheep, however, the vasoconstriction is less than in the prepregnant state.

Alpha-agonists vasoconstrict the uterine artery. If used at all in parturients, they should be used cautiously, in small titrated doses to increase maternal systemic blood pressure. Ephedrine remains the vasopressor of choice for the treatment of hypotension in pregnancy.[29] Ephedrine has a sparing effect on uterine blood flow while effectively increasing maternal arterial pressure.

The effects of maternal hyperventilation on uterine blood flow may be very important in the neurosurgical patient. The effects are controversial and will be addressed in the section on the treatment of increased intracranial pressure (ICP).

Fetal Monitoring During Neurosurgical Procedures

Fetal monitoring, by abdominal ultrasound, by external tocodynametric measurement of uterine tone, by intermittent fetal heart rate (FHR) auscultation, or by continuous electronic monitoring of the FHR may be appropriate in many surgical settings. Signs of fetal distress in a viable fetus may mandate urgent delivery. At the least, appropriate measures should be taken to maximize placental perfusion and fetal oxygenation. Such steps as changing maternal position, correcting hypovolemia or hypotension, inhibiting uterine contractions (tocolysis), and increasing maternal oxygen administration should be considered. Even in a pre-viable fetus, monitoring may be appropriate to allow similar measures to be undertaken to allow the fetus to safely reach a more mature status. The decision of whether or not to continuously monitor the FHR is often based on the proposed site of surgery, the presence or absence of maternal obesity, and the gestational age of the fetus. Monitoring during abdominal surgery is difficult, if not impossible, but would often be possible in neurological surgery. Although often possible at 18 weeks' gestation, FHR monitoring may not be reliable until 22 weeks' gestation.[6,24]

FHR variability is an important indicator of fetal well being. In the absence of drug effects, a decrease in FHR variability may be an indicator of fetal distress. Healthy fetuses, beyond 28 weeks' gestation, are felt to exhibit beat-to-beat variability.[6] Electronic FHR monitoring with a scalp electrode requires ruptured membranes. The external Doppler device is less reliable for assessment of beat-to-beat FHR variability.[6] Another caveat when interpreting FHR variability is the suppressing effect of various drugs, including anesthetic agents. It is beyond the scope of this chapter to list the effects of each of these drugs on FHR variability, although in general they make it unreliable as a mode of fetal assessment.[24] During general anesthesia, the most important changes to be aware of are sudden increases or decreases in basal FHR. Since changes in fetal position may artifactually produce changes in the FHR, it is best to confirm the change by auscultation prior to making any management decisions.

The early postoperative period is a time of increased risk of premature labor. This is especially true if the abdominal cavity has been entered, such as in some peritoneal shunting procedures. Therefore it is prudent, where possible, to continue fetal monitoring into the postoperative setting. It is not possible to give specific guidelines for the duration of postoperative monitoring, although 24 hours seems reasonable.

Specific Neurosurgical Conditions and Their Anesthetic Implications

Brain Neoplasms

While the incidence of brain tumors is not influenced by pregnancy,[4] the water retention that can occur[1] may cause increased brain swelling and unmask a previously unrecognized mass. Many of these tumors can be surgically removed after completion of pregnancy. Mass effects can be minimized by modest fluid restriction and the use of steroids. Steroid use is relatively safe in pregnancy.[2] If surgery is necessary, patients will often have advanced disease with evidence of raised ICP. The principle anesthetic concerns are anesthetic induction technique and the management of elevated ICP. Fetal monitoring should be undertaken and is discussed elsewhere.

Cerebrovascular Diseases

The epidemiology and surgical management of these conditions (i.e., intracranial aneurysms and arteriovenous malformations) is dealt with elsewhere. Standard neuroanesthetic concerns for these conditions apply. Particular fetal issues confronted in this type of surgery are management of elevated ICP, induced hypotension, and induced hypothermia. These are dealt with in turn.

Management of Increased Intracranial Pressure During Pregnancy

Barbiturates, with their ability to suppress brain metabolic activity, can reduce blood flow and ICP. Often, large doses of thiopental or phenobarbital are required to suppress brain activity to isoelectricity, thus producing the maximal reduction in ICP. The effects on the fetus of such large doses of barbiturates are largely unknown. In one study, high-dose thiopental (8 mg/kg compared to a usual induction dose of 3-5 mg/kg) was associated with neonatal depression.[16]

Osmotic diuretics such as mannitol are discussed in Chapter 1. Osmotic diuretics increase plasma osmotic pressure and cause a net movement of water from the brain. This can shrink the brain and relieve intracranial hypertension. In rabbits, mannitol has been shown to cross the placenta and raise the fetal plasma osmotic pressure.[8] In that study a net flow of water from the fetus to the mother was demonstrated, leading to decreased fetal blood volume, total body water, and extracellular fluid volume. This resulted in severe fetal dehydration. However, the clinical significance of these findings is unclear since in these animals the osmotic pressure was increased from 300 to >400 mOsm/kg. In clinical practice osmotic pressures >320 mOsm/kg are rarely effective or indicated. Indeed they are undesirable and potentially harmful. Battaglia et al[5] administered 200 g of mannitol to pregnant women at term 1 hour prior to delivery and increased their osmotic pressure from 290 to 320 mOsm/kg water. The fetal osmotic pressure rose less sharply to 312 mOsm/kg water. Moderate doses of mannitol (100 g) have been used without adverse fetal outcome.[21] While reliable clinical data are lacking, it seems reasonable that moderate doses of mannitol (<1.0 g/kg maternal body weight) can be given safely during pregnancy, although there are potential adverse fetal effects.

Maternal hyperventilation decreases $PaCO_2$ and, in the presence of normal cerebral blood flow-CO_2 coupling, leads to a reduction of cerebral blood flow. This in turn leads to decreased cerebral blood volume and a reduction in ICP. The cerebral blood volume response to changes in $PaCO_2$ is brisk and clinically significant. The effect of marked maternal hypocapnia on uterine blood flow has been controversial. Severe maternal hypocapnia ($PaCO_2 \leq 17$ mm Hg) is said to be associated with decreased uterine blood flow. This has been alleged to be due to direct uterine artery vasoconstriction.[30] A classic study by Levinson et al[23] demonstrated that mechanical ventilation can account for the changes in uterine blood flow, since the addition of inhaled CO_2 to maintain normocapnia did not prevent the decrease in uterine blood flow. The effects of positive pressure mechanical ventilation on venous return and cardiac output may mediate this change.

Safe guidelines for the use of hypocapnia to reduce ICP in pregnancy have not been established and it seems reasonable to use this method sparingly. It should be remembered that the normal maternal $PaCO_2$ in pregnancy is 32 mm Hg; therefore, the useful range of hypocapnia is reduced. FHR monitoring may indicate when safe limits have been exceeded, although this cannot be relied on. If hyperventilation cannot be avoided and fetal distress is suspected, judicial use of a vasopressor such as ephedrine may maintain uterine blood flow.

Induced Hypotension

It is occasionally necessary to induce controlled hypotension in a pregnant patient undergoing a craniotomy for vascular lesions. This may reduce the likelihood of vascular rupture or bleeding if rupture occurs. Uterine perfusion is not autoregulated and therefore will be reduced in situations of maternal hypotension. This should be well tolerated by the healthy fetus if the degree or duration of hypotension is not severe. However, safe guidelines cannot be recommended. Hypotension from maternal hemorrhage has been demonstrated in chronically instrumented fetal sheep to be associated with severe (80-90%) reductions in uterine blood flow and progressive fetal acidosis.[36] This was rapidly fatal to the fetus if not reversed. Induced hypotension in pregnancy has been used successfully but the reported use is limited to isolated case reports[13,34] and small case series.[40] Success is often measured by a living fetus or live birth with no assessment of fetal neurological status or pediatric follow-up.

The most commonly used agents to induce hypotension are isoflurane, sodium nitroprusside, and nitroglycerin. These will be discussed in turn. Isoflurane anesthesia, 0.5-1.5 MAC, is not associated with significant reductions in uterine blood flow.[35] In nonpregnant patients it can be used effectively to induce hypotension.[33] There are few reports of its use for this purpose in pregnancy but it has been used effectively without obvious fetal compromise.[33]

Sodium nitroprusside is widely used for inducing hypotension in neurosurgical patients.[25,26] There are several reports of nitroprusside use for this purpose in pregnant patients.[13,40] Nitroprusside metabolism releases cyanide.[45] This is not normally a problem in small doses, since the cyanide is combined with thiol compounds such as thiosulfate to produce thiocyanate. Thiocyanate is relatively nontoxic and is excreted renally. The production of thiocyanate is catalyzed by the enzyme rhodenase. Theoretically, decreased fetal thiosulfate levels or rhodenase activity may lead to greater fetal toxicity of nitroprusside. In pregnant sheep given sodium nitroprusside, peak fetal arterial cyanide levels are significantly higher than those in the mother.[32] Of concern in that study is that five of eight sheep had fetal deaths, and in each of those excessive doses of nitroprusside were required to produce the desired degree of hypotension. These sheep demonstrated early tachyphylaxis in response to nitroprusside, suggesting that sheep may not accurately model the human response to nitroprusside. Despite this, it may be safest to discontinue nitroprusside at the first suggestion of impending tachyphylaxis in response to its hypotensive effects.

I am not aware of any adverse fetal or neonatal effects of nitroglycerin use in pregnant women. Its effects on the uterine vasculature have been compared and contrasted with nitroprusside in pregnant sheep.[49] In that study nitroglycerin (and nitroprusside) were shown to be effective in reducing norepinephrine-induced hypertension. Both drugs were capable of reducing maternal mean arterial pressure (MAP) by 20% without changing uterine blood flow. Nitroglycerin has few adverse side effects and its effects are rapidly reversed if the infusion of drug is discontinued.

Trimethaphan is not currently in favor for induced hypotension. It may have a greater hypotensive effect on pregnant than nonpregnant women.[41] A minor additional problem with trimethaphan is that it prolongs the action of succinylcholine by inhibiting plasma pseudocholinesterase. It may also impair neurological assessment in the postoperative period by causing pupillary dilatation.

Hypothermia

Moderate hypothermia decreases cerebral metabolic requirements and is neuroprotective in the adult[17] and the immature brain during hypoxic-ischemic episodes.[46] Although there are numerous reports of purposeful hypothermia during cardiac surgery within pregnancy, there are only a handful that concern intracranial surgery.[27,44] The lowest maternal temperature achieved in those studies was 26.5° to 28°C. There is little if any conclusive data on the effectiveness of hypothermia for neuroprotection during surgery in humans. There are even fewer data upon which to base guidelines for its application during pregnancy.

Fetal Effects of Positioning for Neurosurgical Procedures

The importance of avoiding aortocaval compression by applying left uterine displacement has been mentioned previously. Due to venous pooling in the lower extremities and the potential for exacerbation of aortocaval obstruction, it may be inadvisable to operate on pregnant patients in the sitting position. However, I am currently unaware of any data to suggest that this is absolutely contraindicated.

Miscellaneous Neurosurgical Procedures During Pregnancy

Among the conditions that may require CSF shunting is pseudotumour cerebri. Pseudotumor cerebri, so-called benign intracranial hypertension, has four cardinal features: elevated cerebrospinal fluid (CSF) pressure, normal CSF composition, normal level of consciousness, and absence of intracranial abnormality.[3] It is not uncommon to have a worsening of symptoms during pregnancy. If carbonic anhydrase inhibitors fail, therapy usually consists of either serial lumbar punctures to remove CSF or placement of a lumboperitoneal shunt. The anesthetic implications are the same as for any surgical procedure during pregnancy.

The presence of a lumboperitoneal shunt presents a dilemma when faced with providing epidural or spinal anesthesia for labor and delivery. In addition to the risk of introducing infection, it is conceivable that the shunt may be entered, allowing the local anesthetic solution to pass into the peritoneal cavity. Although epidural anesthesia has been safely performed, it is recommended that spinal anesthesia be avoided in this situation.[3]

Specific Effects of Anesthetic Techniques and Agents

General Anesthesia

As a general rule most of the induction and maintenance drugs administered to the mother also cross the placenta rapidly and in appreciable quantities to the fetus. The general exception to this is the muscle relaxants, which are charged compounds and as such cross the placenta in only nonsignificant amounts. In circumstances where the fetus is in an acidotic state, some drugs, such as most of the local anesthetics, exist in the fetal circulation as the charged species. It is possible that the concentration of that drug will increase relative to the mother, a phenomenon termed "ion-trapping."

Induction Agents

Thiopental has been the primary intravenous (IV) induction drug in obstetrics for many years. It is also a very useful induction drug in neurosurgical patients. While thiopental use may be associated with hypotension, especially in hemodynamically compromised patients, at usual induction doses of 4 mg/kg there is little if any adverse effect on the fetus. In hypovolemic patients, ketamine may be a better choice. Thiopental rapidly crosses the placenta and concentrations peak in the umbilical venous circulation 1 minute after maternal IV administration.[22]

Ketamine has little effect on uterine blood flow, uterine tone, and neonatal behavior at dosages of 0.25-1.0 mg/kg.[39] At doses greater than 1.0 mg/kg, there is a report of transiently lower newborn neurobehavioral assessments when compared to thiopental.[18] Ketamine has a sympathomimetic activity that tends to maintain blood pressure in hypovolemic patients, but in profound hypovolemia its inherent myocardial depressant properties can produce hypotension. These same sympathomimetic properties would make it a poor choice if hypertension is to be avoided, such as in intracranial aneurysm patients. In situations of reduced intracerebral compliance ketamine can increase ICP, a situation that can be mostly attenuated or prevented by prior hyperventilation. Thus, ketamine remains a potentially useful drug that can be used effectively if the above factors are taken into consideration.

Propofol is a drug that may allow more rapid emergence from anesthesia when used alone for induction or as a complete anesthetic. This could be an advantage in neurosurgical patients. It has been used successfully in pregnancy although there are conflicting reports of its hypotensive effects in this group of patients.[39] Recently, there has been a randomized prospective trial in which patients receiving propofol had lower pregnancy rates than a group of patients receiving thiopental-isoflurane anesthesia.[47] Without a clear indication of its superiority to other agents, it remains to be seen if propofol finds a use in pregnant neurosurgical patients.

Etomidate can be used to induce anesthesia with minimal hemodynamic compromise even in hypovolemic patients. It produces pain upon IV injection and often leads to myoclonic jerks.[39] Etomidate use is limited due to its tendency to suppress serum cortisol production, including that in neonates.[38] Despite these potential side effects, its favorable cardiovascular properties may make it a useful drug. I am unaware of any reports of its use in pregnant neurosurgical patients.

Benzodiazepines

Benzodiazepines such as diazepam and midazolam are used occasionally as adjuncts to general anesthesia or as sedatives during monitored anesthetic care. Like most of the general anesthetics, even small doses decrease beat-to-beat variability. A small dose of midazolam (5 mg) administered just before delivery may cause fetal and newborn depression, which can be greater than that seen with thiopental.[7] This is not likely to be of much consequence since there was no associated fetal or neonatal acidosis and the behavioral differences were undetectable by 4 hours of age.

Opioids

Meperidine is one of the most commonly used analgesics during labor, having peak analgesia at 40 to 50 minutes when given intramuscularly (IM) or 5 to 10 minutes if given IV. The total duration is usually 3 to 4 hours. Peak neonatal respiratory depression occurs at 2 to 3 hours and should not be a problem if administered <1 hour or >4 hours prior to delivery.[48] It is not currently in vogue as an anesthetic drug during neurosurgery.

Fentanyl has a peak IV effect within 3 to 5 minutes and is typically effective for 30 to 60 minutes. Doses of 50 to 100 μg or 25 to 50 μg IV, if given within 15 minutes of delivery, have no detectable neonatal effects.[48] Slightly higher doses may have some detectable neurobehavioral changes at 4 hours but are not detectable 24 hours following delivery.

Morphine causes greater respiratory depression at equi-analgesic doses than does meperidine. Its peak effect is at 20 minutes given IV or 2 hours given IM. Analgesia typically lasts 4 to 6 hours.[48]

Nalbuphine (10-20 mg) and butorphanol (1-2 mg) are partial agonists at the opiate receptor and produce analgesia but have a ceiling effect on respiratory depression at high dosages.[48] They are moderately effective analgesics for labor and have significant sedative properties.

Epidural opioids such as fentanyl or sufentanil should have minimal effects on the fetus, especially if the total dose of sufentanil is kept at <30 μg and that for fentanyl ≤600 μg. In labor, combinations of local anesthetics and opioids in low doses (i.e., fentanyl (1-2 μg/ml) or sufentanil (0.1-0.2 μg/ml)) by infusion at 10-15 ml/hr showed no adverse fetal effects or loss of beat-to-beat variability. This is in contrast to systemic opioids, which may reduce FHR variability.[48] This is not much of an additional problem during neurological surgery under general anesthesia since FHR variability is usually unreliable.

Inhalational Anesthetics

All of the halogenated inhalational anesthetics relax uterine smooth muscle in a dose-related manner.[31] Uterine blood flow is maintained with commonly used doses (0.5-1.5 MAC) of halothane, enflurane, isoflurane, desflurane, or sevoflurane.[15,35] At very high doses these agents may cause cardiac depression with hypotension and may markedly reduce uterine blood flow. Even so, 1.5% to 2.0% isoflurane has been used to induce hypotension in a parturient during cerebral aneurysm surgery without any apparent fetal complications.[34] From the fetal point of view there seems to be little to choose from in selecting a particular agent. Maternal or neurosurgical factors will determine the best choice. It is important to mention that the use of these potent agents during combined cesarean section and emergency neurosurgery (e.g., ruptured aneurysm or head trauma) may complicate patient care. The profound uterine relaxation that can be induced with clinical doses of these agents may lead to postpartum hemorrhage from uterine atony. Vaginal bleeding may be occult (i.e., under the surgical drapes) and should be checked periodically.

Nitrous oxide is a useful adjunct to many neuroanesthesia regimes and is very commonly used (inspired concentrations of 50%) in obstetrical anesthesia. It is only an effective analgesic at relatively high concentrations (≥ 50% inspired concentrations; MAC approximately 102%). For this reason it needs to be used with other anesthetic agents to provide complete anesthesia. The drawback is that it limits the percentage of oxygen that may be administered to the patient. During prolonged neurosurgical procedures there is a theoretical problem with nitrous oxide because it inhibits methionine synthetase, an enzyme essential for DNA synthesis.[11] Prolonged exposure in humans may inhibit the bone marrow apparatus and produce signs of pernicious anemia.[20]

Regional Anesthesia

Major conduction anesthesia such as epidural or spinal (subarachnoid or intrathecal) techniques will not often be useful in neurological surgery. Both techniques have a very long record of safety for mother and fetus if basic principles of anesthesia are followed. However, uncorrected hypotension from excessively high levels of sympathetic blockade can lead to fetal hypoxia and acidosis.[37]

Guidelines for Minimizing the Risks of Anesthesia for Pregnant Neurosurgical Patients

1. Whenever possible, surgery should be postponed until 4-6 weeks postpartum.
2. Careful maternal positioning to maximize fetal oxygenation.
3. Administration of high maternal oxygen concentrations.
4. Prompt treatment of maternal hypovolemia, hemorrhage, or hypotension. Ephedrine is the vasopressor of choice.
5. All parturients have a "full stomach" and should receive pulmonary aspiration precautions and rapid sequence intubations whenever possible.
6. Fetal heart rate and uterine activity monitoring should be instituted whenever fetal maturity and surgical circumstances permit. This monitoring should continue into the postoperative period.
7. A team approach between neurosurgeons, anesthesiologists, obstetricians, neonatologists, and nurses is essential to the smooth and effective management of these challenging patients.

References

1. Abad J, Alvarez F, Manrique M, et al: Cerebral arteriovenous malformations. Comparative results of surgical vs conservative treatment in 112 cases. **J Neurosurg Sci 27:**203-210, 1983
2. Abouleish E: Neurologic disease, in James FM III, Wheeler AS, Dewan DM (eds): **Obstetric Anesthesia: The Complicated Patient.** Philadelphia, PA: FA Davis, 1988
3. Abouleish E, Ali V, Tang RA: Benign intracranial hypertension and anesthesia for cesarean section. **Anesthesiology 63:**705-707, 1985
4. Aronson NI, Kaplaw S, Goldstein PJ: Brain tumors during pregnancy, in Goldstein PJ (ed): **Neurological Disorders of Pregnancy.** Mt Kisco, NY: Futura, 1986
5. Battaglia F, Prystowsky H, Smisson C, et al: Fetal blood studies. XIII. The effect of the administration of fluids intravenously to mothers upon the concentrations of water and electrolytes in plasma of human fetuses. **Pediatrics 25:**2-10, 1960
6. Biehl DR: Foetal monitoring during surgery unrelated to pregnancy. **Can Anaesth Soc J 32:**455-459, 1985
7. Bland BAR, Lawes EG, Duncan PW, et al: Comparison of midazolam and thiopental for rapid sequence anesthetic induction for elective cesarean section. **Anesth Analg 66:**1165-1168, 1987
8. Bruns PD, Linder RO, Drose VE, et al: The placental transfer of water from fetus to mother following the intravenous infusion of hypertonic mannitol to the maternal rabbit. **Am J Obstet Gynecol 86:**160-167, 1963
9. Cheek TG, Gutsche BB: Maternal physiologic alterations during pregnancy, in Shnider SM, Levinson G (eds): **Anesthesia for Obstetrics, 3rd ed.** Baltimore, MD: William & Wilkins, 1993, pp 3-17
10. Chestnut DH (ed): **Obstetric Anesthesia: Principles and Practice.** St Louis, MO: Mosby-Year Book, 1994, 1040 pp
11. Cohen SE: Nonobstetric surgery during pregnancy, in Chestnut DH (ed): **Obstetric Anesthesia: Principles and Practice.** St Louis, MO: Mosby-Year Book, 1994, pp 273-293
12. Conklin KA: Physiologic changes of pregnancy, in Chestnut DH (ed): **Obstetric Anesthesia: Principles and Practice.** St Louis, MO: Mosby-Year Book, 1994, pp 17-42
13. Donchin Y, Amirav B, Sahar A, et al: Sodium nitroprusside for aneurysm surgery in pregnancy. Report of a case. **Br J Anaesth 50:**849-851, 1978
14. Duncan PG, Pope WDB, Cohen MM, et al: Fetal risk of anesthesia and surgery during pregnancy. **Anesthesiology 64:**790-794, 1986
15. Eisenach JC: Uteroplacental blood flow, in Chestnut DH (ed): **Obstetric Anesthesia: Principles and Practice.** St Louis, MO: Mosby-Year Book, 1994
16. Finster M, Mark LC, Morishima HO: Plasma thiopental concentrations in the newborn following delivery under thiopental-nitrous oxide anesthesia. **Am J Obstet Gynecol 95:**621-629, 1966
17. Ginsberg MD, Sternau LL, Globus MYT, et al: Therapeutic modulation of brain temperature: relevance to ischemic brain injury. **Cerebrovasc Brain Metab Rev 4(3):**189-225, 1992
18. Hodgkinson R, Marx GF, Kim SS, et al: Neonatal neurobehavioral tests following vaginal delivery under ketamine, thiopental, and extradural anesthesia. **Anesth Analg 56:**548-553, 1977
19. Koblin DD: Mechanisms of action, in Millar RD

(ed): **Anesthesia.** New York, NY: Churchill Livingstone, 1994

20. Koblin DD, Waskell L, Watson JE, et al: Nitrous oxide inactivates methionine synthetase in human liver. **Anesth Analg 61:**7578, 1982
21. Kofke WA, Wuest HP, McGinnis LA: Cesarean section following ruptured cerebral aneurysm and neuroresuscitation. **Anesthesiology 60:**242-245, 1984
22. Kosaka Y, Takahashi T, Mark LC: Intravenous thiobarbiturate anesthesia for cesarean section. **Anesthesiology 31:**489-506, 1969
23. Levinson G, Shnider SM, Delorimier AA, et al: Effects of maternal hyperventilation on uterine blood flow and fetal oxygenation and acid-base status. **Anesthesiology 40:**340-347, 1974
24. Liu PL, Warren TM, Ostheimer GW, et al: Foetal monitoring in parturients undergoing surgery unrelated to pregnancy. **Can Anaesth Soc J 32:**525-532, 1985
25. Maktabi M, Warner D, Sokoll M: The effects of hypotension induced by sodium nitroprusside and isoflurane on serum catecholamines and plasma renin activity. **Anesthesiology 65 (Suppl):**A578, 1986 (Abstract)
26. Maktabi M, Warner DS, Sokoll MD, et al: Comparison of nitroprusside, nitroglycerin, and deep isoflurane anesthesia for induced hypotension. **Neurosurgery 19:**350-355, 1986
27. Matsuki A, Oyama T: Operation under hypothermia in a pregnant woman with an intracranial arteriovenous malformation. **Can Anaesth Soc J 19:**184-191, 1972
28. Mazze RI, Källén B: Reproductive outcome after anesthesia and operation during pregnancy: a registry study of 5405 cases. **Am J Obstet Gynecol 161:**1178-1185, 1989
29. McGrath JM, Chestnut DH, Vincent RD, et al: Ephedrine remains the vasopressor of choice for treatment of hypotension during ritodrine infusion and epidural anesthesia. **Anesthesiology 80:** 1073-1081, 1994
30. Morishima HO, Daniel SS, Adamsons Jr K, et al: Effects of positive pressure ventilation of the mother upon the acid-base state of the fetus. **Am J Obstet Gynecol 93:**269-273, 1965
31. Munson ES, Embro WJ: Enflurane, isoflurane, and halothane and isolated human uterine muscle. **Anesthesiology 46:**11-14, 1977
32. Naulty J, Cefalo RC, Lewis PE: Fetal toxicity of nitroprusside in the pregnant ewe. **Am J Obstet Gynecol 139:**708-711, 1981
33. Newman B, Gelb AW, Lam AM: The effect of isoflurane-induced hypotension on cerebral blood flow and cerebral metabolic rate for oxygen in humans. **Anesthesiology 64:**307-310, 1986
34. Newman B, Lam AM: Induced hypotension for clipping of a cerebral aneurysm during pregnancy: a case report and brief review. **Anesth Analg 65:** 675-678, 1986
35. Palahniuk RJ, Shnider SM: Maternal and fetal cardiovascular acid-base changes during halothane and isoflurane anesthesia in the pregnant ewe. **Anesthesiology 41:**462-472, 1974
36. Penning DH, Chestnut DH, Dexter F, et al: Glutamate release from the ovine fetal brain during maternal hemorrhage. A study using chronic *in utero* cerebral microdialysis. **Anesthesiology 82:**521-530, 1995
37. Ralston DH, Shnider SM: The fetal and neonatal effects of regional anesthesia in obstetrics. **Anesthesiology 48:**34-64, 1978
38. Reddy BK, Pizer B, Bull PT: Neonatal serum cortisol suppression by etomidate compared with thiopentone, for elective caesarean section. **Eur J Anaesthesiol 5:**171-176, 1988
39. Reisner LS, Lin D: Anesthesia for cesarean section, in Chestnut DH (ed): **Obstetric Anesthesia: Principles and Practice.** St Louis, MO: Mosby-Year Book, 1994, pp 459-486
40. Rigg D, McDonagh A: Use of sodium nitroprusside for deliberate hypotension during pregnancy. **Br J Anaesth 53:**985-987, 1981
41. Rosen MA: Anesthesia for neurosurgery during pregnancy, in Shnider SM, Levinson G (eds): **Anesthesia for Obstetrics, 3rd ed.** Baltimore, MD: Williams & Wilkins, 1993, pp 551-561
42. Rosen MA: **Physiologic Alterations of Pregnancy: Anesthetic Implications.** 1994 Annual Refresher Course Lectures, American Society of Anesthesiologists, 1994, 174 pp
43. Shnider SM, Levinson G (eds): **Anesthesia for Obstetrics, 3rd ed.** Baltimore, MD: Williams & Wilkins, 1993, 744 pp
44. Stånge K, Halldin M: Hypothermia in pregnancy. **Anesthesiology 58:**460-461,1983
45. Tinker JH, Michenfelder JD: Sodium nitroprusside: pharmacology, toxicology and therapeutics. **Anesthesiology 45:**340-354, 1976
46. Towfighi J, Housman C, Heitjan DF, et al: The effect of focal cerebral cooling on perinatal hypoxic-ischemic brain damage. **Acta Neuropathol 87:** 598-604, 1994
47. Vincent RD, Syrop CH, Van Voorhis BJ, et al: An evaluation of the effect of anesthetic technique on reproductive success after laparoscopic pronuclear stage transfer. **Anesthesiology 82:**352-358, 1995
48. Wakefield ML: Systemic analgesia: opioids, ketamine, and inhalational agents, in Chestnut DH (ed): **Obstetric Anesthesia: Principles and Practice.** St Louis, MO: Mosby-Year Book, 1994, pp 340-352
49. Wheeler AS, James FM III, Meis PJ, et al: Effects of nitroglycerin and nitroprusside on the uterine vasculature of gravid ewes. **Anesthesiology 52:**390-394, 1980

CHAPTER 4

CHANGES IN CARDIOVASCULAR AND CEREBROVASCULAR FUNCTION DURING PREGNANCY

DALE M. SWIFT, MD

Normal pregnancy induces dramatic adaptations in cardiovascular function. These changes, exemplified by the "plethora" of pregnancy, have been recognized since antiquity. Pregnancy may also be associated with various forms of cerebrovascular disease, including intracerebral and subarachnoid hemorrhage. The relationship between pregnancy and cerebrovascular diseases remains obscure despite much conjecture. With the exception of encephalopathy and intracerebral hemorrhage associated with hypertensive disorders of pregnancy (e.g., eclampsia), a causal relationship remains to be demonstrated. Understanding cardiovascular changes associated with pregnancy may assist in managing patients with cerebrovascular disease either caused by, influenced by, or coincident with pregnancy.

This chapter summarizes the hemodynamic changes accompanying normal pregnancy as well as some of the changes seen during pathological pregnancy. A brief discussion of the current state of knowledge regarding cerebrovascular function in pregnancy follows.

CARDIOVASCULAR CHANGES IN PREGNANCY

As the ability to accurately measure various hemodynamic parameters has evolved, so has the knowledge regarding changes in these parameters, and therefore cardiovascular physiology, occurring during pregnancy. The well-known parameters of blood volume, blood pressure, heart rate, and cardiac output all demonstrate characteristic adaptations to pregnancy and are described below.

Blood Volume

Total red cell mass and plasma volume constitute the whole-blood volume. The most reliable measurements to date indicate that whole-blood volume increases an average of 1600 ml (40%-50%) during normal pregnancy.[20,21,23] Plasma volume increases an average of 1200 ml (45%-50%) while total red cell mass increases by 250 to 450 ml (20%-30%).[16] This differential increase accounts for the physiological anemia seen in pregnancy. Hemoglobin concentration and hematocrit reach their nadir in the middle of the third trimester, with hemoglobin concentrations not usually falling below 11 g/dl.[16] In women receiving iron supplements the increase in red cell mass is significantly greater (400 vs. 240 ml) and the anemia less severe.[16] The relative anemia associated with pregnancy decreases blood viscosity and has been postulated to provide some defense[20] against thrombosis.

Plasma volume begins to increase at approximately 8 weeks' gestation, expanding progressively to reach a plateau at 32 weeks.[23] The degree to which the plasma volume expands is increased in multiple pregnancies and with second or subsequent pregnancies.[25] In addition, the amount of increase in plasma volume correlates with birth weight.[2] Early reports described a diminution in plasma volume during the end of the third trimester. This conclusion is now considered erroneous, however, owing to measurements of plasma volume having been made in the supine position. In the supine position, compression of the vena cava by the gravid uterus may cause a significant decrease in venous blood return to the heart. This phenomenon may significantly alter measurements of blood volume, blood pressure, and cardiac output.

The stimulus to increase plasma volume during pregnancy is not precisely known. It may be due to normal or enhanced mechanisms of fluid conservation in the setting of diminished peripheral vascular resistance. Peripheral vascular resistance decreases in normal pregnancy, in part due to the addition of the low-resistance utero-placental vasculature to the circulatory system.[24] Another important factor is systemic vasodilatation apparently resulting from direct influences of progesterone and prostacyclins on the vasculature. This vasodilatation is thought to be responsible for the decrease in systemic blood pressure observed in normal pregnancy (see below).

Increased plasma and red cell volumes help prevent hypotension during pregnancy and also serve as an important buffer against the inevitable blood loss accompanying delivery. Average estimated blood loss during vaginal delivery of a single neonate is >500 ml. With cesarean delivery or vaginal delivery of twins, blood loss averages 1000 ml.[16] Whole-blood volume returns to normal prepregnancy values several weeks after delivery or sooner, depending upon the amount of blood lost at delivery. Plasma volume is lost due to diuresis and red cells are lost more slowly due to normal senescence. Postpartum diuresis is maximal between the second and fifth day, at which time hemoglobin concentrations and hematocrit may rise above normal.[15] Complete return to normal cardiovascular function occurs gradually by 12 weeks' postpartum.[6]

Blood Pressure

Systemic arterial blood pressure declines somewhat during the middle of normal pregnancy, rising again to prepregnancy levels toward term. Mean arterial pressure is decreased by approximately 10% by the seventh week, with little change throughout the remainder of pregnancy.[5,17] Systolic pressure decreases less than diastolic, thus widening the pulse pressure. The maximum decrease in diastolic pressure is typically 10 to 20 mm Hg and is achieved by 28 weeks' gestation.[20,21,29]

Again, care must be taken in documenting the position of the subject during measurement of various hemodynamic parameters during pregnancy. This is especially true when measuring blood pressure. Up to 11% of pregnant women will demonstrate a significant decrease in arterial blood pressure in the supine position due to compression of the vena cava. Aortic compression may also occur, compromising utero-fetal blood flow, while maternal arterial blood pressure measured at the brachial artery actually increases.[21]

The etiology of the observed diminution in systemic blood pressure appears to be a decrease in systemic vascular resistance for which increased cardiac output fails to compensate sufficiently to maintain normal prepregnancy pressures. There appears to be a relative resistance to angiotensin II in pregnancy. Thus, despite relatively high levels of renin, angiotensin, and aldosterone, blood pressure remains normal or subnormal.[21]

Elevation of arterial blood pressure >90 mm Hg diastolic may occur during pregnancy.

Hypertension associated with pregnancy is divided into four categories: pre-eclampsia/eclampsia, transient hypertension of pregnancy, chronic hypertension (pre-existing), and pre-eclampsia superimposed on chronic hypertension.[7] Pre-eclampsia, especially when superimposed on chronic hypertension, represents the greatest risk to the mother and fetus. Eclampsia is defined when generalized seizures occur. Severe hypertension or eclampsia may result in encephalopathy or intracerebral hemorrhage.

In the hypertensive states of pregnancy, especially pre-eclampsia/eclampsia, there is a lack of the normal pregnancy-induced resistance to vasopressor substances such as catecholamines and angiotensin.[11] In fact there may be intense sensitivity to vasoactive hormones resulting in cerebral and systemic vasospasm.[4,26]

Cardiac Output

Maternal cardiac output increases markedly during pregnancy. Heart rate and stroke volume, the determinants of cardiac output, increase 29% and 18%, respectively, producing an increase in cardiac output of up to 50%.[17] Cardiac output during pregnancy has been determined by a variety of techniques with varying results. Recently, using Doppler echocardiography, cardiac output has been shown to progressively increase up to term.[17] Previous reports, however, suggest that cardiac output reaches a plateau at 24 weeks' gestation.[9] The calculation of cardiac index is similar to cardiac output but standardized for body-surface area. Cardiac index increases less than cardiac output during pregnancy due to increases in body-surface area associated with pregnancy.

The dynamics of labor are reflected in the cardiac output. During the first stage of labor cardiac output increases approximately 12%.[24] With each uterine contraction cardiac output increases another 20% to 30%.[25] Valsalva maneuvers add to this effect. By the time of delivery there is a cumulative 30% to 40% increase in cardiac output.[24,25] Anesthesia administered during labor may blunt these changes.

Cardiac output remains elevated postpartum as venous return to the heart is increased. Emptying of the uterine contents decompresses the vena cava and returns a significant vascular volume from the previously highly vascular uteroplacental circulation. Elevated cardiac output persists through the second postpartum day, thereafter rapidly decreasing to normal prepregnancy values by 2 to 6 weeks.[9] It is therefore during the early postpartum period that the mother is most at risk to develop cardiac failure.

Anatomical Vascular Changes in Pregnancy

Generalized dilatation of the arterioles occurs during pregnancy, especially in the arterioles of the uterus, kidney, and skin. Vasodilatation is thought to be a direct effect of progesterone, estrogen, and prostacyclins on vascular smooth muscle.[15] Relaxin, the pregnancy hormone which allows lengthening of the interpubic ligament in preparation for parturition, also has been implicated in causing vasodilatation during pregnancy.[14]

In addition to dilatation, anatomical changes occur in blood vessel wall structure during pregnancy.[3] These changes may be due to the hemodynamic stresses imparted by pregnancy or to the direct effects of the hormones of pregnancy. Intimal hyperplasia of both arteries and veins has been observed in pregnancy and in nonpregnant women receiving oral estrogens.[13,18,22] Changes in the vessel media include thickening, reticular fragmentation, and loss of normal elastic corrugation.[18] It has been suggested that hormonal changes compounded by increased hemodynamic stress account for the increased incidence of dissecting aortic and ruptured renal aneurysms seen in pregnancy.[3]

Cerebrovascular Changes in Pregnancy

Although cardiovascular adaptations to pregnancy have been studied extensively, relatively little is known about specific cerebrovascular changes during pregnancy. After an early publication by McCall[19] in 1949 describing cerebral blood flow (CBF) in normal and toxemic pregnant women, there has been a paucity of published literature on the subject. Given concerns regarding cerebrovascular events during pregnancy, measurement of cerebrovascular parameters remains important. Recently Doppler studies of the cerebrovascular system have been performed in both normal and complicated pregnancies. Doppler studies provide noninvasive, albeit limited, assessment of the cerebrovasculature and are presumed safe for both mother and fetus. Two reports of single photon emission computed tomography (SPECT) measurements of CBF during pregnancy have now been published.[1,11] The conclusions drawn by these preliminary studies remain to be substantiated.

Doppler studies of the internal carotid artery performed serially during normal pregnancy have shown a decrease in peak systolic and mean velocities after 28 weeks.[12] Transcranial Doppler ultrasound of the middle cerebral artery by the same authors revealed transient increases in mean and peak systolic velocities from 8 to 27 weeks' gestation.[10] Other authors have observed a decrease in middle cerebral artery velocities at 25 to 36 weeks' gestation.[27] In patients with pre-eclampsia, transcranial Doppler ultrasound reveals higher flow velocities than those seen in normal pregnancy.[28] Thus, despite a lack of agreement regarding the nature and time course of middle cerebral artery flow velocity changes in pregnancy, transcranial Doppler studies may be of benefit in assessing intracranial vascular changes in pregnancies complicated by hypertension.

CBF has rarely been measured during normal pregnancies. McCall,[19] in 1949, reported normal CBF measured by nitrous oxide technique during otherwise normal pregnancies in nine women. More recently, Ikeda et al[10] have given evidence that regional CBF (rCBF) is increased during normal pregnancy. Using ^{133}Xe SPECT technique they found increases in rCBF varying from 5.6% to 16.7% in 10 women during the 7th to the 19th week of pregnancy. The women served as their own controls 17 to 67 days after elective abortion. The greatest increase in rCBF was seen in the cerebellum (16.7%), followed by the temporal lobe (12.9%), parietal lobe (9.8%), and frontal lobe (9.1%). The smallest increase was observed in the occipital lobe (5.6%) and was not statistically significant.

Interestingly, the observed increase in rCBF during early pregnancy occurred despite a concomitant decrease in $PaCO_2$. Maternal hypocapnia in pregnancy is well recognized and thought to result from progesterone-induced hyperventilation.[8] Citing evidence that rCBF may be increased in women during their reproductive years or during administration of progesterone, Ikeda et al[10] postulated that estrogen or progesterone may act to increase rCBF.

In conclusion, it must be said that it is not definitively known whether there are consistent changes in cerebrovascular physiology during normal pregnancy. Reported alterations, when confirmed, may be the result of hormonal influences upon the cerebral vasculature or effects transmitted from the systemic circulation. The effect of pregnancy on cerebrovascular autoregulation remains to be determined. Ultimately, accurate assessment of cerebrovascular function may help predict those women at risk to develop intracranial complications during pregnancy.

REFERENCES

1. Akutsu T, Sakai F, Hata T, et al: [Neurological and neuroimaging studies of eclampsia.] **Rinsho Shinkeigaku** 32:701-707, 1992 (Jpn)
2. Arias F: Expansion of intravascular volume and fetal outcome in patients with chronic hypertension and pregnancy. **Am J Obstet Gynecol 123**:610-616, 1975
3. Barrett JM, Van Hooydonk JE, Boehm FH: Pregnancy-related rupture of arterial aneurysms. **Obstet Gynecol Surv 37**:557-566, 1982
4. Barton JR, Sibai BM: Cerebral pathology in eclampsia. **Clin Perinatol 18**:891-910, 1991
5. Capeless EL, Clapp JF: Cardiovascular changes in early phase of pregnancy. **Am J Obstet Gynecol 161**: 1449-1453, 1989
6. Capeless EL, Clapp JF: When do cardiovascular parameters return to their preconception values? **Am J Obstet 165**:883-886, 1991
7. Cunningham FG, Lindheimier MD: Hypertension in pregnancy. **N Engl J Med 326**:927-932, 1992
8. DeSwiet M: Diseases of the respiratory system, in DeSwiet M (ed): **Medical Disorders in Obstetric Practice, 2nd ed.** Oxford: Blackwell Scientific, 1989, p 74
9. Hunter S, Robson SC: Adaptation of the maternal heart in pregnancy. **Br Heart J 68**:540-543, 1992
10. Ikeda T, Ikenoue T, Mori N: Maternal cerebrohemodynamics assessed by internal carotid and middle cerebral artery pulsed Doppler velocimetry. **J Cardiovasc Technol 10**:55-63, 1991
11. Ikeda T, Ikenoue T, Mori N, et al: Effect of early preg-

nancy on maternal regional cerebral blood flow. **Am J Obstet Gynecol 168:**1303-1308, 1993
12. Ikeda T, Mori N: Assessment of cerebral hemodynamics in pregnant women by internal carotid artery pulsed Doppler velocimetry. **Am J Obstet Gynecol 163:**494-498, 1990
13. Irey NS, Norris HJ: Intimal vascular lesions associated with female reproductive steroids. **Arch Pathol 96:**227-234, 1973
14. Kakouris H, Eddie LW, Summers RJ: Relaxin: more than just a hormone of pregnancy. **Trends Pharmacol Sci 14:**4-6, 1993
15. Lee W: Cardiorespiratory alterations during normal pregnancy. **Crit Care Clin 7:**763-775, 1991
16. Lietsky EA: Blood volume, haematinics, anaemia, in DeSwiet M (ed): **Medical Disorders in Obstetric Practice, 2nd ed.** Oxford: Blackwell Scientific, 1989, pp 48-52
17. Mabie WC, DiSessa TG, Crocker LG, et al: A longitudinal study of cardiac output in normal human pregnancy. **Am J Obstet Gynecol 170:**849-856, 1994
18. Manalo-Estrella P, Barker AE: Histopathologic findings in human aortic media associated with pregnancy. A study of 16 cases. **Arch Pathol 83:**336-341, 1967
19. McCall ML: Cerebral blood flow and metabolism in toxemias of pregnancy. **Surg Gynecol Obstet 89:**715-721, 1949
20. Monga M, Creasy RK: Cardiovascular and renal adaptation to pregnancy, in Creasy RK, Resnik R (eds): **Maternal-Fetal Medicine: Principles and Practice, 3rd ed.** Philadelphia, PA: WB Saunders, 1994, pp 758-763
21. Myers SA, Gleicher N: Physiologic changes in normal pregnancy, in Gleicher N (ed): **Principles and Practice of Medical Therapy in Pregnancy, 2nd ed.** Norwalk, CT: Appleton & Lange, 1991, pp 35-40
22. Osterholzer HO, Grillo D, Kruger PS: The effect of oral contraceptive steroids on branches of the uterine artery. **Obstet Gynecol 49:**227, 1977
23. Pritchard JA: Changes in the blood volume during pregnancy and delivery. **Anesthesiology 26:**393-399, 1965
24. Robson SC, Hunter S, Boys RJ, et al: Serial study of factors influencing changes in cardiac output during human pregnancy. **Am J Physiol 256:**H1060-H1065, 1989
25. Rovinsky JJ, Philipp EE: Blood volume and the hemodynamics of pregnancy, in Barnes J, Newton M (eds): **Scientific Foundations of Obstetrics and Gynaecology.** Chicago, IL: Yearbook Medical, 1977, pp 455-466
26. Sadeh M: Action of magnesium sulfate in the treatment of preeclampsia-eclampsia. **Stroke 20:**1273-1275, 1989
27. Williams K, Wilson S: Maternal middle cerebral artery blood flow velocity variation with gestational age. **Obstet Gynecol 84:**445-448, 1994
28. Williams KP, McLean C: Peripartum changes in maternal cerebral blood flow velocity in normotensive and preeclamptic patients. **Obstet Gynecol 82:** 334-337, 1993
29. Wilson M, Morganti AA, Zervoudakis I, et al: Blood pressure, the renin-aldosterone system, and sex steroids throughout normal pregnancy. **Am J Med 68:**97-104, 1980

CHAPTER 5

HEMOSTASIS AND THROMBOSIS CONSIDERATIONS IN PREGNANCY

JOHN D. OLSON, MD, PHD

Hemostasis is the mechanism by which we protect ourselves from death due to exsanguination following an injury. The normal hemostatic mechanism is a complex interaction among blood vessels (particularly the endothelium), platelets, and plasma proteins which promotes and regulates coagulation and fibrinolysis. For ease of discussion, we will review these three components separately; however, their activation in vivo occurs simultaneously and in a mutually interdependent fashion.

NORMAL HEMOSTASIS

Platelet Function

Platelet functions which support hemostasis involve reaction with plasma proteins, blood vessels, inflammatory cells, and other platelets. Platelets are sticky when activated and adhere to virtually all surfaces except normal endothelium.[81] They also stick to each other, upon activation.[24] These functions are mediated by exposure of membrane receptors (e.g., glycoproteins IIb-IIIa, Ib-IX, and P-selectin) and their corresponding ligands in the plasma and subendothelium (e.g., von Willebrand factor, fibrinogen, fibronectin, and vitronectin) as well as on other inflammatory cells. When activated, platelets release a variety of vasoactive amines, nucleotides, proteins (pro- and anticoagulant), and growth factors into the microenvironment.[111] These released compounds induce further platelet activation, promote plasma coagulation, stimulate the vasculature at the site of the injury, and activate inflammatory cells at the site, initiating the inflammatory response at the site.[57] Platelets form filapodia when activated, the ends of which concentrate receptors and bind to fibrin.[45] The filapodia contain contractile proteins, the action of which leads to the retraction of the clot, helping to close the gap between the edges of the injured tissue.[40,113] Platelets do not adhere to normal endothelium, but when the endothelium is damaged, the platelet appears to adhere to and fuse with the endothelial cell, apparently providing support to the damaged cell.[51]

Plasma Coagulation

In its simplest form, plasma coagulation can be thought of as the process of changing the blood from a liquid to a solid. The soluble molecule, fibrinogen, is changed to an insoluble molecule, fibrin, at the site of an injury and only at the site of an injury. The biochemistry of this process is complex and presents a particularly interesting problem. The molecules required

TABLE 1

Effect of "Cofactors" on the Rate of Prothrombin Activation*

Activation Components	Relative Rate of Activation
Factor Xa	1
Factor Xa; phospholipid; Ca^{2+}	50
Factor Xa; factor Va; Ca^{2+}	350
Factor Xa; factor Va; phospholipid; Ca^{2+}**	20,000
Factor Xa; platelets; Ca^{2+}	300,000

* Data from Nesheim et al.[76] In each reaction, the rate of thrombin generation is compared to the rate of factor Xa alone, which is assigned the relative rate of 1.

** Data from Miletich et al.[72]

(proteins, lipids, and ions) are present in plasma in very low concentrations (with the possible exception of fibrinogen at 10 μM).[42] The activation of the enzyme cascade and the inhibition of excess activated enzymes must occur at rates which, in many cases, cannot be supported by the limited concentration of the components. Consider a similar analogy of linking two railroad boxcars. Spinning about randomly in space, the specific coupling would be nearly impossible. Take the same cars to the surface and the coupling becomes much easier, but is still difficult. Now add the "cofactor" (a railroad track) to the surface, mount the boxcars on the track, and the coupling occurs without failure and in short time. Enzymes, substrates, and their cofactors are faced with a similar, but more difficult, problem. In solution, with the random motion of all components in three dimensions, high concentrations are required to bring components together in the exact conformation for binding. The problem appears to be solved by changing the three-dimensional binding situation to a two-dimensional one.

The principle of the assembly of enzyme activation complexes on membrane surfaces has been demonstrated by several investigators in the assembly of the prothrombinase complex, the enzyme and substrate binding to the cofactor on the surface of the platelet.[66,77] The dramatic effect of this assembly of the complex on the rate of generation of thrombin is shown in Table 1.[72,76,102]

Platelets and inflammatory cells are delivered to the site of an injury in high numbers and provide the surfaces for activation of both intrinsic and extrinsic coagulation. In addition, plasminogen circulates in association with fibrinogen; at the time of the formation of fibrin, plasminogen is bound to the fibrin, providing a surface for the generation of plasmin.[22]

The mechanisms by which the coagulation cascade is initiated have been the source of considerable debate. Severe deficiency of contact factors (factor XII, prekallikrein, and high-molecular weight kininogen) causes marked prolongation of coagulation tests with no corresponding bleeding disorder, a discrepancy which is still not well explained. It now appears that factor VII-tissue factor generated at the site of an injury can activate both factor X and factor IX. In addition, factor XI is activated by thrombin. This mechanism is depicted in Figure 1.[13] The relationship of contact activation to thrombin generation appears to be of importance only in understanding abnormal coagulation times.

When endothelial cells are stimulated by agonists (e.g., thrombin bound to thrombomodulin), tissue-type plasminogen activator (tPA) is released.[8,112] TPA is one of the endogenous activators of fibrinolysis. Activation of plasminogen to plasmin by tPA requires fibrin as a cofactor (an unusual situation in which the substrate of the enzyme is a required cofactor for the enzyme's generation). This reaction takes place on a fibrin surface (Figure 2). The other endogenous activator of plasminogen is urokinase. Urokinase-type plasminogen activator (uPA) is produced in a single-chain inactive form by connective tissue cells, endothelial cells, and other cells.[11,59] Activation of urokinase to the active two-chain form is facilitated by binding to a urokinase-specific receptor found on monocytes and other cells.[23,83] When bound it can be cleaved by plasmin, kallikrein, two-chain urokinase, and other proteases.[49,83] The role of uPA in fibrinolysis and metastasis continues to be defined. TPA and uPA, along with streptokinase in varying forms, are now used pharmacologically to induce fibrinolysis.

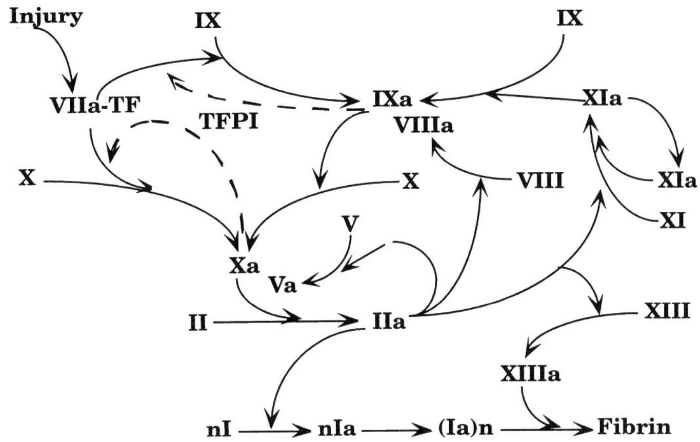

Figure 1: Mechanism of plasma coagulation. A schematic representation of an alternative mechanism of coagulation emphasizing the role of tissue factor-factor VII complex and TFPI.[13]

Vascular Contribution and Inhibition of Active Enzymes

The inhibition of the active enzymes generated at the site of an injury and released into the circulation and the down-regulation of the system are also dependent upon the surface of cells. As the vasculature proceeds to the capillary bed, the surface area is increased to such a degree that virtually all cells and molecules traversing the capillary bed will contact the endothelial surface (Figure 3).[17] The surface of the endothelial cell has many receptors, among them thrombomodulin. As thrombin is released into the circulation, it travels to the capillary bed and binds to thrombomodulin.[26,30] When bound it changes its enzymatic specificity, no longer able to cleave fibrinogen, but effectively activating protein C (Figure 4). Activated protein C is among the most potent inhibitors of coagulation due to its proteolytic cleavage of factor Va and VIIIa. In addition, the binding of activated coagulation factors to one of the primary inhibitors, antithrombin III, also appears

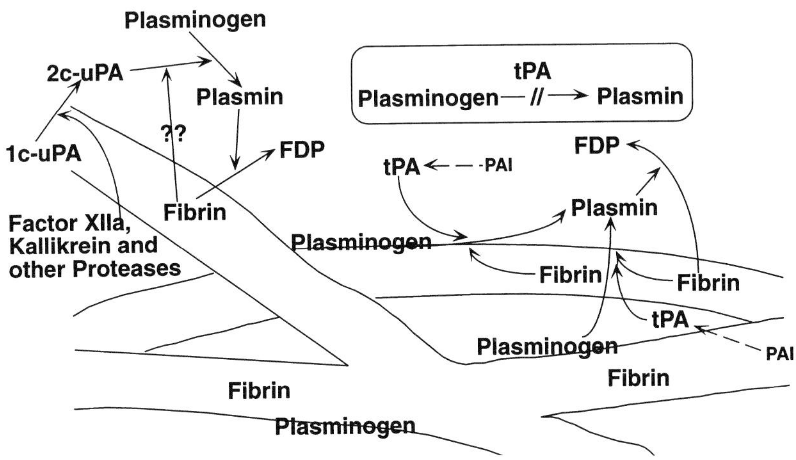

Figure 2: Activation of plasminogen. Plasminogen is activated to plasmin by tPA or uPA. Activation by tPA requires fibrin as a cofactor for the reaction. In the two-chain form uPA is not fibrin-specific; however, conversion of single-chain uPA (inactive) to two-chain uPA may be fibrin-specific.[22,23,79]

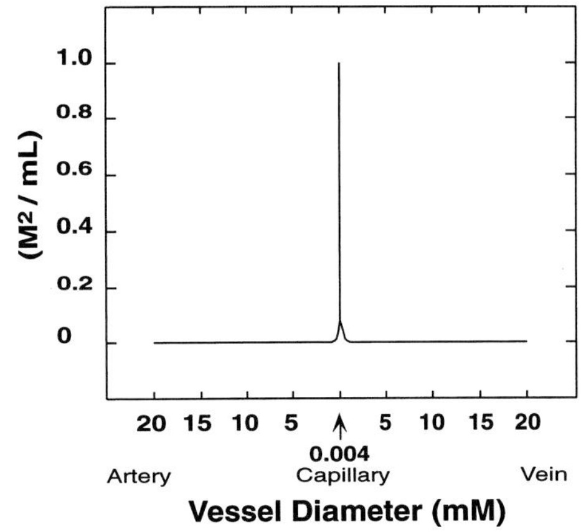

Figure 3: Relationship of the blood volume to the endothelial surface area in the vascular system. Calculation of the surface area and volume assumes cylindrical shape of the vessel.[18,79]

to take place at the capillary endothelial cell surface, accelerated by the heparinoids in the endothelial membrane (Figure 3).[18,43] Another recently described inhibitor, the tissue factor pathway inhibitor (TFPI), circulates in association with lipoprotein. It binds to factors Xa and IXa, inactivating them; the inhibitory complex can bind to factor VII-tissue factor complex, competitively inhibiting further activation of factor Xa or IXa (Figure 5).[14]

Hemostatic Changes Expected in Pregnancy

Humorist Garrison Keillor once referred to the sport of jogging as "mindless gerbil activity." In fact it does appear that only rodents and people run for enjoyment. In nature, the physical exercise of running is punctuated by a bleeding episode. Physiology recognizes this and rapidly prepares the body for the hemorrhagic event by producing a hypercoagulable state. Pregnancy appears to do a similar thing in slow motion. The delivery of a child can be complicated by severe hemorrhage, an event which is prevented in the majority of cases by the preparation of the hemostatic mechanism. An understanding of these changes is useful in evaluating the complications of hemorrhage and thrombosis seen in pregnant and postpartum women. Changes in many of the components of the hemostatic mechanism induced by pregnancy are reviewed briefly below. Table 2 summarizes changes in hemostatic factors induced by pregnancy.[25,39,42,99,105]

In populations of normal pregnant women, the mean platelet count remains normal during the course of pregnancy.[31,99] There is, however, a greater range in counts seen; particularly in the third trimester, the lower limits in pregnant

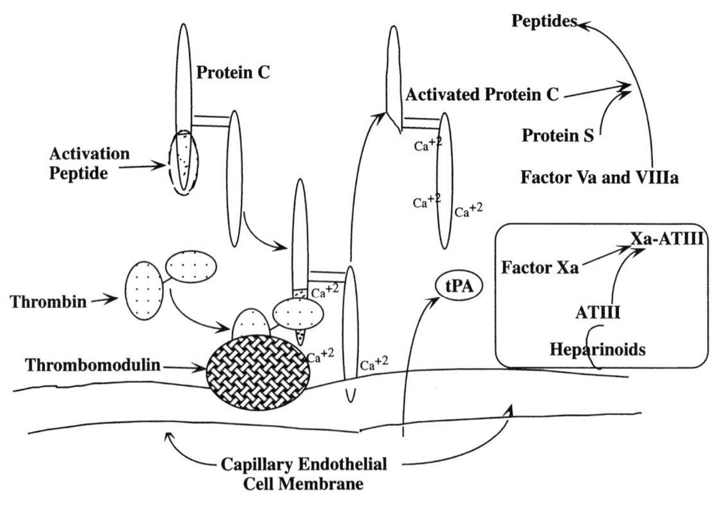

Figure 4: Hypothetical model of the activation of protein C. Thrombin in the circulation binds to the thrombomodulin on the membrane of the capillary endothelial cell. When bound to thrombomodulin, thrombin changes its enzyme specificity, no longer recognizing fibrinogen and activating protein C. Protein C, which binds to the thrombin, thrombomodulin, and the phospholipid membrane complex on the cell, is then activated.[30,79]

women are considerably lower at ≈100,000/μl when compared to nonpregnant adults.[99] Indirect evidence implies that there is an increased turnover of platelets in late pregnancy. Platelet function and platelet vessel interaction are normal in pregnancy and the bleeding time is not changed.[87,110] The metabolite of prostacyclin increases in the third trimester.[60]

The data in Table 2 indicate that most coagulation factors are not substantially changed during pregnancy. Factors X, VII, prekallikrein, high-molecular weight kininogen (HMWK), VIII, von Willebrand factor (vWF), vWF:Ag, and fibrinogen do rise substantially, particularly in the third trimester. Factors VIII, vWF, vWF:Ag, and fibrinogen are known to be acute phase reactant and to rise progressively through pregnancy. They are also increased in the stress reaction seen following exercise or surgery.

It is of interest that despite a common dependence on vitamin K, factors II, VII, IX, and X and proteins C and S do not rise or fall in concert during pregnancy. Factors II and IX and protein C are essentially unchanged, factors X and VII rise significantly, and protein S falls to less than one-half the normal levels.[25,26,99,105]

The components involved in fibrinolysis also rise in the latter part of pregnancy. Prekallikrein and HMWK may rise as a result of other prostaglandin stimulation that results from uterine contractions.[50,93,101] In addition, tPA and plasminogen activator inhibitors 1 and 2 increase.[39,99] The balance of all of these changes is reflected in an increase in the clot lysis times, both euglobulin and whole blood.[3,10,67]

The net effect of these changes (rise in coagulation factors and fall in coagulation inhibition) is a hemostatic mechanism prepared for the hemorrhagic challenge of the delivery of the child. It also provides a background for the easy precipitation of intravascular coagulation or thrombosis, which frequently complicate pregnancy.

Disorders of Hemostasis in Pregnancy

All of the disorders of hemostasis that affect adult women can occur during pregnancy or, on occasion, as a complication of pregnancy. The discussion below reviews the disorders of hemostasis and thrombosis with a focus on the pregnant woman and the way that these disorders may lead to complications requiring neu-

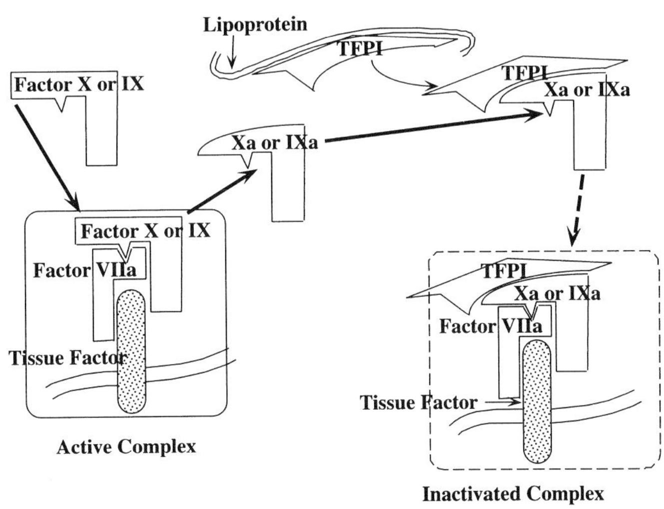

Figure 5: Extrinsic pathway activation and inhibition. Tissue factor in the membrane of monocytes and other tissue cells binds and activates factor VII. Factor X or IX binds the complete the activation complex and are activated. Factors Xa and IXa bind to TFPI forming an inactive complex which can compete with factors X and IX for the VII-tissue factor complex.[14,79]

TABLE 2

CHANGES IN HEMOSTATIC FACTORS DURING PREGNANCY*

Factor	1st Trimester	2nd Trimester	3rd Trimester	Postpartum
Fibrinogen (g/l)	3.63	3.65	4.23	4.61
Range	1.64-5.00	2.53-5.26	2.90-6.15	2.98-7.14
Prothrombin (%)	125	125	115	112
Range	70-224	73-214	68-194	74-170
Factor V (%)	93	82	85	91
Range	46-188	36-185	39-184	36-233
Factor VII (%)	111	150	171	134
Range	60-206	80-280	87-336	70-255
Factor VIII (%)	122 ± 57	141	212	206
Range	53-283	44-453	79-570	74-569
Factor IX (%) (range)	79-105	110-205	72-120	—
Factor X (%)	103	115	127	117
Range	61-169	74-177	72-208	72-191
Factor XI (%)	83 ± 23	74 ± 15	70 ± 18	81 ± 20
Factor XII (%)	130 ± 24	142 ± 43	127 ± 28	110 ± 18
Prekallikrein (%)	120	130	160 ± 30	104 ± 20
Range	60-150	60-150		
High-molecular weight kininogen (%)	@ 105	@ 150	@ 160	@ 100
VWF (%)	—	168	171	—
Range		142-199	146-199	
VWF:Ag (%)	133	167	262	165
Range	56-318	66-427	95-718	
Platelet count ($10^3/\mu l$)	207	228	199	222
Range	128-285	125-331	91-308	91-352
Antithrombin III (%)	102 ± 11	106 ± 10	103 ± 11	103 ± 10
Protein C (%)	63.6 ± 12.8	79.6 ± 17.8	78.8 ± 10.2	72.3 ± 10.2
Protein S (tot) (%)	—	—	68 ± 10.7	—
Protein S (func) (%)	68	38 ± 17	33	—
C4 binding protein (%)	—	—	100 ± 16.9	—
Plasminogen (%)	144 ± 16	149 ± 17	139 ± 10	141 ± 11
TPA (ng/ml)	5.5 ± 1.6	5.8 ± 1.3	11.7 ± 3.7	7.2 ± 3.4
PAI 1 (ng/ml)	25.3 ± 15.2	47.1 ± 22.5	79.3 ± 19.7	28 ± 10
PAI 2 (ng/ml)	20.5 ± 13.4	50.5 ± 18.9	183 ± 37.5	2.8 ± 7.0

*Values are mean ± standard deviation or range. Data from Comp et al,[26] Halligan et al,[39] Hathaway and Bonnar,[42] Stirling et al,[99] and Walker.[105]

rosurgical intervention or which may complicate neurosurgery. The management of these requires a team approach, including obstetrician, hematologist, and neurosurgeon, working with sound laboratory support.

THROMBOCYTOPENIA

The pathogenesis of thrombocytopenia is easily thought of in terms of two primary mechanisms: 1) rapid peripheral destruction with shortened platelet half-life as seen in immune-mediated thrombocytopenias, thrombotic thrombocytopenic purpura, post-transfusion purpura, intravascular coagulation with fibrinolysis, or hypersplenism; or 2) suppression of platelet production in the bone marrow as seen in hypoplastic anemia, vitamin deficiency primary bone marrow malignancy, or metastatic malignancy involving the bone marrow, commonly as the result of chemotherapy or disorders of ineffective hematopoiesis.

Rapid Peripheral Destruction of Platelets

Immunological Platelet Destruction

Idiopathic thrombocytopenic purpura (ITP) is a disorder of immune-mediated platelet destruction. Patients with chronic ITP can present with mild to severe thrombocytopenia. The diagnosis of ITP involves the exclusion of other possible etiologies of thrombocytopenia in which the bone marrow demonstrates normal to increased megakaryocytes, indicating adequate to increased platelet production. In 30% to 90% of cases, laboratory tests can confirm the presence of immunoglobulin on the platelet surface.[95] In chronic ITP, the antibody may be an autoantibody which is directed toward a platelet antigen. In ITP, the development of spontaneous intracranial hemorrhage is unusual, ranging from 1% to 3% of cases in chronic ITP.[12] The occurrence of intracerebral hemorrhage is related to the severity of the thrombocytopenia, being rare in patients with platelet counts exceeding 10,000/μl.[36] The general mortality rate due to acute ITP is <1% and death is most frequently caused by intracerebral hemorrhage. The risk of fetal hemorrhage in the pregnant woman is only slightly higher than in the nonpregnant patient. The rate of mortality due to ITP in pregnancy is reported to be one in 88, with postpartum hemorrhage occurring in six of 90 patients.[53]

Chronic ITP most frequently (in approximately 90% of cases) requires therapy and, in many instances, therapy must be maintained chronically in order to raise and maintain the platelet count.[54,106] Therapy for ITP would include glucocorticoids or intravenous gamma globulin in the acute phase. The most uniformly effective method for raising platelet count in a short period of time is splenectomy, an option rarely used in pregnant women because of the risk to the fetus. However, with an intracerebral event, consideration may be given to removal of the spleen.[12,48] Combining the therapy mentioned, with the addition of plasma exchange, has been reported in the successful management of intracranial hemorrhage in ITP.[47] Plasma exchange to remove antibody (in this case antiplatelet antibody) has been used with some limited success.[9,82] Finally, in refractory patients, recent studies indicate that staphylococcal protein-A immunoabsorption may induce remission in 46% of patients, with long-term remission in 36%. Data on treatment of pregnant women by this method are not available.[96]

Concerning platelet transfusion in acute or chronic ITP, it is important to realize that the survival of platelets which are transfused will parallel the survival of the patient's own platelets, making the effectiveness of platelet transfusion generally very poor. Therefore, prophylactic platelet transfusion in an attempt to prevent catastrophic hemorrhage such as intracerebral hemorrhage is not advocated. In the event of life-threatening hemorrhage, platelet transfusions should be administered. Platelets transfused for managing intracerebral hemorrhage or for a surgical procedure designed to evacuate hematoma will have a half-life that is very short. Preoperative transfusion is likely to be ineffective. The role of platelet transfusion is best reserved for arresting hemorrhage (or controlling it), while other approaches to raising the patient's platelet count are employed.[12]

Drug-induced immune-mediated thrombocytopenia is an additional etiology for profound decrease in platelets.[6] More than 150 medications from virtually all classes of drugs have been associated with immunologically mediated thrombocytopenia. In all patients in whom thrombocytopenia occurs concurrent with underlying illness and medication, the possibility of drug-mediated thrombocytopenia should be considered. In general, patients who develop thrombocytopenia should be taken off all medications. If medication is absolutely required, an alternative medication should be sought in order to determine if the thrombocytopenia is being mediated by a drug. Management of drug-induced thrombocytopenia requires removing the drug. Recovery of the platelet count following cessation of the drug may be rapid, but in some cases it may require many weeks or even longer. The use of glucocorticoids and intravenous gamma globulin has been shown to be effective in some cases. If the drug has been cleared, transfusion of platelets may be effective; however, the response is not predictable in most cases and requires monitoring of transfusion with post-transfusion platelet counts.

Post-transfusion purpura is a rare complication of transfusion in which antibody to platelet-specific antigens, most frequently human platelet antigen (PLA) 1, already present in the patient, leads to profound thrombocytopenia. The actual mechanisms by which these antibodies lead to thrombocytopenia remain obscure.[5] The thrombocytopenia can be severe and spontaneous hemorrhagic complications are not uncommon, with intracranial hemorrhage occurring in 10% of reported cases. Glucocorticoids have been used with some effectiveness; however, dramatic responses are not common. Intravenous immunoglobulin has also been helpful at times. The use of plasma exchange transfusion has been reported to have induced dramatic improvement in several cases and should be considered in situations where life-threatening hemorrhage is occurring.[58] In this situation, as with other immune-mediated thrombocytopenias, the transfusion of platelet concentrates is generally not effective and in some cases the administration of platelet concentrates has led to life-threatening transfusion reaction.[4]

Isoimmune thrombocytopenia is a rare condition in adults; however, mothers may occasionally have isoantibodies which recognize platelet-specific antigens not present on their platelets or they may have chronic ITP with circulating antibody. In these cases, when the woman becomes pregnant, it is possible for antibody to cross the placenta to the fetus, leading to thrombocytopenia in the fetus and subsequently the neonate.[46] The diagnosis of fetal thrombocytopenia due to either passively transfused iso- or autoantibody from the mother is generally made by testing the mother and by umbilical vein sampling. This is an important issue in intracranial hemorrhage in the neonate but is rarely a problem for the mother.

Nonimmunological Platelet Destruction

Thrombotic thrombocytopenic purpura (TTP) is a syndrome which presents with some combination of the classically described pentad of fever, renal insufficiency, neurological findings, microangiopathic hemolytic anemia, and thrombocytopenia. In the pregnant woman, differentiation from the HELLP (hemolysis, elevated liver enzymes, and low platelets) syndrome and pre-eclampsia may be difficult. TTP occurs in acute, intermittent, and chronic relapsing forms and can affect patients of all ages. The etiology and mechanism of platelet destruction in the syndrome remain obscure. It does appear that vWF-mediated platelet aggregation may be of importance in the intermittent and chronic relapsing varieties of TTP. Unusually large forms of vWF have been identified in these patients.[73] Such evidence has not yet been described in individuals with acute TTP, and the etiology in those cases is less well defined. Prior to the advent of plasma exchange transfusion in the late 1970s, more than 80% of patients with TTP died, many of them due to complicating intracerebral hemorrhage.[2] The advent of plasma exchange with plasma transfusion has reversed this trend so that currently 80% to 90% of patients recover.[61,94] The response to exchange transfusion, reflected by the rise in platelet count, generally takes several days. This is also a disease in which platelet transfusion is not indicated and would be reserved only for life-threatening hemorrhage. It should be pointed out that a case has been reported of a patient having rapid progression of the TTP syndrome concomitant with the transfusion of platelets in which there was ultimately a fatal outcome.[15,41] Other modalities such as intravenous immunoglobulin have been attempted in TTP but have not as yet demonstrated efficacy comparable to plasma exchange and/or a plasma transfusion. TTP in pregnancy is associated with high rates of morbidity and mortality. In one report of 62 patients with TTP in pregnancy (pre-eclampsia carefully excluded), only 17 mothers survived.[20]

Hypersplenism. Thrombocytopenia due to rapid peripheral destruction can also be due to accelerated consumption of platelets (discussed briefly below) and hypersplenism. A number of other etiologies can lead to peripheral destruction of platelets but are rarely the cause of severe thrombocytopenia. Hypersplenism has many possible origins, ranging from passive congestion secondary to liver or cardiac disease to infiltrative processes and hematological malignancies. The severity of thrombocytopenia is rarely severe enough to lead to a hemorrhagic diathesis.

Decreased Platelet Production

The etiologies of decreased platelet production are numerous and include: rare congenital and inherited syndromes; neonatal problems related to infection, drugs, or infiltrative diseases; aplastic anemia and other primary hematological diseases; hematological malignancies (addressed briefly below); radiation of the bone marrow and chemotherapeutic agents which suppress the bone marrow; metastatic malignancy infiltrating the bone marrow; a variety of other drugs which can suppress bone marrow production; and the nutritional deficiency of vitamin B_{12}, folic acid, or iron. Many of these conditions are associated with mild thrombocytopenia. By far the most common cause of severe thrombocytopenia in the medical center relates to the radiation and chemotherapy given to patients with hematological and solid tumor malignancies, conditions which can occur during pregnancy. The ablative therapy used in these situations leads to severe depression of the bone marrow with concomitant leukopenia, anemia, and severe thrombocytopenia. Two to three decades ago when the treatment of acute leukemia with chemotherapy was being developed, the thrombocytopenia leading to intracerebral hemorrhage was a common mechanism of death during the induction-phase therapy. The ability to more effectively manage the chemotherapy and the supportive care of these patients has significantly reduced this complication; however, intracerebral hemorrhage as a complication of chemotherapy remains significant.

The risk of spontaneous hemorrhage complicating severe thrombocytopenia in response to bone marrow suppression increases inversely with the platelet count. This complication is unusual in patients with platelet counts >10,000/μl and occurs with increasing frequency in patients who have platelet counts of ≤5,000/μl.[36] Hemostatic effectiveness in the bleeding patient who has thrombocytopenia is generally felt to occur at platelet counts approaching 50,000/μl.[4] Therefore, the patient with severe thrombocytopenia and hemorrhage should be transfused with platelet concentrates, attempting to achieve platelet counts above 50,000/μl when managing patients with intracranial hemorrhage.

In relation to the problem of severe thrombocytopenia and the potential development of intracranial hemorrhage, it would be appropriate to address the question of whether or not this catastrophic complication can be prevented by the prophylactic use of platelet transfusion to raise the patient's platelet count. This practice is common in medical centers; however, the effectiveness of prophylactic platelet transfusion remains to be conclusively demonstrated.[52,100] Available evidence would indicate that minor bleeding episodes can be reduced with the use of platelet transfusion; however, the rate at which life-threatening hemorrhage occurs in patients receiving chemotherapy is not significantly altered by the use of prophylactic platelet transfusion. The usefulness of prophylactic platelet transfusion in profoundly thrombocytopenic patients continues to be debated.

Incidental Thrombocytopenia of Pregnancy

Only after all other etiologies of thrombocytopenia have been excluded can one make the diagnosis of incidental thrombocytopenia of pregnancy.[16] Thrombocytopenia which is mild (75,000-1,500,000 platelets/μl) usually occurs in the third trimester. Its etiology remains obscure. The condition presents no risk to mother or fetus and requires no therapy.[7,16]

Disorders of Platelet Function

Inherited Disorders of Platelet Function

Von Willebrand's Disease

Von Willebrand's disease is a unique inherited bleeding disorder because it represents a genetic abnormality in which protein in the plasma is produced in reduced amounts or in an abnormal form, leading to abnormal function of the platelet. Among the inherited bleeding disorders, von Willebrand's disease is possibly the most common[89] and is clearly the most common in women. Many varieties of von Willebrand's disease have been described. In its most frequent form, Type I, bleeding tends to be mild to moderate, usually requiring therapy only at the time of trauma or surgical procedures. In Type I disease, the laboratory and clinical findings normalize during the third trimester, making therapy at the time of delivery unnecessary in most patients.[42] The vWF levels and bleeding time should be followed sequentially to confirm the expected rise. Because the rise is late in pregnancy, bleeding events (such as abortion) may require therapy if they occur earlier in pregnancy.[98] Levels in vWF fall rapidly postpartum in patients with Type I disease, often requiring infusion of factor or use of desmopressin acetate (DDAVP).

Other types either do not improve during pregnancy or are inconsistent, making therapeutic intervention much more likely. Rare forms affect the platelets as well as plasma proteins. The patients have normal platelet counts, and function of the platelets in these patients is generally normal as reflected in usual platelet function studies. In general, however, the disease is best thought of as an abnormality in the platelet protein.[75]

Spontaneous intracerebral hemorrhage in patients with von Willebrand's disease is a rare complication. Certainly, patients with this disease are at increased risk for the development of intracerebral hemorrhage in the event of injury, other intracranial lesions, or hypertensive complications of pregnancy leading to the onset of hemorrhage.

The management of patients with von Willebrand's disease who are having hemorrhagic complications is by transfusion of vWF. At the current time, the most satisfactory source of vWF is in commercial concentrates which have been heat-treated;[35,57] however, the emergency transfusion of cryoprecipitate is still effective. DDAVP has been used effectively for the treatment of mild hemophilia and mild von Willebrand's disease. In addition, DDAVP may cause hyponatremia in the fetus and should be reserved for use in the postpartum period.[56,75] The use of DDAVP, however, is most effective in the management of mild hemorrhagic complications or in the prevention of significant hemorrhage with minor surgery and in the postpartum period; however, DDAVP would not be considered appropriate in the management of major hemorrhagic complication except as an adjunct to transfusion by vWF concentrate or cryoprecipitate.[91] The transfusion of platelets into patients with von Willebrand's disease is not indicated unless the patient has complications which have led to significant thrombocytopenia, the patient has severe (Type III) von Willebrand's disease, or the patient is known to have a rare platelet type of von Willebrand's disease.

Other Inherited Platelet Function Disorders

Inherited platelet function disorders generally fall into the categories of disorders in which platelet membrane glycoproteins are either missing or produced in abnormal form, as is seen in the Bernard-Soulier syndrome and Glanzmann's thrombasthenia or in the abnormalities of the ability of the platelet to appropriately store and release its granular contents. These disorders generally present with mild to moderate bleeding disorders. They require sophisticated laboratory testing in order to confirm the specific diagnosis. In the event of hemorrhage, in the management of surgical procedures, or in the event of delivery, the appropriate therapy is the transfusion of platelet concentrates.

Acquired Platelet Function Disorders

Uremia

Uremia may be complicated by either spontaneous hemorrhage or hemorrhage following procedures or trauma.[27] Defects in all phases of platelet function (adhesion, aggregation, and release and the support of plasma coagulation of platelets) have been described in platelets from uremic patients, and studies indicate that there may be multiple possible mechanisms for the development of these lesions. Some of these abnormalities can be explained by dialyzable organic acids (such as phenolic acids and guanidinosuccinic acid), which may be retained in the plasma of uremic patients.[28,85,97] In addition, patients with uremia frequently have complicating conditions requiring treatment with drugs which may also influence platelet function and they are often exposed chronically to heparin in the course of hemodialysis. All of these and other more poorly defined factors contribute to the abnormal hemostasis observed in patients with uremia.

The management of the pregnant patient with uremia who has developed significant spontaneous bleeding is difficult. In general, the bleeding or potential for bleeding in these patients is monitored using the skin bleeding time, although its effectiveness in predicting hemorrhage has not been demonstrated.[90] In many patients who have bleeding related to uremia, the skin bleeding time will have corrected and hemorrhagic complication improved as a result of intensive dialysis; it continues to be the treatment of choice in this condition.[88] Desmopressin will shorten the bleeding time in 50% to 75% of patients with uremia and in emergency situations has been used successfully to control hemorrhage for procedures.[68] Its use in pregnancy is limited because of potential effects on the fetus.[56,75] Uncontrolled studies have shown an improvement in uremic hemorrhage in response to the transfusion of cryoprecipitate. The risk of transfusion outweighs this benefit as a first-line therapy; however, in patients in whom other modes have failed, the transfusion of cryoprecipitate may merit a trial.[52,103] Correction of significant anemia with red blood cell transfusion[33] or treatment with erythropoietin[74] has also been associated with correction of the skin bleeding time. Because the hemorrhagic abnormality in patients with uremia appears to be caused by retained chemicals in the blood which affect platelets and their function, these retained components will have an equivalent effect on any transfused platelets. Therefore, the transfusion of platelet concentrates into patients with significant uremia is not usually effective unless the patient also suffers from significant thrombocytopenia.

Medications

There are a large number of medications from a broad spectrum of drug classes that may affect platelet function. Drugs affect platelet function by: interfering with platelet cyclo-oxygenase; binding to the surface membrane; interfering with activation by agonists; and increasing or decreasing platelet cyclic adenosine monophosphate levels. In general, patients who are hemostatically normal can take these drugs without bleeding complications because there is considerable redundancy in overall platelet function. However, when these drugs are taken by the patient who has thrombocytopenia, another abnormality in hemostasis (either inherited or acquired), or if multiple drugs are being used at the same time, each of which affect different aspects of platelet function, then hemorrhagic complications may ensue.[21,64] The appropriate approach to the patient who develops bleeding while taking these drugs is to take the patient off the drug or to change to a medication which will have equal therapeutic effect but not affect platelet function.

Coagulation Factor Deficiencies

In general, the inherited disorders of coagulation (the hemophilias) result in the deficiency of a single coagulation factor. In contrast, the acquired disorders will result in multiple factor deficiencies and, frequently, in platelet and vessel dysfunction as well. The inherited and acquired disorders of coagulation are addressed below.

Inherited Factor Deficiency

Patients with hemophilia are susceptible to both spontaneous and post-traumatic intracranial hemorrhage. The severity of the complication varies greatly depending not only upon the location of the hemorrhage but also the rate at which the hemorrhage develops and the efficacy of the therapy that can be rendered. In patients who suffer from hemophilia, the bleeding may occur spontaneously and does not relate directly to the severity of the trauma.

Because of the sex-linked inheritance, severe factor VIII and factor IX deficiency is rare in females. Bleeding due to deficiency of these factors has been reported in carriers of hemophilia. The deficiency in these cases is usually mild (<5% factor level) and is thought to be due to extreme lyonization. Cases of severe factor VIII and factor IX deficiency in females have been reported;[38,65] of four reported cases of pregnancy among these women, one bled at delivery. Intracranial hemorrhage in this setting is a risk, but has not been reported.

Other inherited coagulation factor deficiencies are autosomally inherited and occur with equal frequency in men and women. Severe deficiency states can be complicated at any time by spontaneous intracranial hemorrhage. This complication occurring in pregnancy has not been reported.

Management in cases of inherited coagulation factor deficiency requires replacement of the deficient factor. Sterile, commercial concentrates of factors VIII and IX are available. Other conditions require infusion of (or replacement with) fresh frozen plasma. Women with mild or moderate factor VIII deficiency may also respond to DDAVP in the postpartum period.

Acquired Disorders of Coagulation

Factor Inhibitors

Inhibitors can complicate hemophilia or may occur spontaneously in individuals who do not have hemophilia. These inhibitors are antibodies that recognize a specific procoagulant. By far the most frequently described are those against factor VIII; however, factor IX inhibitors occur at a similar frequency in those factor IX-deficient patients who have severe disease. In addition, inhibitors to coagulation factors XI, V, and vWF, although rare, have been described. Spontaneously occurring inhibitors in patients who do not have hemophilia are directed at the factor VIII molecule with rare exception.[32] Spontaneous inhibitors of factor VIII can complicate pregnancy, leading to a severe hemorrhagic diathesis. Antibodies and hemorrhage have been reported at the onset of pregnancy,[104] in the third trimester,[70] in the puerperium,[86] or may not appear until weeks or months postpartum.[86]

Management of the patient who has an inhibitor presents a unique and extremely difficult challenge. The therapeutic modalities available for addressing the problem of inhibitors are numerous, an indication that no uniformly effective method is available. In patients in whom the titer and responsiveness of the antibody are low, it is possible to transfuse very large doses of factor VIII concentrates and achieve hemostatic levels of the procoagulant. The factor inhibitor can be "bypassed" by the use of prothrombin concentrates or activated prothrombin complexes. These therapies are effective in some patients; however, they are difficult to monitor in the laboratory so their effectiveness can only be judged on a clinical basis. Newer activated factor VII complexes are currently in clinical trials.[44] In the case of factor VIII inhibitors, the antibody occasionally recognizes specifically human factor VIII, and for a short period of time patients can be effectively treated utilizing factor VIII which has been isolated from porcine plasma. These patients almost uniformly will develop a porcine inhibitor within 5-14 days following the initiation of therapy; however, the therapy can be very effective in this "window" of time, allowing for procedures which are absolutely necessary.[55,71] Intravenous immunoglobulin has been used with varying effectiveness in these patients and can effect a fall in the antibody titer in as short a time as 48 hours. Intravenous immunoglobulin has been used by some investigators in both hemophiliacs with inhibitors as well as nonhemophiliacs. In contrast, others have found intravenous immunoglobulin not to be effective.

Disseminated Intravascular Coagulation with Fibrinolysis

Disseminated intravascular coagulation (DIC) is a secondary mechanism of disease in which there is an intravascular generation of thrombin and plasmin activity. The presence of these activating enzymes leads to accelerated coagulation and fibrinolytic activity; this can lead to the generation of active thrombosis, particularly in the microvasculature, and the consumption of coagulation factors and platelets resulting in a hemorrhagic diathesis. It is not rare for patients to manifest hemorrhagic and thrombotic complications simultaneously. Etiological factors which may lead to intravascular clotting and fibrinolysis are numerous and include: the complications of pregnancy; infections, particularly those caused by Gram-negative bacilli; malignancy, particularly mucin-producing adenocarcinomas and the acute leukemias of the granulocytic and monocytic lines; trauma (with particular importance of central nervous system (CNS) trauma); hypotension of any etiology; and moderate to severe liver disease. The bleeding diathesis which complicates severe acute DIC may predispose to spontaneous intracerebral hemorrhage which is usually fatal. Patients may develop chronic intravascular clotting and fibrinolysis accompanying chronic underlying conditions (malignancy, infection, and others). In this state of chronic intravascular clotting and fibrinolysis, the patient may be at increased risk for the development of hemorrhage or thrombosis.[92]

As with other conditions, events which precipitate intravascular coagulation and fibrinolysis can occur in pregnant women. Because of the relative hypercoagulable state existing in pregnancy, the risk of developing DIC may be increased. Therefore, pregnant women suffering from unrelated head injury,[80] other trauma, malignancy, or other disorders[69] merit close monitoring for the development of a consumptive coagulopathy. Specific complications of pregnancy which may lead to intravascular coagulation and fibrinolysis are listed in Table 3.[42] The resulting syndrome of DIC in pregnant women can be severe and acute, or may be chronic in its presentation. As indicated in Table 3, the etiological factors are varied, depending on the condition. The principles of management, outlined below, are the same as for other adults, with the ever-complicating factor of the desire to salvage the pregnancy, if possible, despite the pregnancy being the major etiological factor. The management of intravascular clotting and fibrinolysis involves four approaches which are used in concert with one another. 1) Of greatest importance is the appropriate treatment of the underlying cause of the DIC, in this case the complication of pregnancy. All other therapy planned and described briefly below is of value only in providing time in which the treatment of the primary problem can be accomplished. 2) Anticoagulation in an effort to arrest or slow the generation of thrombin is frequently helpful. As a general rule, full anticoagulation with heparin is attempted only in patients in whom there is no active bleeding. In patients who are bleeding, anticoagulation may carry an unacceptable risk. Currently, the utilization of

TABLE 3
COMPLICATIONS OF PREGNANCY WHICH MAY LEAD TO INTRAVASCULAR COAGULATION AND FIBRINOLYSIS*

Possible Etiology	Complication of Pregnancy
Endothelial damage	Eclampsia and pre-eclampsia HELLP syndrome Shock
Neoplasm	Hydatidiform mole Degenerating fibroma
Tissue damage/necrosis	Abruptio placenta Amniotic fluid embolism Induced abortion Retained dead fetus Placenta accreta Uterine rupture Chronic tubal pregnancy
Incompatible blood	Incompatible transfusion Fetomaternal transfusion
Infection	Septic abortion Intrauterine infection

*Modified from Hathaway and Bonnar.[42]

heparin in low doses (low enough so that the activated partial thromboplastin time is not prolonged) may be sufficient to control the intravascular generation of thrombin. 3) Transfusion therapy is administered in the form of fresh frozen plasma for coagulation factors, cryoprecipitate to replace fibrinogen, and platelet concentrates to manage thrombocytopenia. The dosing of these transfusion products can be guided by the use of the prothrombin time, fibrinogen assay, and the platelet count, respectively. 4) The use of inhibitors of fibrinolysis in the treatment of DIC is controversial. Epsilon aminocaproic acid (Amicar), a competitive inhibitor of the enzyme plasmin, is used in the treatment of DIC only if evidence of profound fibrinolysis is present and the patient is adequately anticoagulated with heparin.[69]

Liver Disease in Pregnancy

The function of the liver is key in maintaining an appropriate balance of coagulation factors, naturally occurring coagulation inhibitors, and components involved in fibrinolysis. When there is significant liver dysfunction, many aspects of hemostasis can be affected, including: decreased synthesis of coagulation factors; decreased synthesis of natural coagulation inhibitors; decreased synthesis of plasminogen and α-2 antiplasmin; decreased clearance of fibrin degradation products; decreased clearance of activated factors and complexes of inhibitors and activated factors; and synthesis of dysfibrinogens. A combination of these events leaves the patient at risk for the development of a significant hemorrhagic diathesis which may be complicated by intravascular clotting and fibrinolysis.

When severe liver failure occurs in pregnancy without evidence of underlying preeclampsia or hemolytic-uremic syndrome or evidence of infectious hepatitis or ingestion of hepatotoxins, the condition is referred to as acute fatty liver of pregnancy. This severe liver failure is accompanied by severe coagulopathy and thrombocytopenia and is often associated with severe deficiency of antithrombin III.[84] Cases are frequently complicated by associated coagulation activation, and treatment with antithrombin III concentrates may be of some benefit.[62,109]

Although the direct linkage between liver disease and the development of spontaneous intracerebral hemorrhage remains to be well demonstrated and has not been discussed in relation to pregnancy, analysis of patients with spontaneous intracranial hemorrhage without a vascular lesion will show as many as 30% with evidence of abnormal liver function.[78] Of these, nearly one-half will have an abnormality of hemostasis which may be related to the liver disease or complicating intravascular clotting and fibrinolysis. In addition, nearly 80% of patients with spontaneous intracerebral hemorrhage will also suffer from hypertension. These data would indicate the increased risk of the development of intracerebral hemorrhage when the combination of liver disease (with or without alcoholism) and hypertension exists. The difficulty in management of patients with this combination of problems is demonstrated by the frequency (5%) of those patients who will demonstrate recurrent intracerebral bleeding postoperatively. The simultaneous presentation of DIC and hypertension with liver failure in pregnancy would be expected, increasing the risk of CNS hemorrhage.

Hypercoagulability and Thrombosis in Pregnancy

Deep venous thrombosis (DVT) is the most common vascular complication in pregnancy, occurring in 0.11% to 0.36% of pregnancies,[107] and pulmonary embolus (PE) is a leading cause of death.[29,42] In a study of 2,475 maternal deaths, 11% were attributed to PE, the second most common cause of death.[29] As mentioned above, there is a natural development of hypercoagulability during pregnancy. This, combined with the vascular compression in the pelvis, provides a setting in which any additional insult may precipitate DVT. Several specific etiological factors were described by Hathaway and Bonnar.[1,42]

- Method of delivery – There is a five-fold increased risk of thromboembolism after cesarean section.

- Age and parity – Risk of death from PE increases with age and parity.
- Obesity – One of three women dying of PE weigh in excess of 76 kg.
- Hospitalization – The requirement of hospitalization and bed rest because of other complications during pregnancy increases risk.
- Operative procedures – Any operative procedure in the puerperium or during pregnancy increases risk.
- Prior history of thrombosis – As with nonpregnant patients, prior thrombosis increases risk for recurrence.
- Inherited thrombotic disorder – Deficiency of antithrombin III, protein C, protein S, or dysfibrinogenemia increases risk during pregnancy.
- Lupus-type anticoagulant – Lupus-type anticoagulants are associated with increased thrombosis and with recurrent fetal demise.

Diagnosis of DVT or PE often requires consideration of radiation exposure to the fetus. Issues of diagnosis and treatment of DVT and PE in pregnancy have been recently reviewed.[29] Heparin is the treatment of choice and is usually well tolerated. Long-term therapy can be complicated by osteoporosis. In addition, some patients may develop heparin-induced thrombocytopenia requiring alternative therapy. Because of the risk to the fetus, particularly in Weeks 6-12 of gestation, warfarin is avoided during pregnancy. Newer low-molecular weight heparins, heparinoids, or hirudin may offer treatment alternatives in the future.

Arterial thrombosis, stroke, and myocardial infarction are rare in women of childbearing age. The risk of stroke, however, is 13 times as great in pregnant compared to nonpregnant women, occurring in one in every 3,000 pregnancies.[34] The causes of these strokes are numerous, as in nonpregnant women. It is possible that the increased rate is related to the general hypercoagulable condition of the patient, added to the numerous other risk factors for arteriovascular disease. These issues are covered in greater detail elsewhere in this book.

Hypertensive Disorders of Pregnancy and Coagulopathy

These disorders include: 1) pre-eclampsia and eclampsia; 2) chronic hypertension; 3) chronic hypertension with pre-eclampsia; and 4) transient hypertension.[63] Available studies, using sensitive coagulation assays, demonstrate increased thrombin generation in pregnant women with hypertension.[108] Although not well understood, it is apparent that the etiology is damage to the vascular endothelium; this can then lead to activation of coagulation and consumption of platelets. There appears to be a decrease in fibrinolytic activity with increased fibrinolytic inhibitors,[39] and vWF is increased.[42] Thrombin-antithrombin complexes are higher and antithrombin III levels are reduced.[19,108] These findings make the frequent development of DIC in these patients expected. In addition, the coupling of hypertension with the resulting coagulopathy increases the risk of CNS hemorrhage.

References

1. Ament LA: Anticardiolipin antibodies. A review of the literature. **J Nurse Midwifery 39:**19-24, 1991
2. Amorosi EL, Ultmann JE: Thrombotic thrombocytopenic purpura: report of 16 cases and review of the literature. **Medicine 45:**139-159, 1966
3. Arias F, Andrinopoulos G, Zamora J: Whole-blood fibrinolytic activity in normal and hypertensive pregnancies and its relation to placental concentration of urokinase inhibitor. **Am J Obstet Gynecol 133:**624-629, 1979
4. Aster R, Chairman (Consensus Development Panel): Platelet transfusion therapy. **JAMA 257:**1777-1780, 1987
5. Aster RH: "Gestational" thrombocytopenia. A plea for conservative management. **N Engl J Med 323:** 264-266,1990
6. Aster RH: Post-transfusion purpura, in Engelfreit CP, von dem Borne AEG (eds): **Balliere's Clinical Immunology and Allergy.** Philadelphia, PA: Balliere, Tindall, 1987
7. Aster RH, George JN: Thrombocytopenia due to enhanced platelet destruction by immunologic mechanisms, in Williams WJ, Beutler E, Erslev AJ, et al (eds): **Hematology, 4th ed.** New York, NY: McGraw-Hill, 1990, pp 1370-1398
8. Bachmann F, Kruithof IEKO: Tissue plasminogen activator: chemical and physiological aspects. **Semin**

Thromb Hemost 10:6-17, 1984
9. Blanchette VS, Hogan VA, McCombie NE, et al: Intensive plasma exchange therapy in ten patients with idiopathic thrombocytopenic purpura. **Transfusion 24:**388-394, 1984
10. Bonnar J, McNicol GP, Douglas AS: Fibrinolytic system enzymes and pregnancy. **Br Med J 3:**387-381, 1969
11. Booyse FM, Scheinbuks J, Radek J, et al: Immunological identification and comparison of plasminogen activator forms in cultured normal human endothelial cells and smooth muscle cells. **Thromb Res 24:**495-504, 1981
12. Brenner B, Guilburd JN, Tatarsky I, et al: Spontaneous intracranial hemorrhage in immune thrombocytopenic purpura. **Neurosurgery 22:**761-764, 1988
13. Broze GJ Jr: The role of tissue factor pathway inhibitor in a revised coagulation cascade. **Semin Hematol 29:**159-169, 1992
14. Broze GJ Jr, Girard TJ, Novotny WF: The lipoprotein-associated coagulation inhibitor. **Prog Hemost Thromb 10:**243-268, 1991
15. Bukowski RM, Hewlett JS: Reimer RR, et al: Therapy of thrombotic thrombocytopenic purpura: an overview. **Semin Thromb Hemost 7:**1-8, 1981
16. Burrows RF, Kelton JG: Incidentally detected thrombocytopenia in healthy mothers and their infants. **N Engl J Med 319:**142-145, 1988
17. Busch C, Cancilla PA, DeBault LE, et al: Methods in laboratory investigation. Use of endothelium cultured on microcarriers as a model for the microcirculation. **Lab Invest 47:**498-504, 1982
18. Busch C, Owen WG: Identification *in vitro* of an endothelial cell surface cofactor for antithrombin III. Parallel studies with isolated perfused rat hearts and microcarrier cultures of bovine endothelium. **J Clin Invest 69:**726-729, 1982
19. Cadroy Y, Grandjean H, Pichon J, et al: Evaluation of six markers of haemostatic system in normal pregnancy and pregnancy complicated by hypertension or pre-eclampsia. **Br J Obstet Gynaecol 100:**416-420, 1993
20. Caggiano V, Fernando LP, Schneider JM, et al: Thrombotic thrombocytopenic purpura: report of the fourteen cases–occurrence during pregnancy and response to plasma exchange. **J Clin Apheresis 1:** 17-85, 1983
21. Chesebro JH, Fuster V, Elveback LR, et al: Trial of combined warfarin plus dipyridamole or aspirin therapy in prosthetic heart valve replacement: danger of aspirin compared to dipyridamole. **Am J Cardiol 51:**1537-1541, 1983
22. Collen D: On the regulation and control of fibrinolysis. Edward Kowalski Memorial Lecture. **Thromb Haemost 43:**77-89, 1980
23. Collen D: Tissue-type plasminogen activator (t-PA) and single chain urokinase-type plasminogen activator (scu-PA): potential for fibrin-specific thrombolytic therapy. **Prog Hemost Thromb 8:**1-18, 1986
24. Colman RW, Walsh PN: Mechanisms of platelet aggregation, in Colman RW, Hirsh J, Marder VJ, et al (eds): **Hemostasis and Thrombosis: Basic Principles and Clinical Practice, 2nd ed.** Philadelphia, PA: JB Lippincott, 1987, pp 594-605
25. Comp PC: Hereditary disorders predisposing to thrombosis. **Prog Hemost Thromb 8:**71-102, 1986
26. Comp PC, Thurnau GR, Welsh J, et al: Functional and immunologic protein S levels are decreased during pregnancy. **Blood 68:**881-885, 1986
27. Couch P, Stumfp JL: Management of uremic bleeding. **Clin Pharm 9:**673-681, 1990 and **Clin Pharm 10:**429, 1991
28. Davis JW, McField JR, Phillips PE, et al: Guanidinosuccinic acid on human platelet. Effects of exogenous urea, creatinine, and aggregation *in vitro.* **Blood 39:**388-397, 1972
29. Demers C, Ginsberg JS: Deep venous thrombosis and pulmonary embolism in pregnancy. **Clin Chest Med 13:**645-656, 1992
30. Esmon CT: The regulation of natural anticoagulant pathways. **Science 235:**1348-1352, 1987
31. Fay RA, Hughes AO, Farron NT: Platelets in pregnancy: hyperdestruction in pregnancy. **Obstet Gynecol 61:**238-240, 1983
32. Feinstein D: Immune coagulation disorders, in Colman RW, Hirsch J, Marder VJ, et al (eds): **Hemostosis and Thrombosis: Basic Principles and Clinical Practice, 3rd ed.** Philadelphia, PA: JB Lippincott, 1994, pp 881-905
33. Fernandez F, Goudable C, Sie P, et al: Low haematocrit and prolonged bleeding time in uraemic patients: effect of red cell transfusions. **Br J Haematol 59:**139-148, 1985
34. Fox MW, Harms RW, Davis DH: Selected neurologic complications of pregnancy. **Mayo Clin Proc 65:** 1595-1618, 1990
35. Fukui H, Nishino M, Terada S, et al: Hemostatic effect of a heat-treated factor VIII concentrate (Haemate P) in von Willebrand's disease. **Blut 56:** 171-178, 1988
36. Gaydos LA, Freireich EJ, Mantel N: The quantitative relation between platelet count and hemorrhage in patients with acute leukemia. **N Engl J Med 266:** 905-909, 1962
37. Goudemand J, Mazurier C, Marey A, et al: Clinical and biological evaluation in von Willebrand's disease of a von Willebrand factor concentrate with low factor VIII activity. **Br J Haematol 80:**214-221, 1992
38. Guy GP, Baxi LV, Hurlet-Jensen A, et al: An unusual complication in a gravida with factor IX deficiency: case report with review of the literature. **Obstet Gynecol 80:**502-505, 1992
39. Halligan A, Bonnar J, Sheppard B, et al: Haemostatic, fibrinolytic and endothelial variables in normal pregnancies and pre-eclampsia. **Br J Obstet Gynaecol 101:**488-492, 1994
40. Hantgan RR, Taylor RG, Lewis JC: Platelets interact with fibrin only after activation. **Blood 65:** 1299-1311, 1985
41. Harkness DR, Byrnes JJ, Lian ECY, et al: Hazard of platelet transfusion in thrombotic thrombocytopenic purpura. **JAMA 246:**1931-1933, 1981
42. Hathaway WE, Bonnar J: **Hemostatic Disorders of the Pregnant Woman and Newborn Infant.** New York, NY: Elsevier, 1987
43. Hatton MWC, Berry LR, Regoeczi E: Inhibition of thrombin by antithrombin III in the presence of certain glycosaminoglycans found in the mammalian aorta. **Thromb Res 13:**655-670, 1978
44. Hedner U, Kisiel W: Use of human Factor VIIa in the treatment of two hemophilia A patients with high-

titer inhibitors. **J Clin Invest 71**:1836-1841, 1983
45. Hensler ME, Frojmovic M, Taylor TG, et al: Platelet morphologic changes and fibrinogen receptor localization. Initial responses in ADP-activated human platelets. **Am J Pathol 141**:707-719, 1992
46. Herman JH, Jumbelic MI, Ancona RJ, et al: *In utero* cerebral hemorrhage in alloimmune thrombocytopenia. **Am J Pediatr Hematol Oncol 8**:312-317, 1986
47. Hoots WK, Huntington D, Devine D, et al: Aggressive combination therapy in the successful management of life-threatening intracranial hemorrhage in a patient with idiopathic thrombocytopenic purpura. **Am J Pediatr Hematol Oncol 8**:225-230, 1986
48. Humphreys RP, Hockley AD, Freedman MH, et al: Management of intracerebral hemorrhage in idiopathic thrombocytopenic purpura. Report of four cases. **J Neurosurg 45**:700-704, 1976
49. Ichinose A, Fujikawa K, Suyama T: The activation of pro-urokinase by plasma kallikrein and its inactivation by thrombin. **J Biol Chem 261**:3486-3489, 1986
50. Ito R, Statland BE, Sher G, et al: Assaying plasma prekallikrein (PPK) by chromogenic based method: analytical considerations and reference values in healthy adults, the pregnant women, and the neonate. **Adv Exp Med Biol 156**:205-223, 1983
51. Johnson SA, Balboa RS, Dessel BH, et al: The mechanism of endothelial supporting function of intact platelets. **Exp Molec Pathol 3**:115-127, 1964
52. Juhl A: DDAVP, cryoprecipitate, and highly 'purified' factor VIII concentrate in uremia. **Nephron 43**: 305-306, 1986
53. Kelton JG: Management of the pregnant patient with idiopathic thrombocytopenic purpura. **Ann Intern Med 99**:796-800, 1983
54. Kelton JG, Ali AM: Platelet transfusions–a critical appraisal. **Clin Oncol 2**:549-585, 1983
55. Kernoff PBA, Thomas ND, Lilley PA, et al: Clinical experience with polyelectrolyte-fractionated porcine Factor VIII concentrate in the treatment of hemophiliacs with antibodies to factor VIII. **Blood 63**:31, 1984
56. Kojima T, Isozaki Y, Hirata Y, et al: Urinary arginine vasopressin excretion and hyponatremia in the sick neonates. **Am J Perinatol 9**:329-333, 1992
57. Larsen E, Celi A, Gilbert GE, et al: PADGEM protein: a receptor that mediates the interaction of activated platelets with neutrophils and monocytes. **Cell 59**: 305-312, 1989
58. Lau P, Sholtis CM, Aster RH: Post-transfusion purpura: an enigma of alloimmunization. **Am J Hematol 9**:331-336, 1980
59. Levin EG, Loskutoff DJ: Cultured bovine endothelial cells produce both urokinase and tissue-type plasminogen activators. **J Cell Biol 94**:631-636, 1982
60. Lewis PJ, Boylan P, Friedman LA, et al: Prostacyclin in pregnancy. **Br Med J 280**:1581-1582, 1980
61. Lichtin AE, Schreiber AD, Hurwitz S, et al: Efficacy of intensive plasmapheresis in thrombotic thrombocytopenic purpura. **Arch Intern Med 147**:2122-2126, 1987
62. Liebman HA, McGehee WG, Patch MJ, et al: Severe depression of antithrombin III associated with disseminated intravascular coagulation in women with fatty liver of pregnancy. **Ann Intern Med 98**:330-333, 1983
63. Lindheimer MD, Katz AI: Hypertension in pregnancy. **N Engl J Med 313**:675-680, 1985
64. Livio M, Benigni A, Viganò G, et al: Moderate doses of aspirin and risk of bleeding in renal failure. **Lancet 1**:414-416, 1986
65. Lusher JM, McMillan CW, the Hemophilia Study Group: Severe factor VIII and factor IX deficiency in females. **Am J Med 65**:637-648, 1978
66. Mann KG: Membrane-bound enzyme complexes in blood coagulation. **Prog Hemost Thromb 7**:1-23, 1984
67. Manning FA, Wodzicki A, Dundar L, et al: The fibrinolytic system in late pregnancy, labor, and the early puerperium. **Am J Obstet Gynecol 110**:900-907, 1971
68. Mannucci PM: Desmopressin (DDAVP) for treatment of disorders of hemostasis. **Prog Hemost Thromb 8**:19-45, 1986
69. Marder VJ, Feinstein D, Francis CW, et al: Consumptive, thrombohemorrhagic disorders, in Colman RW, Hirsch J, Marder VJ, et al (eds): **Hemostosis and Thrombosis: Basic Principles and Clinical Practice, 3rd ed.** Philadelphia, PA: JB Lippincott, 1994, pp 1023-1063
70. Marengo-Rowe AJ, Murff G, Leveson JE, et al: Hemophilia-like disease associated with pregnancy. **Obstet Gynecol 40**:56-64, 1972
71. Mayne EE, Madden M, Crothers IS, et al: Highly purified porcine factor VIII in haemophilia A with inhibitors to factor VIII. **Br Med J 282**:318, 1981
72. Miletich JP, Jackson CM, Majerus PW: Properties of the factor X_a binding site on human platelets. **J Biol Chem 253**:6908-6916, 1978
73. Moake JL, Rudy CK, Troll JH, et al: Unusually large plasma factor VIII: von Willebrand factor multimers in chronic relapsing thrombotic thrombocytopenic purpura. **N Engl J Med 307**:1432-1435, 1982
74. Moia M, Mannucci PM, Vizzotto L, et al: Improvement in the haemostatic defect of uraemia after treatment with recombinant human erythropoietin. **Lancet 2**:1227-1229, 1987
75. Montgomery RR, Coller BS: von Willebrand disease, in Colman RW, Hirsch J, Marder VJ, et al (eds): **Hemostasis and Thrombosis: Basic Principles and Clinical Practice.** Philadelphia, PA: JB Lippincott, 1994, pp 134-168
76. Nesheim ME, Eid S, Mann KG: Assembly of the prothrombinase complex in the absence of prothrombin. **J Biol Chem 256**:9874-9882, 1981
77. Nesheim ME, Hibbard LS, Tracy PB, et al: Participation of Factor Va in prothrombinase, in Mann KG, Taylor FB Jr (eds): **The Regulation of Coagulation.** New York, NY: Elsevier North-Holland, 1980, p 145
78. Niizuma H, Suzuki J, Yonemitsu T, et al: Spontaneous intracerebral hemorrhage and liver dysfunction. **Stroke 19**:852-856, 1988
79. Olson JD: Mechanisms of hemostasis. Effect on intracerebral hemorrhage. **Stroke 24(Suppl 12)**: I109-I114, 1993
80. Olson JD, Kaufman HH, Moake J, et al: The incidence and significance of hemostatic abnormalities in patients with head injuries. **Neurosurgery 24**: 825-832, 1989
81. Packham MA, Mustard JF: Platelet adhesion. **Prog Hemost Thromb 7**:211-288, 1984
82. Patten E: Therapeutic plasmapheresis and plasma

exchange. **Crit Rev Clin Lab Sci 23**:147-75, 1986

83. Ploug M, Behrendt N, Løber D: Protein structure and membrane anchorage of the cellular receptor for urokinase-type plasminogen activator. **Semin Thromb Hemost 17**:183-193, 1991
84. Pockros PJ, Peters RL, Reynolds TB: Idiopathic fatty liver of pregnancy: findings in ten cases. **Medicine 63**:1-11, 1984
85. Rabiner SF, Molinas F: The role of phenol and phenolic acids on thrombocytopathy and defective platelet aggregation in patients with renal failure. **Am J Med 49**:346-351, 1970
86. Reece EA, Romero R, Hobbins J: Coagulopathy associated with factor VIII inhibitor. A literature review. **J Reprod Med 29**:53-58, 1984
87. Reid DE, Frigoletto FD, Tullis JL, et al: Hypercoagulable states in pregnancy. **Am J Obstet Gynecol 111**:493-504, 1971
88. Remuzzi G, Livio M, Marchiaro G, et al: Bleeding in renal failure: altered platelet function in chronic uraemia only partially corrected by haemodialysis. **Nephron 22**:347, 1978
89. Rodeghiero F, Castaman G, Dini E: Epidemiological investigation of the prevalence of von Willebrand's disease. **Blood 69**:454-459, 1987
90. Rodgers RPC, Levin J: A critical reappraisal of the bleeding time. **Semin Thromb Hemost 16**:1-20, 1990
91. Ruggeri ZM, Mannucci PM, Lombardi R, et al: Multimeric composition of factor VIII/von Willebrand factor following administration of DDAVP: implications for pathophysiology and therapy of von Willebrand's disease subtypes. **Blood 59**:1272-1278, 1982
92. Sack GH Jr, Levin J, Bell WR: Trousseau's syndrome and other manifestations of chronic disseminated coagulopathy in patients with neoplasms: clinical, pathophysiologic, and therapeutic features. **Medicine 56**:1-37, 1977
93. Sayama S, Kashiwagi H, Ogawa T, et al: Circulating levels of prekallikrein and kallikrein in pregnancy and labor. **Int J Biol Res Pregnancy 2**:90-94, 1981
94. Shepard KV, Bukowski RM: The treatment of thrombotic thrombocytopenic purpura with exchange transfusion, plasma infusions, and plasma exchange. **Semin Hematol 24**:178-193, 1987
95. Sinha RK, Kelton JG: Current controversies concerning the measurement of platelet-associated IgG. **Transfus Med Rev 4**:1212-1235, 1990
96. Snyder HW Jr, Cochran SK, Balint JP Jr, et al: Experience with protein A-immunoadsorption in treatment-resistant adult immune thrombocytopenic purpura. **Blood 79**:2237-2245, 1992
97. Somer JB, Stewart JH, Castaldi PA: The effect of urea on the aggregation of normal human platelets. **Thrombos Diathes Haemost 19**:64-69, 1968
98. Sorosky J, Klatsky A, Nobert GF, et al: von Willebrand's disease complicating second-trimester abortion. **Obstet Gynecol 55**:253-254, 1980
99. Stirling Y, Woolf L, North WRS, et al: Haemostasis in normal pregnancy. **Thromb Haemost 52**:176-182, 1984
100. Strauss RG: The risks of thrombocytopenia and the standard use of platelet transfusions. **Plasma Ther Transfus Technol 7**:279-285, 1986
101. Suzuki S, Sakamoto W: The kinetics of blood coagulability: fibrinolytic and kallikrein-kinin system at the onset and during labor. **Eur J Obstet Gynecol Reprod Biol 17**:209-218, 1984
102. Tracy PB, Mann KG: A model for assembly of coagulation factor complexes on cell surfaces: prothrombin activation on platelets, in Phillips DR, Shuman MA (eds): **Biochemistry of Platelets.** Orlando, FL: Academic Press, 1986, p 295-318
103. Triulzi DJ, Blumberg N: Variability in response to cryoprecipitate treatment for hemostatic defects in uremia. **Yale J Biol Med 63**:1-7, 1990
104. Voke J, Letsky E: Pregnancy and antibody to factor VIII. **J Clin Pathol 30**:928-932, 1977
105. Walker FJ: Protein S and thrombotic disease. **Proc Soc Exp Biol Med 200**:285-295, 1992
106. Warkentin TE, Kelton JG: Current concepts in the treatment of immune thrombocytopenia. **Drugs 40**: 531-542, 1990
107. Weiner CP: Diagnosis and management of thromboembolic disease during pregnancy. **Clin Obstet Gynecol 28**:107-118, 1985
108. Weiner CP: Preeclampsia-eclampsia syndrome and coagulation. **Clin Perinatol 18**:713-726, 1991
109. Weiner CP, Herrig JE, Pelzer GD, et al: Elimination of antithrombin III concentrate in healthy pregnant and preeclamptic women with an acquired antithrombin III deficiency. **Thromb Res 58**:395-401, 1990
110. Whigham KAE, Howie PW, Drummond AH, et al: Abnormal platelet function in pre-eclampsia. **Br J Obstet Gynaecol 85**:28-32, 1978
111. White JG: Electron microscopic studies of platelet secretion. **Prog Hemost Thromb 2**:49-98, 1974
112. Zhou Q, Zhao Y, Li P, et al: A monoclonal antibody (SZ-53) against thrombomodulin inhibits thrombin-mediated release of t-PA and PGI2 from endothelial cells. **Nouv Rev Fr Hematol 33**:281-286, 1991
113. Zucker-Franklin D, Grusky G: The actin and myosin filaments of human and bovine blood platelets. **J Clin Invest 51**:419-430, 1972

CHAPTER 6

Back Pain in Pregnancy

Steven J. Beer, MD, and Christopher M. Loftus, MD

Back pain in pregnancy affects more than one-half of all pregnant women and ranges from mild to incapacitating. These pain syndromes have been proposed to have various etiologies, ranging from purely structural theories based on requisite changes in posture which occur so as to compensate for the growth of a fetus to more complex mechanisms believed to be of either hormonal or mechanical influence. Therapeutic options, in turn, range from no treatment (considering back pain to be merely a side effect of pregnancy warranting no therapy) to the concept that active intervention may result in a more tolerable experience for women.

We will focus first on the epidemiology of back pain in pregnancy to establish its significance as a neurological problem in pregnancy. We then consider the various proposed pathogenic theories of this pain, which will further identify the complex nature of this problem. An understanding of this, in turn, sets the stage for discussing some of the proposed treatment options for back pain in pregnancy.

Incidence and Characteristics

The incidence of back pain during pregnancy in reported series ranges from 10% to 90%, with an average of 50%.[3,5,12,28,34,42] The many variables in obstetrical back pain make direct comparison of individual studies impossible. As suggested by Hainline,[16] the type of pain, the time of onset during the day and during the pregnancy, the precipitating and palliative features, the relationship to activity, body mechanics, and weight gain, the complications of pregnancy, the previous history of back pain, and multiple other characteristics must be taken into consideration.

Pain syndromes range from isolated low-back symptomatology to pain that radiates into the buttocks and posterior thighs. Classic radicular pain which radiates below the knee is uncommon.[12,28,45] Some authors have suggested localization of pain to the sacroiliac joints.[3,40] Pain often occurs with activity; however, increased back pain with recumbency was noted by a large percentage of pregnant women.[13] Of published studies available, each addresses the problem in a slightly different fashion.

In 1988 Berg et al[3] published a prospective analysis in which 862 women were interviewed by questionnaire during Weeks 20 through 35 of pregnancy. In this series, 49% of patients had some degree of low-back pain. In 9% of patients the pain was so severe that they could not continue normal activities. Factors associated with increased risk of developing pain included physically strenuous activity and an antenatal history of low-back pain.

Mantle et al[28] reviewed in 1977 the experience of 180 women interviewed by questionnaire within 24 hours of delivery. In this study, approximately one-half of the respondents experienced pain and, of these, one-third considered it severe enough to seriously interfere with normal activity. The study specifically addressed the benefit of antenatal low-back pain training, which was generally effective in reducing pain. Furthermore, advancing age and parity were associated with a greater incidence of pain; no correlation existed between weight gain during pregnancy, the birth weight of the child, patient height, and pain severity. Pain was found to commence most often in the sixth and seventh months of pregnancy and to become most symptomatic in the evening.

In a similar study of 99 women assessed at delivery in 1982, Nwuga[34] found a 90% incidence of pain, 10% of which was considered severe. Again, antenatal physiotherapy was found to be beneficial in reducing the incidence of that pain commonly associated with advancing age and parity. Additionally, pain was noted most frequently to occur later in pregnancy, between the sixth and seventh months, with peak symptoms occurring in the evening in 60% and at night in 30%.

Fast et al[12] in 1987 conducted personal interviews of 200 patients within 24 to 36 hours of delivery. In this review, 56% experienced pain; the pain was radicular to the lower extremities in nearly 46%. Contrary to what the authors had expected, neither the patient age, weight of the child, weight gained by mother, nor parity were related to back pain. Pain commenced between the fifth and seventh months of pregnancy and increased toward evening in one-third; in another one-third pain was most severe at night and disturbed sleep. Subsequently, Fast et al[13] reported a 67% incidence of night backache with recumbency; in 36% of 100 women surveyed, pain was severe enough to interfere with sleep.

Ostgaard and Andersson[37] assessed over 800 pregnancies specifically to determine whether a history of back pain in pregnancy would predispose women to pain in future pregnancies. In this study, 429 women had a history of back pain and 375 did not. During the pregnancies, back pain occurred twice as frequently in women with prior histories of low-back pain. Contrary to previously described findings, however, this study showed that younger women have a greater risk of back pain. Ostgaard and Andersson[36] subsequently investigated the prevalence of back pain in the postpartum period in 817 women followed for a minimum of 12 months. In that study, 67% of women reported back pain at the time of delivery, whereas only 37% reported pain at approximately 18 months postpartum (in the majority, pain had lessened compared with the time of delivery). Only 7% of the group had persistent late severe pain. Factors associated with a tendency to have persistent pain included a history of low-back pain prior to pregnancy and a history of physically heavy work. Therefore, in this study pregnancy-related low-back pain in the absence of predisposing factors was for the most part a self-limited event.

The incidence of pregnancy-related low-back pain is lower in retrospective studies. In two such reviews, Biering-Sørensen[5] and Svensson et al[42] noted incidences of low-back pain in 20% of 478 women and 24% of 1760 women, respectively. The discrepancy between retrospective analyses and the studies during pregnancy likely relates to recall bias, as subjects may not remember episodic back pain associated with pregnancy when questioned years later.

In summary, studies to date indicate that about one-half of pregnant women experience some degree of low-back pain during pregnancy, which is severe in about one-third.[3,12,28] Most frequently, pain commences late in pregnancy and late in the day and evening.[12,13,28,34] Patient age,[20,34] parity,[28,34] an antenatal history of low-back pain,[3,37] and physically strenuous activity[3,36] have been positively correlated with an increased incidence. Antenatal low-back pain training has been shown to decrease this incidence.[28,34]

Etiology of Low-Back Pain Related to Pregnancy

Back pain has previously been treated as a side effect of maternity with postural changes deemed responsible for the majority of pain syndromes; even today some authors maintain this view. There are, however, physiological changes that occur during pregnancy which may be implicated as the source of this pain, rather than obvious changes which occur in posture and which may make proactive treatment of pregnancy-related low-back pain now possible.

Posture

In 1940 Williams described the most common cause of back pain in pregnancy to be "faulty body mechanics."[15,47] To compensate for the weight of an enlarging fetus and to offset the progressive anterior displacement of their center of gravity, women shift their posture. In so doing, the lumbar spine assumes a more lordotic configuration and the pelvis tilts forward.[6,11,14] As such, weight-bearing responsibility which normally rests within the column of vertebral bodies shifts toward the posterior articular elements of the spine. Stretch placed on the anterior abdominal wall musculature and the shortening of the paraspinal muscles decrease the mechanical advantage of these muscle groups and further stress the posterior vertebral elements as well as the pelvis and sacroiliac joints.[14] The resultant change in the anatomical configuration of the spine and pelvis results in abnormal mechanics of lifting and ambulation.[33] Back pain, in turn, has been proposed to result from both muscular strain[33] and irritation to the exiting lumbosacral nerves.[6]

Pregnancy-related back pain theories based solely on a postural etiology, however, have been controversial.[12] According to Fast et al,[12] Fahrni supported the postural hypothesis in his review of posture in primitive societies when he noted a zero incidence of back pain in societies in which individuals were forced to maintain a flexed lumbar stature for prolonged periods during the day.[10] On the other hand, Hansson et al[17] found no relationship between the degree of lordosis in individuals with and without back pain.

Sacroiliac Origin of Pain/ Ligamentous Laxity

Other authors have implicated changes primarily in the pelvis and sacroiliac joints as the cause of low-back pain in pregnancy. In 1934 Abramson et al[1] suggested this relationship and in 1958 Sands[40] stated, "the site of origin of the backache of pregnancy is almost exclusively the sacroiliac joints . . . primarily." In support of this mechanism for pain, many authors believe that biomechanical changes related to increased ligamentous laxity in the symphysis pubis and sacroiliac joints contribute to a sacroiliac pain syndrome.[3,25,40] During pregnancy, hormones cause adaptive changes in the pelvis in preparation for the enlarging uterus and eventual descent of the child through the birth canal.[20] The effects of estrogen result in proliferation of connective tissue, and relaxin (secreted by the corpus luteum) causes vascularization and softening of the proliferative connective tissue.[23,43,45]

The effect of ligamentous laxity on the stability of the pelvis and the changes in the configuration of the pelvis both radiographically and clinically have been reviewed in detail.[50] Serum relaxin levels have been shown to correlate with pelvic ligamentous laxity and pelvic pain during pregnancy.[27] Although sacroiliac-related pain can cause a "low-back pain" syndrome with referred pain to the lower extremities, lumbar pain is difficult to distinguish from sacroiliac pain, making a clear cause-and-effect relationship hard to prove.[7,16,24,45] In addition, there is contradictory radiographic evidence in which some women have significant ligamentous laxity without pain whereas others have minimal laxity with significant symptoms.[25,45]

Lumbar Disc Disease and Other Spinal Disorders

In further support of the pain implications of hormonally induced changes which occur during pregnancy, O'Connell[35] in 1960 suggested that relaxin may affect intervertebral joints, rendering them susceptible to stress, and as such, implicated "pregnancy [as] an aetiological factor in the development of lumbar disc protrusions in woman." In this study, 30% of 179 women who had surgically proven lumbar disc disease reported that their symptoms commenced during pregnancy or the puerperium. Kelsey et al[21] in 1975 supported this concept with a case-control epidemiological study which found that a greater number of pregnancies resulting in live births predisposed women to disc herniation. The aforementioned studies, however, did not support a higher rate of disc herniation associated with pregnancy as they suggested.[2] Perhaps more accurately, LaBan and Perrin[25] in 1983 reviewed 48,760 deliveries and found an incidence of lumbar disc herniation to be only 1:10,000. This study supported the earlier conclusion of King[22] in 1950 that disc rupture in pregnancy was a rare occurrence. In 1988, Weinreb et al[46] compared magnetic resonance images (MRIs) of 45 pregnant subjects with 41 nonpregnant asymptomatic women. Fifty-three percent of the pregnant and 54% of the nonpregnant woman had an abnormal disc (bulge or herniation) at one or more lumbar levels. The differences between the groups were not statistically significant.

In addition to concern that hormonal influences may result in an increased propensity for disc herniation, others have addressed potential changes which may occur with spondylitic disease of the spine, scoliosis, and rheumatoid arthritis. Betz et al[4] in 1987, in a case-control study, reviewed 355 patients with scoliosis (175 of whom had been pregnant at least once and 180 who had never been pregnant) and found no change in spinal curvature with pregnancy. In a study of 171 men and 18 "never-pregnant" women compared to 66 "ever-pregnant" women over a 20-year period, Saraste[41] found no significant change in spondylolisthesis associated with pregnancy. Finally, Parke[38] described an improvement in pain resulting from rheumatoid arthritis and an exacerbation of pain related to ankylosing spondylosis during pregnancy.

Night Pain

As mentioned previously, pain with recumbency and pain at night in general affect a significant percentage of pregnant women.[12,13] Fast et al[13] hypothesized that hypervolemia associated with pregnancy and further increased with recumbency, combined with inferior vena cava obstruction by the enlarged uterus and inadequate venous collateral circulation, results in lumbar venous obstruction and overdistention. Increased pressure in the venous channels and vertebral bodies, in turn, leads to stasis of flow around the nerves with associated edema formation and metabolic disturbances, as well as irritation from the direct pressure of the overdistended venous structures.[13] Similar to LaBan and Wesolowski's theory in which venous volume and pressure gradients may exacerbate symptoms of chronic stenosis during congestive heart failure,[26] Fast proposed a plausible mechanism for night pain in pregnancy. In further support of this hypothesis, radiographic evidence of venous distention in pregnancy has been shown[30] and others have suggested a venous obstructive pathophysiology of back pain.[39,48,49]

Direct Pressure and Labor

In addition to the postural and hormonal mechanisms, the direct effect of pressure from the enlarged uterus on intrapelvic and intraabdominal structures likely contributes to "low-back pain" during pregnancy. The lumbosacral plexus, ureters, and great vessels all cross the pelvic brim, making these structures particularly vulnerable to the compressive effects of the uterine mass.[19,22] Nociceptors in this region may in turn cause referred pain to the lumbar and sacral regions,[31] further confounding the source of "back pain." In labor, further pain from these "compressive effects" of the uterine mass as well as from the stress of labor have been described.[31,32] Continuous low-back pain was shown to be present in 74% of 46 women in a review of early labor by Melzack and Schaffelberg.[32] In this study, continuous pain was described by 44% of women to be more intense than back pain associated with contractions, and 33% stated that it was the worst pain of labor. The authors postulated that traction and pressure on the adnexa, parietal peritoneum, bladder, urethra, rectum, and lumbosacral plexus as well as muscle spasm and vasospasm in structures supplied by spinal cord segments also subtending the uterus were responsible for this pain.[31] Additionally, Hainline[16] suggested that Fast's[13] theory for night back pain might also contribute to this pain since inferior vena cava compression and subsequent obstruction likely occurs during labor and the characteristic constant nature of pain correlates with the pain resulting from venous obstructive processes.

Diagnosis and Management

Given the complex nature of back discomfort in pregnancy, treatment must be directed by each individual's symptomatology, taking into consideration the various proposed mechanisms for pain generation.[16] Potential harm to the fetus resulting from both conservative and more aggressive forms of evaluation and treatment must always be remembered. With this in mind, the mainstay of initial evaluation is the medical history and the physical examination. Most frequently, conservative measures will suffice for self-limited cases of back pain. Should signs and symptoms warrant, further limited diagnostic studies may be necessary.

Treatment, however, should commence whenever possible with preventive measures prior to the onset of pregnancy. As mentioned above, antenatal training has been shown to have a beneficial effect in reducing the frequency of back pain in pregnancy.[28,34] Hainline[16] reviewed and described many conservative measures appropriate for antenatal training, including proper posture both sitting and standing, appropriate lifting techniques, exercise activities, and education in the antenatal period as well as stress management and other modalities. In addition, Hainline stressed the importance of counseling women with a history of back pain, given the tendency for recurrence of pain with pregnancy.[16,37] Others have described exercise programs designed to condition women prior to, during, and after pregnancy to reduce back pain.[33] Should preventive measures fail, conservative treatment modalities, which have been reviewed in detail by Alexander and McCormick[2] and others,[8,16, 24,33] may be employed.

Given the self-limited nature of most back pain in pregnancy,[36] simple reassurance with the implementation of further conservative measures usually serves as adequate treatment for symptoms.[8] Conservative measures most frequently employed include the aforementioned preventive techniques as well as bed rest, analgesics, massage and manipulative therapies, local heat, and supportive care.[2,8] Other medical therapies, including the injection of local steroids in the region of low-back and sacroiliac pain, have been suggested,[25] as well as the various systemic medications used for back pain in nonpregnant individuals; however, these entities must be considered seriously given the potential risk to the fetus.[2,8] In patients with night pain, techniques designed to improve venous return and decrease potential inferior vena cava obstruction, such as the utilization of wedge-shaped pillows to support the gravid abdominal pelvic region off midline, have proved successful.[44] These methods may be employed before proceeding to diagnostic evaluation. In cases of severe refractory symptomology, or when progessive neurological deficits result, more detailed evaluation will be necessary.

Similar to evaluating back pain and associated radicular pain in nonpregnant subjects, MRI in pregnant subjects reveals detailed anatomical information without the risk of ionizing radiation to the fetus which accompanies alternative imaging studies such as computed tomography and myelography.[2,46] As pointed out by Alexander and McCormick,[2] the fetal risk associated with MRI has not been established but appears to be acceptable.[18,29] One must then determine whether the risk of surgery warrants intervention if surgical lesions are evident on MRI. In cases of progressive neurological deficit (as, for example, would be associated with a cauda equina syndrome from a large disc herniation), surgical decompression would be mandatory.[9] Although conservative treatment has been for years the mainstay of therapy for less clear-cut cases, the literature lacks detailed studies supporting the safety of discectomy in cases where surgery is believed warranted by pain alone or pain associated with minor neurological deficits.

Conclusion

Back pain in pregnancy complicates approximately 50% of pregnancies, with severe pain noted in about one-third of patients. Etiologies proposed for this pain range from theories of a mechanical nature focused on postural changes which occur with pregnancy to changes in pelvic and spinal stability, to theories in which hormonally induced changes confound the structural phenomena. In most cases the pain is self-limiting and relief occurs with conservative care and preventive measures. On the other hand, rare cases resulting from true neurological compression from disc herniation with concomitant loss of neurological function deserve careful work-up and expedious care. Properly implemented, these approaches to back pain in pregnancy will make pregnancy a more tolerable experience for women.

REFERENCES

1. Abramson D, Roberts SM, Wilson PD: Relaxation of the pelvic joints in pregnancy. **Surg Gynecol Obstet 58:**595-613, 1934
2. Alexander JT, McCormick PC: Pregnancy and discogenic disease of the spine. **Neurosurg Clin North Am 4:**153-159, 1993
3. Berg G, Hammar M, Möller-Nielsen J, et al: Low back pain during pregnancy. **Obstet Gynecol 71:** 71-75, 1988
4. Betz RR, Bunnell WP, Lambrecht-Mulier, et al: Scoliosis and pregnancy. **J Bone Joint Surg (Am) 69:** 90-95, 1987
5. Biering-Sørensen F: A prospective study of low back pain in a general population. I. Occurrence, recurrence and aetiology. **Scand J Rehabil Med 15:**71-79, 1983
6. Bushnell, LF: The postural pains of pregnancy. **West J Surg 57:**123-127, 1949
7. Cailliet R: **Low Back Pain Syndrome.** Philadelphia, PA: FA Davis, 1987
8. Deyo RA: Nonsurgical care of low back pain. **Neurosurg Clin North Am 2:**851-862, 1991
9. Epstein JA: Symposium: Treatment of low back pain and sciatic syndromes during pregnancy. **NY State J Med 59:**1757-1768, 1959
10. Fahrni WH: Conservative treatment of lumbar disc degeneration: our primary responsibility. **Orthop Clin North Am 6:**93-103, 1975
11. Fast A, Floman Y: Low back pain in pregnancy, in Floman Y (ed): **Disorders of the Lumbar Spine.** Rockville, CO: Aspen Publishers, 1990, pp 895-901
12. Fast A, Shapiro D, Ducommun EJ, et al: Low-back pain in pregnancy. **Spine 12:**368-371, 1987
13. Fast A, Weiss L, Parikh S, et al: Night backache in pregnancy. Hypothetical pathophysiological mechanisms. **Am J Phys Med Rehabil 68:**227-229, 1989
14. Fitzhugh ML, Newton M: Posture in pregnancy. **Am J Obstet Gynecol 85:**1091-1095, 1963
15. Goldthwait JE, Brown LT, Swaim LT, et al: **Essentials of Body Mechanics in Health and Disease, 5th ed.** Philadelphia, PA: JB Lippincott, 1956, p 175
16. Hainline B: Low-back pain in pregnancy. **Adv Neurol 64:**65-76, 1994
17. Hansson T, Bigos S, Beecher P, et al: The lumbar lordosis in acute and chronic low-back pain. **Spine 10:** 154-155, 1985
18. Heinrichs WL: Biohazards of magnetic resonance to the female reproductive system, in McCarthy S, Haseltine F (eds): **Magnetic Resonance of the Reproductive System.** Thorofare, NJ: Slack, 1987, p 220
19. Hill EC: Maternal obstetric paralysis. **Am J Obstet Gynecol 83:**1452-1460, 1962
20. Hisaw FL: Corpus lutem hormone: experimental relaxation of the pelvic ligaments of guinea-pig. **Phys Zool 2:**59-79, 1929
21. Kelsey JL, Greenberg RA, Hardy RJ, et al: Pregnancy and the syndrome of herniated lumbar intervertebral disc: an epidemiological study. **Yale J Biol Med 48:** 361-368, 1975
22. King AB: Neurologic conditions occurring as complications of pregnancy. **Arch Neurol Psychiatry 63:** 611-644, 1950
23. Koay ESC, Too CKL, Greenwood FC, et al: Relaxin stimulates collagenase and plasminogen activator secretion by dispersed human amnion and chorion cells *in vitro.* **J Clin Endocrinol Metab 56:**1332-1334, 1983
24. Kuhns JG: Body mechanics in pregnancy. **Publ Health Nursing 34:**308-314, 1942
25. LaBan MM, Perrin JCS, Latimer FR: Pregnancy and the herniated lumbar disk. **Arch Phys Med Rehabil 64:**319-321, 1983
26. LaBan MM, Wesolowski DP: Night pain associated with diminished cardiopulmonary compliance. A concomitant of lumbar spinal stenosis and degenerative spondylolisthesis. **Am J Phys Med Rehabil 67:**155-160, 1988
27. MacLennan AH, Nicolson R, Green RC, et al: Serum relaxin and pelvic pain of pregnancy. **Lancet 2:** 243-245, 1986
28. Mantle MJ, Greenwood RM, Currey HLF: Backache in pregnancy. **Rheumatol Rehabil 16:**95-101, 1977
29. Mattison DR, Angtuaco T, Miller FC, et al: Magnetic resonance imaging in maternal and fetal medicine. **J Perinatol 9:**411-419, 1989
30. McCarthy SM, Stark DD, Filly RA, et al: Obstetrical magnetic resonance imaging: Maternal anatomy. **Radiology 154:**421-425, 1985
31. Melzack R, Bélanger E: Labour pain: correlations with menstrual pain and acute low-back pain before and during pregnancy. **Pain 36:**225-229, 1989
32. Melzack R, Schaffelberg D: Low-back pain during labor. **Am J Obstet Gynecol 156:**901-905, 1987
33. Noble E: **Essential Exercises for the Childbearing Year: A Guide to Health and Comfort Before and After Your Baby is Born, 2nd ed.** Boston, MA: Houghton Mifflin, 1982
34. Nwuga VCB: Pregnancy and back pain among upper class Nigerian women. **Aust J Physiother 28:**8-11, 1982
35. O'Connell JEA: Lumbar disc protrusions in pregnancy. **J Neurol Neurosurg Psychiatry 23:**138-141, 1960
36. Ostgaard HC, Andersson GBJ: Postpartum low-back pain. **Spine 17:**53-55, 1992
37. Ostgaard HC, Andersson GBJ: Previous back pain

and risk of developing back pain in a future pregnancy. **Spine 16**:432-436, 1991
38. Parke AL: Pregnancy and the rheumatic diseases: the arthropathies, in Gleicher N (ed): **Principles of Medical Therapy in Pregnancy.** New York, NY: Plenum Press, 1985, pp 1003-1013
39. Reginald PW, Beard RW, Kooner JS, et al: Intravenous dihydroergotamine to relieve pelvic congestion with pain in young women. **Lancet 2**:351-353, 1987
40. Sands RX: Backache of pregnancy. A method of treatment. **Obstet Gynecol 12**:670-676, 1958
41. Saraste H: Spondylolysis and pregnancy – a risk analysis. **Acta Obstet Gynecol Scand 65**:727-729, 1986
42. Svensson HO, Andersson GBJ, Johansson S, et al: A retrospective study of low-back pain in 38- to 64-year-old women. Frequency of occurrence and impact on medical services. **Spine 13**:548-552, 1988
43. Talmage RV: Changes produced in the symphysis pubis of the guinea pig by the sex steroids and relaxin. **Anat Rec 99**:91-107, 1947
44. Thomas IL, Nicklin J, Pollock H, et al: Evaluation of a maternity cushion (Ozzlo pillow) for backache and insomnia in late pregnancy. **Aust NZ J Obstet Gynaecol 29**:133-138, 1989
45. Walde J: Obstetrical and gynecological back and pelvic pains, especially those contracted during pregnancy. **Acta Obstet Gynecol Scand 41(Suppl 2)**: 11-53, 1962
46. Weinreb JC, Wolbarsht LB, Coven JM, et al: Prevalence of lumbosacral intervertebral disk abnormalities on MR images in pregnant and asymptomatic nonpregnant women. **Radiology 170**:125-128, 1989
47. Williams PC: Low back pain. **Southern Med J 33**:788-797, 1940
48. Wyke B: The neurological basis of thoracic spinal pain. **Rheumatol Phys Med 10**:356-367, 1970
49. Wyke B: The neurology of low back pain, in Jayson MIV (ed): **The Lumbar Spine and Back Pain, 3rd ed.** New York, NY: Churchill Livingstone, 1987, pp 56-99
50. Young J: Relaxation of the pelvic joints in pregnancy: pelvic arthropathy of pregnancy. **J Obstet Gynecol Br Emp 47**:493-524, 1940

CHAPTER 7

CARPAL TUNNEL SYNDROME IN PREGNANCY

JOEL D. SIEGAL, MD, AND SETTI S. RENGACHARY, MD

Compression of the median nerve within the carpal tunnel produces the carpal tunnel syndrome (CTS), consisting of dysesthesias along the distribution of the median nerve to the lateral three and one-half fingers. Patients are characteristically awakened at night by pain and/or a "numb hand" and may only achieve relief by shaking their hand back and forth. Weakness of the thenar muscles also may be present, but this is a late sign and is no longer seen frequently. The precise cause of the compression is unknown, but narrowing of the carpal tunnel diameter through trauma, thickening of the synovial sheaths of the flexor tendons, or arthritic changes in the carpal bones is thought to be responsible in many cases.[6,22,23,28] Edematous tissue during pregnancy also may cause narrowing of the carpal tunnel, triggering the onset of the syndrome, but the precise causative factors relating CTS to pregnancy are still unknown.

This paper reviews CTS in pregnancy from a detailed chronological and historical perspective. Three hypothetical etiologies are offered to explain the development of CTS in pregnancy, and treatment options are discussed.[4,8,10,13,18-20]

HISTORY

Putnam[21] is credited with writing the first description of CTS "... presenting as a common symptom[,] a disturbance of the subjective sensibility of the skin, giving rise to what is known popularly as numbness, recurring periodically, coming on especially at night or very early in the morning, and affecting one or both hands. ..." Putnam stated that the "numbness was often excessively intense so as to amount to real pain in itself. ..." He presented eight case histories selected from a cohort of 31 patients suffering from nocturnal numbness and paresthesias in the median nerve distribution. Of the 31 patients, 28 were women, approximately four of whom he noted to be pregnant. He, therefore, appears to be the first author to have mentioned the possible relationship between CTS and pregnancy.

Marie and Foix[12] gave the earliest gross pathological description of CTS when they documented the enlargement of the median nerve proximal to the transverse carpal ligament during the postmortem examination of a patient with bilateral thenar atrophy. At the conclusion of this paper, Marie and Foix became the first group to suggest transecting the flexor retinaculum or transverse carpal ligament as a therapeutic intervention for CTS.

Learmonth[11] is credited with the initial surgical decompression of the carpal tunnel. In 1930, he divided the "annular ligament" completely in a patient with severe median nerve compression between the transverse carpal ligament and "arthritic outgrowths from the carpal bones."

Brain et al[1] was the first to describe the surgical division of the transverse carpal ligament on patients in whom the symptom complex "arose spontaneously." He reported six patients treated surgically for "bilateral median neuritis" due to median nerve compression by the transverse carpal ligament at the wrist.

Wallace and Cook[31] appear to be the first authors specifically to link CTS to pregnancy and to perform a surgical decompression of the median nerve on a pregnant woman. Their paper describes two case histories focusing on "pressure as a cause of such symptoms." For example, because in one patient "pain was increasingly severe over the volar aspect of the forearm, wrist, and thenar eminence and the lateral three fingers," transection of the carpal ligament was performed. The pain resolved by the day after surgery and the entire symptom complex "had entirely disappeared at six weeks post partum." These authors mentioned "ischemia of the compressed nerve" and "endocrine features" as contributing factors possibly linking pregnancy and CTS, but did not expound on this. They concluded that "greater attention should be paid to detecting and relieving nerve pressure, by whatever means, in the treatment of these symptoms in pregnant women."

Layton[9] treated three patients who suffered from CTS in pregnancy with exogenous estrogens. All three patients obtained significant relief from their classical symptoms. One patient, in particular, had several exacerbations of her symptomatology when the estrogens were weaned and experienced relief when they were restarted. All seven of his patients had spontaneous improvement in symptoms after delivery and were almost normal by 6 weeks. No attempt at an explanation for this relationship between CTS, pregnancy, and relief of symptoms with estrogen treatment was given.

Soferman et al[26] treated 40 pregnant patients suffering from acroparesthesias in pregnancy with estrogens, analgesics, and sedatives "without definite success." They noted that the onset of symptoms was typically during the third trimester, that nocturnal paresthesias were seen in 90% of their patients, and that parity was not a predictor of the occurrence of symptoms. The majority of patients spontaneously became asymptomatic after delivery, but not as a result of medical intervention. One patient, however, did require surgery.

Guly,[7] McCallum,[14] and Wood[32] described their own success using diuretics to treat pregnant edematous women with CTS. These authors believed that salt and water retention caused swelling in the wrist with a resultant narrowing of the carpal tunnel and compression of the median nerve. The symptomatic acroparesthesias were relieved in many of their patients after administering diuretics.

Tobin,[29] however, observed that diuretic therapy did not give "dramatic" relief in most cases of CTS in pregnancy. Nevertheless, he concluded that because of the tendency for fluid retention in pregnancy ". . . it seems logical to attack this theoretical consideration [that edematous tissue causes carpal tunnel compromise], even if pitting edema is not present. [Therefore], diuretic therapy is in order as a therapeutic trial in every case of carpal tunnel in pregnancy." Of the 42 cases that he accumulated, all eventually obtained complete relief: 85% spontaneously and 15% surgically. He concluded that "no particular trimester of pregnancy seems to be a factor in the occurrence of the carpal tunnel syndrome. . . ."

Nicholas et al[17] also believed that weight gain with fluid retention may be one factor contributing to CTS in pregnancy. In addition, Nicholas' group was one of the first to suggest that the hormone relaxin may cause relaxation of the transverse carpal ligament with flattening of the bony arch and compression of the median nerve and thereby cause CTS. No scientific evidence was offered to explain these hypotheses. Nicholas et al further attempted to establish the true incidence of CTS in pregnancy. By interviewing and examining 100 consecutive pregnant patients they determined that 18% had signs or symptoms of median nerve compression at the wrist. Of the control group, 3% (100 nonpregnant student nurses) had CTS. Nerve conduction delay was not present in any subject nor did any need to undergo surgical treatment; all had relief of symptoms within 3 weeks of delivery.

Melvin et al[16] were the earliest group to study

median nerve conduction by electromyography (EMG) in pregnant women and they concluded that there is a 7% incidence of CTS in pregnancy. Of the 58 pregnant women randomly referred to their clinic, 31% complained of symptoms of "numbness and tingling in the hand" and only 7% had significant electrical abnormalities. Of the 15 pregnant patients referred specifically because of CTS symptomatology, all had some EMG abnormality, including sensory latencies >3.5 msec and motor latencies >5 msec. The findings on EMG usually returned to normal after delivery. Two of the 15 patients did require surgery, but no results of postoperative EMG were published.

Gould and Wissinger[5] studied 100 consecutive obstetric patients without EMG analysis in order to determine the incidence of CTS in pregnancy. All had delivered within the 3 days prior to the interview and 21% of the women interviewed reported ". . . paresthesias or hypesthesia in the median nerve distribution during pregnancy." The majority of symptomatic patients had the onset of symptoms in the third trimester. All had resolution of their clinical symptoms spontaneously within 3 months after delivery. Potential causes of pain in CTS were not mentioned.

Snell et al[25] were the first to publish case reports describing CTS developing in the puerperium and to link the onset of symptoms to breast-feeding and the resolution of symptoms to the termination of breast-feeding. They suggested that ". . . fluid retention due to the action of a hormone or hormones stimulated by lactation led to the development of symptoms. Prolactin is a candidate for this role."

Voitk et al[30] interviewed 1,000 consecutive postpartum patients with questionnaires to establish the incidence of CTS in pregnancy. No physical examination was performed. Of the patients questioned, 34% had hand symptoms: 25% with CTS, 2% with ulnar nerve compression, and 7% with ill-defined symptomatology. Maternal age, weight gain, and parity did not correlate with the presence of symptoms; however, there was a correlation between pre-eclamptic and eclamptic abnormalities and the rate of ring removal due to local swelling with the occurrence of CTS. These authors, therefore, believed that ". . . fluid retention in pregnancy is often sufficient to lead to nerve compression in the wrist." Treatment included restriction of salt intake, rest, diuretics, splints, arm movement, analgesics, and sedatives. Only 46% of the symptomatic patients reported their symptoms to their physician and ". . . less than half the patients treated judged their treatment to be of help, no matter what type it was."

McLennan et al[15] studied a large enough cohort of both control and pregnant patients to draw meaningful conclusions regarding hand symptoms in pregnancy. They retrospectively studied 1,216 pregnancies and 132 control patients who were nonpregnant, premenopausal nursing staff members. Thirty-five percent of the pregnant women and 30% of the control group reported hand symptoms, although the severity of the hand symptoms in the nonpregnant women was much less than that of the pregnant women. The majority of the pregnant patients' symptoms was bilateral, commenced in the third trimester, and resolved after pregnancy. A significant correlation existed between hand symptoms and the presence of pre-eclampsia, tight rings, body weight at confinement, birth weight, and a history of premenstrual bloating. "There was no association with age, the medical history . . . the contraceptive history, parity, antenatal complications other than pre-eclamspia, weight gain, breast-feeding or gestational diabetes." Because of the similar incidence in hand symptoms between the pregnant cohort and the control group, the authors determined that ". . . hand symptoms in pregnancy may be due to an aggravation of a relatively mild pre-existing condition by one or more mechanisms." None of the symptomatic patients required surgical intervention, but the long term follow-up was not clear.

Ekman-Ordeberg et al[3] were the first group to conduct a prospective study on CTS in pregnancy, although it was nonrandomized and uncontrolled. In their study of 2,358 pregnant women, 56 (2.4%) had experienced CTS. Paresthesias and nocturnal pain were the most common subjective complaints. Of these patients, 82% became asymptomatic following wrist splinting. Three women required surgical decompression because of failed conservative management. Several women received suboptimal relief with medical management but were not offered surgery because the estimated time to parturition was short. The authors also noted that symptoms were bilateral in most of their patients and all had generalized edema.

Stevens et al[27] performed the largest retrospective analysis of comorbid conditions and risk factors for patients who had the diagnosis of CTS between 1961 and 1980 in Rochester, Minnesota. Of the 1,016 men and women studied, 57% had a comorbid condition identified. The most frequently associated conditions were trauma, rheumatoid arthritis, hormonal agents or oophorectomy, diabetes mellitus, and, in men, repetitive hand movements. Pregnancy was seen in only 47 of the patients analyzed. They calculated the standardized morbidity ratio for women 15 to 44 years old to be 2.5, which meant that "... CTS occurs 2.5 times more often among pregnant women than among nonpregnant women...." Unfortunately, the authors' analyses did not mention the overall incidence of CTS in pregnancy.

Hypothetical Etiologies

The factors that produce CTS in pregnancy are not known and can only be surmised. Some hypothetical causes include relaxin, water retention, and musculoskeletal changes.

Relaxin is a two-chained protein hormone secreted by the corpus luteum of pregnancy and possibly by the uterine decidua during pregnancy. Unlike progesterone, relaxin is secreted throughout the entire pregnancy; however, its role is not defined and it is not essential to the maintenance of human pregnancy. In animal experiments relaxin has been shown to affect uterine relaxation during pregnancy, softening and effacement of the uterine cervix, changes in symphysis mobility, and remodeling of connective tissues. Relaxin may induce alterations in the transverse carpal ligament so that the carpal tunnel is narrowed enough to cause CTS by compressing the median nerve in some pregnant women.[24]

Increased water retention is thought to be mediated by a resetting of osmotic thresholds for thirst and vasopressin secretion. The minimum amount of extra water retained during an average pregnancy is 6.5 liters. One hypothesis attributes the onset of CTS to the accumulation of this extracellular fluid within the structures of the carpal tunnel, causing a narrowing of its diameter with subsequent median nerve compression. Atrial natriuretic peptide rapidly increases in concentration during the first few postpartum days. This results in a natriuresis, probably due to shifts of fluid from the extravascular space into the vascular compartment. Pregnant women with CTS often obtain relief soon after delivery, perhaps because of this aggressive physiological natriuresis.

Several authors believe that the administration of exogenous estrogens offers symptomatic relief to some women with CTS. Estrogens have been shown to indirectly stimulate the expansion of blood volume that accompanies normal pregnancy by stimulating the hepatic synthesis of angiotensinogen.[21] It is possible that the exogenous administration of pharmacological doses of estrogens triggers a negative feedback pathway which inhibits the normal volume expansion. The resulting relative decrease in volume may be enough to relieve the compression of the median nerve in a tight carpal tunnel and thereby offer symptomatic relief.

Postural changes during late pregnancy include marked lordosis with anterior flexion of the neck and slumping of the shoulder girdle. These musculoskeletal alterations may cause aching, numbness, and weakness of the upper extremities because of traction on the brachial plexus and the ulnar and median nerves.[24]

Conclusion

CTS in pregnancy is now appreciated as a well-known clinical entity, although its cause is still unknown. The overall incidence is disputed and ranges from 2.3% to 35%.[3,5,15-17,30] In most pregnant patients who develop CTS, the symptoms are present in both hands and are first noted during the third trimester.

Controversial interventions include diuretics and estrogen therapy. The successful use of exogenous estrogens to relieve CTS symptomatology in pregnant women is disputed. Layton,[9] for example, believed that his patients gained significant relief from the use of estrogen medications; however, Soferman et al[26] were not convinced that this form of therapy offered significant benefit.

Similarly, the role of water retention in the development of CTS during pregnancy has not been delineated clearly. The proponents of this etiology for CTS have not established a correlation between total weight gain and the onset of CTS; however, they do suggest a relationship between the pre-eclamptic state, the rate of ring removal, and the onset of CTS.[15,30] Yet, the therapeutic benefit of diuretic administration remains unproven.

The overwhelming majority of patients obtain spontaneous relief in the immediate postpartum period. Recognized conservative treatments include physical therapy, wrist splints, a low-salt diet, nonsteroidal anti-inflammatory agents, and hydrocortisone injections. Surgery is rarely indicated as a therapeutic intervention, but can be considered when other forms of conservative treatment have failed.

References

1. Brain WR, Wright AD, Wilkinson M: Spontaneous compression of both median nerves in the carpal tunnel. Six cases treated surgically. **Lancet 1:**277-282, 1947
2. Casey ML, Macdonald PC, Simpson ER: Endocrinological changes of pregnancy, in Wilson JD, Foster DW (eds): **Williams Textbook of Endocrinology, 7th ed.** Philadelphia, PA: WB Saunders, 1985, pp 422-437
3. Ekman-Ordeberg G, Sälgeback S, Ordeberg G: Carpal tunnel syndrome in pregnancy. A prospective study. **Acta Obstet Gynecol Scand 66:**233-235, 1987
4. Godfrey CM: Carpal tunnel syndrome in pregnancy. **Can Med Assoc J 129:**928, 1983 (Letter)
5. Gould JS, Wissinger HA: Carpal tunnel syndrome in pregnancy. **South Med J 71:**144-145, 1978
6. Greenberg MS: **Neurosurgery.** Lakeland, FL: Greenberg Graphics, 1994, pp 413-419
7. Guly PJ: Carpal tunnel syndrome. **Br Med J 1:**1184, 1959 (Letter)
8. Hudson AR: Carpal tunnel syndrome in pregnancy. **Can Med Assoc J 128:**1348-1349, 1983 (Letter)
9. Layton KB: Acroparaesthesia in pregnancy and the carpal tunnel syndrome. **J Obstet Gynecol 65:**823-825, 1958
10. Leach RE, Odom JA Jr: Systemic causes of carpal tunnel syndrome. **Postgrad Med 44(2):**127-131, 1968
11. Learmonth JR: The principle of decompression in the treatment of certain diseases of peripheral nerves. **Surg Clin North Am 13:**905-913, 1933
12. Marie P, Foix C: Atrophie isolee de l'erninence thenar d'origine nevritique. Role du ligament annulaire anterieur du carpe dans la pathogenie de la lesion. **Rev Neurol 26:**647-649, 1913
13. Massey EW: Carpal tunnel syndrome in pregnancy. **Obstet Gynecol Surv 33:**145-148, 1978
14. McCallum MJ: Acroparaesthesia in pregnancy. **Br Med J 2:**1095, 1959 (Letter)
15. McLennan HG, Oats JN, Walstab JE: Survey of hand symptoms in pregnancy. **Med J Aust 147:**542-544, 1987
16. Melvin JL, Burnett CN, Johnson EW: Median nerve conduction in pregnancy. **Arch Phys Med Rehabil 50:**75-80, 1969
17. Nicholas GG, Noone RB, Graham WP: Carpal tunnel syndrome in pregnancy. **Hand 3:**80-83, 1971
18. Noronha A: Neurologic disorders during pregnancy and the puerperium. **Clin Perinatol 12:**695-713, 1985
19. Nygaard IE, Saltzman CL, Whitehouse MB, et al: Hand problems in pregnancy. **Am Fam Physician 39(6):**123-126, 1989
20. Pilar S: Carpal tunnel syndrome in pregnancy. **Can Med Assoc J 129:**536, 1983 (Letter)
21. Putnam JJ: A series of cases of paresthesiae–mainly of the hands–of periodic occurrence and possibly of vasomotor origin. **Arch Med 4:**147-151, 1880
22. Rengachary SS: Entrapment neuropathies, in Rengachary SS, Wilkins RH (eds): **Principles of Neurosurgery.** London: Wolfe Publishing, 1994, pp 23.1-23.12
23. Rengachary SS: Entrapment neuropathies, in Wilkins RH, Rengachary SS (eds): **Neurosurgery.** St Louis, MO: McGraw-Hill, 1985, pp 1771-1777
24. Scott JR, Disaia PJ, Hammond CB, et al: **Danforth's Obstetrics and Gynecology, 19th ed.** Philadelphia, PA: JB Lippincott, 1994
25. Snell NJC, Coysh HL, Snell BJ: Carpal tunnel syndrome presenting in the puerperium. **Practitioner 224:**191-193, 1980
26. Soferman N, Weissman SL, Haimov M: Acroparesthesias in pregnancy. **Am J Obstet Gynecol 89:** 528-531, 1964
27. Stevens JC, Beard CM, O'Fallon WM, et al: Conditions associated with carpal tunnel syndrome. **Mayo Clin Proc 67:**541-548, 1992
28. Tindall SC: Chronic injuries of peripheral nerves by entrapment, in Youmans JR (ed): **Neurological Surgery.** Philadelphia, PA: WB Saunders, 1990, pp 2519-2525
29. Tobin SM: Carpal tunnel syndrome in pregnancy. **Am J Obstet Gynecol 97:**493-498, 1967
30. Voitk AJ, Mueller JC, Farlinger DE, et al: Carpal tunnel syndrome in pregnancy. **Can Med Assoc J 128:**277-281, 1983
31. Wallace JT, Cook AW: Carpal tunnel syndrome in pregnancy. A report of two cases. **Am J Obstet Gynecol 73:**1333-1336, 1957
32. Wood EC: Acroparaesthesia in pregnancy. **Br Med J 2:**1254, 1959 (Letter)

CHAPTER 8

PITUITARY TUMORS AND SHEEHAN'S SYNDROME IN PREGNANT WOMEN

NELSON M. OYESIKU, MD, PHD

PITUITARY DISORDERS AND PREGNANCY

The pituitary gland undergoes complex changes during pregnancy. These physiological transitions make women harboring pituitary tumors more vulnerable to complications. For instance, the pituitary gland enlarges significantly during pregnancy (primarily from the proliferation of prolactin-secreting cells). After parturition the lactotrophs involute, returning the gland to its pregestational state. Similarly, pituitary tumors may expand significantly during pregnancy, resulting in symptoms of mass effect (e.g., headaches and visual defects) or hormone deficiencies. These symptoms are more likely during the second half of pregnancy when the pituitary gland is largest. In addition to pituitary tumors, two other pituitary lesions, Sheehan's syndrome (pituitary necrosis in association with massive postpartum hemorrhage) and lymphocytic hypophysitis, occur predominantly in pregnant women. Either condition may result in life-threatening hypopituitarism, requiring urgent treatment. In addition to these anterior lobe lesions, pregnancy may also worsen the predominant disorder of the posterior lobe, diabetes insipidus.

PHYSIOLOGICAL CHANGES IN THE PITUITARY GLAND DURING PREGNANCY

Adenohypophysis

During pregnancy the volume of the pituitary gland increases by 70% to 100%.[18,19,25,50] This is accompanied by a progressive increase in serum prolactin,[48] with an approximately 10-fold increase by the end of gestation which prepares the breasts for lactation.[47] Despite this dramatic increase, the lactotroph maintains a physiological response to thyrotropin-releasing hormone (TRH), its releasing hormone, unlike the situation in patients with prolactinomas in whom this response is blunted or absent.

Other physiological changes during pregnancy that are of endocrinological importance[29] include: 1) lower gonadotropin concentrations and a diminished response to gonadotropin-releasing hormone (GnRH); 2) attenuated growth hormone response to insulin and arginine; and 3) elevated adrenocorticotropic hormone (ACTH) concentrations, despite a rise in plasma cortisol. The diurnal variation of cortisol is altered but preserved in pregnancy. Thyrotropin, free thyroxine, and tri-iodothyronine concentrations are virtually unchanged during pregnancy; however, total serum thyroxine and tri-iodothyronine concentrations increase due to doubling of thyroxine-binding globulin levels.

Neurohypophysis

Vasopressin regulates plasma osmolarity and blood volume, and is released in response to elevated plasma osmolarity. Early in pregnancy, plasma osmolarity decreases by 5 to 10 mOsm/kg below the mean of 285 mOsm/kg in nonpregnant women.[15] However, plasma levels of vasopressin and the response of vasopressin to water loading and dehydration are normal, indicating a resetting of the threshold (i.e., vasopressin is secreted at a lower plasma osmolarity). Similarly, the plasma osmolarity at which thirst is experienced is lowered during pregnancy.[14] The other posterior lobe hormone, oxytocin, is involved in the process of parturition (although its precise role in initiating labor is unclear) and in suckling. Suckling initiates a neurogenic reflex which is transmitted to the hypothalamus, resulting in oxytocin release from the neurohypophysis. Oxytocin in turn induces milk ejection.[36]

Pituitary Tumors

Adenomas may be functional (75%) or nonfunctional (25%). Of the functional adenomas, prolactinomas account for about to 60% to 70%, and growth hormone, adrenocorticotropic, and thyrotropic hormone adenomas constitute the remainder.

Prolactinomas are the most common pituitary tumor encountered in pregnancy. Interestingly, previously unrecognized nonpituitary parasellar tumors such as craniopharyngiomas or meningiomas may become evident during pregnancy because the enlarging pituitary gland may precipitate symptoms of mass effect in the presence of other masses in the parasellar region.

Most patients with microadenomas have uncomplicated pregnancies, but a significant number of patients with untreated macroadenomas have symptomatic tumor enlargement during pregnancy.[43,52] The natural history of the effect of pregnancy on pituitary tumors has been reported on by Magyar and Marshall,[33] who studied women with previously untreated pituitary adenomas who desired pregnancy (ovulation was spontaneous in only 9%; bromocriptine was used to induce ovulation in the other 91%). In their review of case reports in the literature through 1978, they analyzed 73 women and recorded the incidence of symptoms necessitating therapy during pregnancy. Headaches were experienced by 23% of the pregnant patients, and visual disturbances were found in 25%. Headache usually manifested during the first trimester, whereas visual disturbances occurred equally throughout the pregnancy. In 61% of the 91 pregnancies, patients had no symptoms of headache or visual disturbance. In 35 patients (39 pregnancies), there was pituitary enlargement and symptoms were severe enough to warrant surgical or radiation therapy in 14 patients. An additional seven patients received surgical or radiation therapy during the puerperium because of radiological evidence of progressive tumor growth, increasing prolactin, or progressive visual loss despite medical therapy.[33]

These authors also reviewed the effects of prior pituitary surgery or radiotherapy on subsequent pregnancies. During 78 pregnancies in 73 women, they found that headache occurred in 4% and disturbance of vision in 5%. Only one patient required a subsequent operation during pregnancy for headache and visual disturbance resistant to medical therapy.[33]

Prolactinoma

Hyperprolactinemia from prolactinoma significantly influences ovarian and mammary function and usually results in amenorrhea and galactorrhea.[35] During pregnancy this situation is compounded by hyperplasia of the lactotrophs, which on its own can increase serum prolactin levels about 10-fold. Furthermore, an elevated estrogen level during pregnancy also stimulates prolactin secretion.[38] Despite physiological impediments, successful pregnancies can result from restoring normal gonadal function in these women.

The cornerstone of medical therapy for

hyperprolactinemia is bromocriptine. The primary goal of therapy is to reduce prolactin levels so that the patient achieves a normal menstrual/ovulatory cycle, allowing conception to occur. Bromocriptine is an ergot derivative with potent dopamine receptor agonist activity; however, its effects usually last only for the duration of treatment.[49]

There are numerous reports of successful therapy with bromocriptine. Crosignani et al[13] examined the effect of bromocriptine on ovarian function in 115 women with hyperprolactinemia. Of these patients, 61 had hyperprolactinemia secondary to a prolactinoma. Of the 36 women with microadenomas, 11 became pregnant and 31 ovulated or menstruated. Of 25 patients with macroadenomas, 16 had an improvement in gonadal function and five conceived.

Mornex et al[39] administered bromocriptine to 16 women with hyperprolactinemia. Ovulation was restored in 15 patients, and 13 of 14 patients who desired pregnancy conceived. In their review of the literature, Vance and Thorner[50] noted pregnancy rates varying between 37.5% and 81% in hyperprolactinemic women treated with bromocriptine.

Despite earlier fears of teratogenicity suggested by animal studies, studies have yielded no evidence to date that bromocriptine causes an increased risk of fetal anomalies or that it induces higher rates of occurrence of other obstetric complications in humans even when it is administered throughout pregnancy. Bromocriptine also does not appear to increase the risk of spontaneous abortion, multiple pregnancy, or congenital malformations.[12,25,28,38,39]

Visual Symptoms and Pregnancy

Visual deterioration may occur during pregnancy because of growth of a prolactinoma after cessation of bromocriptine or enlargement of the pituitary gland in the presence of a prolactinoma.[46] Most patients with microadenomas have uncomplicated pregnancies (in that pregnancy in the patient with a prolactin-secreting microadenoma is generally safe and visual deterioration is unusual), whereas a significant number of patients with untreated macroadenomas experience symptomatic tumor enlargement.[43,52] Albrecht and Betz[2] noted that of 352 pregnancies in patients with untreated microadenomas, eight (2.3%) developed visual disturbances, 17 (4.8%) developed headaches, and two (0.6%) had diabetes insipidus. Thus, bromocriptine could be used in a female patient with a microprolactinoma with moderate elevation of serum prolactin (e.g., <250 ng/ml) in whom pregnancy is desired. Once pregnancy is achieved, the drug can be discontinued since there is little chance that vision will be compromised as a result of tumor enlargement during pregnancy.

However, in the patient with a macroprolactinoma, enlargement of the tumor during pregnancy could jeopardize vision. Thus, the use of bromocriptine to suppress prolactin and induce pregnancy in a patient harboring a macroprolactinoma would be risky. In a review of 144 pregnant women with macroadenomas (>10 mm in size), visual disturbances developed in 22 (15.3%), headaches in 22 (15.3%), and diabetes insipidus in two (1.4%)

Based on these data, patients with macroprolactinomas planning pregnancies should be advised to have treatment before pregnancy. Surgery is the preferred treatment, especially if the tumor is associated with suprasellar extension. An alternative would be to maintain the patient on bromocriptine throughout pregnancy, given the paucity of known side effects of bromocriptine in pregnancy and its efficacy in shrinking the volume of pituitary tumors.[10,38] Glucocorticoids may also be given to expedite recovery of visual defects.[30]

Breast-Feeding

A patient with a prolactinoma may safely nurse her child. In one study of 14 women with microadenomas who breast-fed for 6 to 14 months, the serum prolactin concentration was not significantly higher than prepregnancy.[52] Another study noted that the increase in prolactin associated with suckling was absent in women with pathological hyperprolactinemia.[3] If the patient does not wish to lactate, bromocriptine is the treatment of choice, with a dose of approximately 2.5 mg three times daily usually being appropriate. Estrogens should not be used to inhibit lactation, as such treatment may result in tumor growth.[46]

Management of the Postpartum Patient

Ophthalmological and radiological evaluation and determination of serum prolactin concentrations are performed 6 to 8 weeks postpartum. Usually, the gland will involute and prolactin levels will decrease.

Acromegaly

Acromegaly is a syndrome resulting from excessive growth hormone secretion in adults. The biological effect of growth hormone is mediated through somatomedin-C; consequently, the serum concentration of somatomedin-C is a more effective measure of growth hormone secretion and biological activity.[11]

Pregnancy may influence growth hormone dynamics and, conversely, acromegaly may contribute to female endocrinological dysfunction. For instance, somatomedin-C concentrations may be spuriously elevated during pregnancy; therefore, results should be interpreted cautiously.[16] Menstrual irregularity or amenorrhea is an extremely frequent finding in acromegalic women; however, women with acromegaly may become pregnant. Pregnancy may then result in significant tumor expansion.[1]

Treatment of acromegaly before conception is preferred in patients with acromegaly desiring pregnancy. The preferred choice of treatment is surgery, although bromocriptine is sometimes effective in the treatment of acromegaly and patients can achieve pregnancy during bromocriptine therapy. Furthermore, bromocriptine can be continued during pregnancy and can be effective in limiting tumor expansion.[5,32]

Cushing's Disease

Cushing's disease is a state of hypercortisolism secondary to a hyperfunctioning pituitary tumor. As with other pituitary tumors, pregnancy may influence cortisol dynamics and, conversely, Cushing's disease may contribute to female endocrinological dysfunction.

Pregnancy is uncommon in patients with Cushing's disease because it is associated with a high incidence of menstrual disturbances and ovulation.[4] The diagnosis of Cushing's syndrome in pregnancy may be difficult because weight gain, hypertension, striae, and edema also occur in normal pregnancy. More specific signs of Cushing's syndrome, such as thinning of the skin, spontaneous bruising, and muscle weakness, should aid in establishing the diagnosis. The laboratory diagnosis of Cushing's syndrome may be confounded by physiological changes in adrenal activity during pregnancy. For instance, plasma cortisol is elevated and the usual diurnal variation is diminished during pregnancy.[7] Because urinary free cortisol is elevated during pregnancy, a prolonged low-dose dexamethasone suppression (2 mg/d for 8 days) with measurement of urinary steroids is the appropriate test for diagnosis. A failure to suppress will support the diagnosis of Cushing's syndrome. To determine if hypercortisolemia is caused by a pituitary tumor (i.e., Cushing's disease), a prolonged high-dose dexamethasone suppression test is recommended (2 mg/d for 8 days). Significant (≥50%) suppression of plasma cortisol is indicative of Cushing's disease.

Cushing's syndrome may precipitate adverse events in pregnant women. In a review of 35 pregnancies in 31 women with Cushing's syndrome, there were five abortions (one therapeutic), one neonatal birth, three stillbirths, and 26 successful births.[21] Preterm labor was also common. Neonatal adrenal insufficiency in association with Cushing's syndrome has been reported[31] and may be the result of fetal hypothalamic-pituitary-adrenal axis suppression from transplacental transport of excess maternal cortisol. Therefore, the baby should be monitored carefully for adrenal insufficiency.

In patients with Cushing's disease, therapeutic options include surgery or medication. The preferred option is surgery and complete resection of the adenoma. Mitotane is an inhibitor of 11-β-hydroxylation in the pathway of steroidogenesis and is commonly given to achieve adrenal blockade in Cushing's disease.

The drug tends to accumulate in adipose tissue, and serum levels are detectable for up to 1 year after cessation of treatment. Because of its delayed elimination kinetics and its uncertain effects on teratogenesis, it is recommended that patients not become pregnant during the first 2 years after discontinuing mitotane. Metyrapone, another inhibitor of 11-β-hydroxylation, has been given for control of Cushing's disease during gestation with a resulting normal infant, although one with deficient urinary estriol excretion.

Sheehan's Syndrome

In 1937, Sheehan described a syndrome in which postpartum hemorrhage was associated with anterior pituitary necrosis.[45] The syndrome rarely occurs with other situations of hemorrhagic shock or peripheral vascular collapse. Presumably, in pregnancy, the hyperplastic pituitary gland with its increased metabolic demand is more vulnerable to an inadequate blood supply. The incidence of Sheehan's syndrome is approximately 3.6% based on a retrospective survey of pregnant patients admitted for hemorrhagic collapse.[24] There is apparently some correlation between the severity of hemorrhage and the occurrence of Sheehan's syndrome, but it appears that a significant portion of the pituitary must be compromised before symptoms become evident.[24,41]

An established pregnancy is not evidence against the diagnosis of Sheehans's syndrome.[23] Therefore, the possibility should be entertained even in a patient with a previous history of postpartum hemorrhage. Hypopituitarism may be masked during pregnancy because symptoms such as nausea, vomiting, and fatigue are common both in hypopituitarism and in normal pregnancy.

The clinical presentation includes altered menstrual pattern in about 50% of patients, diminished or absent lactation, fatigue, altered level of consciousness, cold intolerance, hypothyroidism, and genital atrophy. The interval between the inciting event to diagnosis is typically more than 10 years. In nonpregnant patients suspected of having Sheehan's syndrome, the diagnosis of hypopituitarism and the extent of pituitary damage can be determined by evaluation of target organ function (e.g., thyroid function tests and cortisol level) as well as tests of pituitary reserve (GnRH test of gonadotropin reserve, a TRH test of thyroid-stimulating hormone (TSH) and prolactin reserve, and an insulin tolerance test to assess growth hormone and ACTH reserves). In the evaluation of pituitary function during pregnancy, it is important to remember that gonadotropin concentrations remain low in normal pregnancy. Furthermore, any attempt at induction of hypoglycemia is undesirable; instead, growth hormone concentrations can be determined after sleep or exercise. Likewise, TRH testing is usually unnecessary, since the finding of a low serum thyroxine and low-normal TSH is in keeping with secondary hypothyroidism. In the adrenal axis, low cortisol concentrations (compared with those of normal pregnant women) and failure of cortisol and ACTH to increase during times of stress are indicative of diminished ACTH reserve.

Although pregnancy in hypopituitary patients is rare, failure to establish the diagnosis and institute proper therapy if pregnancy occurs may have serious consequences for both the mother and the fetus. Pregnancies may terminate as spontaneous abortions. Prompt institution of hormone replacement therapy can result in satisfactory outcomes.[23] In a review of 25 patients with Sheehan's syndrome receiving hormone replacement therapy, the outcomes of pregnancy indicate that 87% of patients had live births and 13% had abortions; there were no stillbirths or maternal deaths in 15 pregnancies. However, when hormone replacement therapy was not provided, as in 24 pregnancies among another 11 women, the rates of adverse outcome were significantly higher. In that group, there were 58% live births, 42% abortions, one stillbirth, and three maternal deaths.[23]

Treatment of pituitary insufficiency during pregnancy is quite simple. Oral l-thyroxine (0.1-0.2 mg/d) and cortisol (20 mg a.m. and 10 mg p.m.) or prednisone (5 mg a.m. and 2.5 mg p.m.) are administered. Mineralocorticoids are not required. As in nonpregnant patients, glucocorticoid requirements may increase during episodes of intercurrent illness. During labor a good state of hydration should be maintained and parenteral glucocorticoids should be administered. The dose may be adjusted as appropriate for the patient's state, ranging from 25 to 75 mg of hydrocortisone every 6 hours. After delivery, parenteral glucocorticoids should be continued, in smaller doses, for a few days along with intravenous fluids.

Lymphocytic Hypophysitis

In 1962, Goudie and Pinkerton[22] described a 22-year-old woman who died of circulatory collapse 8 hours postappendectomy. She was 14 months postpartum following normal pregnancy and delivery, but had subsequently developed secondary amenorrhea. Her autopsy revealed lymphocytic infiltration of the pituitary and the thyroid, and the authors postulated an autoimmune mechanism to explain both. Since then, approximately 25 pathologically confirmed cases have been found, 24 of which have been in women. In most cases the disease occurred in relation to a pregnancy.[22,34] Typically, the patient presents postpartum or during pregnancy. Exacerbation of the disease postpartum, even when it initially presents in pregnancy, has also been described.[37] The diagnosis should be considered in women of reproductive age presenting with signs and symptoms of partial or complete hypopituitarism, antepartum and postpartum (especially in the absence of significant bleeding during labor). Symptoms include headache, lethargy, weight loss, hyperprolactinemia, or galactorrhea.[17] Most patients have some evidence of an autoimmune disorder.[6] This is not suprising since exacerbation of autoimmune disease processes in the postpartum period is a well-known phenomenon;[51] on the contrary, given the immunological tolerance during pregnancy, the occurrence of lymphocytic hypophysitis during pregnancy is less well explained. The condition can be serious enough to be life-threatening but is a treatable disease once recognized. If vision is not compromised, patients can be treated medically with hormone replacement and followed clinically and radiologically by magnetic resonance imaging.

Disorders of the Posterior Lobe

Vasopressin and oxytocin are produced in the supraoptic and paraventricular nuclei of the hypothalamus and are released into the posterior lobe and then into the circulation. No disease process has yet been described with oxytocin deficiency or excess. However, lack of vasopressin results in diabetes insipidus, and this is usually a secondary manifestation of sellar or suprasellar tumors.[40] The main symptoms of diabetes insipidus are polyuria, polydipsia, and low urinary specific gravity. The diagnosis is made by water deprivation, demonstrating increasing serum osmolality in the face of a low urine osmolality and a return toward normal after vasopressin therapy.

With regard to pregnancy, the prior existence of diabetes insipidus in a woman does not appear to alter fertility, the course of an established pregnancy, the effectiveness of labor, or lactation.[26] Although oxytocin is produced in the same hypothalamic nuclei as vasopressin, it is surprising that labor is normal in most patients with diabetes insipidus.[20]

During pregnancy, patients with diabetes insipidus may experience worsening (58%), improvement (20%), or no change (15%) in their disease severity.[27] Placental destruction of vasopressin and its failure may be possible explanations for the worsening of diabetes insipidus and its improvement with preeclampsia.[9]

Diabetes insipidus can be effectively treated with L-deamino-8-D-arginine vasopressin (DDAVP, desmopressin acetate), a synthetic analog of vasopressin, which is administered intranasally. Dosages range from 10 to 25 mg given once or twice daily. Because of lack of information, DDAVP has not been recommended in pregnancy, but the drug has been used successfully in a few pregnant women.[42,44] Available evidence indicates that in patients on the usual dosage regimen, breast milk concentrations showed little change, suggesting that nursing mothers may breast-feed without jeopardizing the infant.[8]

References

1. Abelove WA, Rupp JJ, Paschkis KE: Acromegaly and pregnancy. **J Clin Endocrinol Metab 14:**32-44, 1954
2. Albrecht BH, Betz G: Prolactin-secreting pituitary tumors and pregnancy. **Contemp Issues Endocrinol Metab 2:**195-218, 1986
3. Andersen AN, Tabor A, Hertz JB, et al: Abnormal prolactin levels and pituitary-gonadal axis in the puerperium. **Obstet Gynecol** 57:725-729, 1981
4. Anderson K, Walters W: Cushing's syndrome and pregnancy. **Aust NZ J Obstet Gynaecol 16:**225-230, 1976
5. Bigazzi M, Ronga R, Lancranian I, et al: A pregnancy in an acromegalic woman during bromocriptine treatment: effects of growth hormone and prolactin in the maternal, fetal, and amniotic compartments. **J Clin Endocrinol Metab 48:**9-12, 1979
6. Bottazo GF, Doniach D: Pituitary autoimmunity: a review. **J R Soc Med 71:**433-436, 1978
7. Burrow GN: Pituitary and adrenal disorders, in Burrow GN, Ferris TF (eds): **Medical Complications During Pregnancy, 3rd ed.** Philadelphia, PA: WB Saunders, 1988, pp 254-270
8. Burrow GN, Wassenaar W, Robertson GL, et al: DDAVP treatment of diabetes insipidus during pregnancy and the post-partum period. **Acta Endocrinol 97:**23-25, 1981
9. Campbell JW: Diabetes insipidus and complicated pregnancy. **JAMA 243:**1744-1745, 1980
10. Chiodini P, Liuzzi A, Cozzi R, et al: Size reduction of macroprolactinomas by bromocriptine or lisuride treatment. **J Clin Endocrinol** 53:737-743, 1981
11. Clemmons DR, Van Wyk JJ, Ridgway EC, et al: Evaluation of acromegaly by radioimmunoassay of somatomedin-C. **N Engl J Med 301:**1138-1142, 1979
12. Corenblum B: Successful outcome of ergocryptine-induced pregnancies in twenty-one women with prolactin-secreting pituitary adenomas. **Fertil Steril 32:**183-186, 1979
13. Crosignani PG, Ferrari C, Luizzi A, et al: Treatment of hyperprolactinemic states with different drugs: a study with bromocriptine, metergoline, and lisuride. **Fertil Steril 37:**61-67, 1982
14. Davison JM, Gilmore EA, Dürr J, et al: Altered osmotic thresholds for vasopressin secretion and thirst in human pregnancy. **Am J Physiol 246:** F105-F109, 1983
15. Davison JM, Vallotton MB, Lindheimer MD: Plasma osmolality and urinary concentration and dilution during and after pregancy: evidence that lateral recumbency inhibits maximal urinary concentrating ability. **Br J Obstet Gynaecol 88:**472-479, 1981
16. Furlanetto RW, Underwood LE, Van Wyk JJ, et al: Serum immunoreactive somatomedin-C is elevated late in pregnancy. **J Clin Endocrinol Metab 47:** 695-698, 1978
17. Gal R, Schwartz A, Gukovsky-Oren S, et al: Lymphoid hypophysitis associated with sudden maternal death: report of a case and review of the literature. **Obstet Gynecol Surg 41:**619-621, 1986
18. Goluboff LG, Ezrin C: Effect of pregnancy on the somatotroph and the prolactin cell of the human adenohypophysis. **J Clin Endocrinol 29:**1533-1538, 1969
19. Gonzalez GJ, Elizondo G, Saldivar D, et al: Pituitary gland growth during normal pregnancy: an *in vivo* study using magnetic resonance imaging. **Am J Med 85:**217-220, 1988
20. Gordon G, Bradford W: Pregnancy in a patient with diabetes insipidus following induction of ovulation with clomiphene. **J Obstet Gynaecol 77:**467-469, 1970
21. Gormley MJJ, Hadden DR, Kennedy TL, et al: Cushing's syndrome in pregnancy—treatment with metyrapone. **Clin Endocrinol 16:**283-293, 1982
22. Goudie RB, Pinkerton PH: Anterior hypophysitis and Hashimoto's disease in a young woman. **J Pathol Bacteriol 83:**584-586, 1962
23. Grimes HG, Brooks MH: Pregnancy in Sheehan's syndrome. Report of a case and review. **Obstet Gynecol Surv 35:**481-488, 1980
24. Hall MRP: The incidence of anterior pituitary deficiency following post-partum haemorrhage: cases reviewed from the Oxfordshire and Buckinghamshire area. **Proc R Soc Med 55:**468-470, 1962
25. Hammond CB, Haney AF, Land MR, et al: The outcome of pregnancy in patients with treated and untreated prolactin-secreting pituitary tumors. **Am J Obstet Gynecol 147:**148-155, 1983
26. Hendricks CH: The neurohypophysis in pregnancy. **Obstet Gynecol Surv 9:**323-341, 1954
27. Hime MC, Richardson JA: Diabetes insipidus and pregnancy. Case report, incidence and review of literature. **Obstet Gynecol Surv 33:**375-379, 1978
28. Imura H, Kato Y, Oseko F, et al: Pharmacological treatment of hyperprolactinemia, in Linfoot JA (ed): **Recent Advances in the Diagnosis and Treatment of Pituitary Tumors.** New York, NY: Raven Press, 1979, pp 355-363
29. Itskovitz J, Rosenwaks Z: Pituitary disease in pregnancy, in Brody SA, Ueland K (eds): **Endocrine Disorders in Pregnancy.** Norwalk, CT: Appleton & Lange, 1989, pp 123-150
30. Jewelewicz R, Zimmerman EA, Carmel PW, et al: Conservative management of a pituitary tumor during pregnancy following induction of ovulation with gonadotropins. **Fertil Steril 28:**35-40, 1977
31. Kreines K, DeVaux WD: Neonatal adrenal insufficiency associated with maternal Cushing's syndrome. **Pediatrics 47:**516-519, 1971
32. Luboshitzky R, Dickstein G, Barzilai D, et al: Bromocriptine-induced pregnancy in an acromegalic patient. **JAMA 244:**584-586, 1980
33. Magyar DM, Marshall JR: Pituitary tumors and pregnancy. **Am J Obstet Gynecol 132:**739-751, 1978
34. McGrail KM, Beyerl BD, Black PM, et al: Lymphocytic adenohypophysitis of pregnancy with complete recovery. **Neurosurgery 20:**791-793, 1987
35. McNeilly A: Prolactin and ovarian function, in Müller MR, MacLeod RM (ed): **Neuroendocrine Perspectives.** New York, NY: Elsevier, 1984, Vol 3, pp 279-316
36. McNeilly AS, Robinson ICA, Houston MJ, et al: Release of oxytocin and prolactin in response to suckling. **Br Med J 286:**257-259, 1983
37. Meichner RH, Riggio S, Manz HJ, et al: Lymphocytic adenohypophysitis causing pituitary mass. **Neurology 37:**158-161, 1987
38. Molitch ME: Pregnancy and the hyperprolactinemic woman. **N Engl J Med 312:**1364-1370, 1985

39. Mornex R, Orgiazzi J, Hughes B, et al: Normal pregnancies after treatment of hyperprolactinemia with bromoergocryptine, despite suspected pituitary tumors. **J Clin Endocrinol Metab 47**:290-295, 1978
40. Moses AM, Notman DD: Diabetes insipidus and syndrome of inappropriate antidiuretic hormone secretion (SIADH). **Adv Intern Med 27**:73-100, 1982
41. Moszkowski EF: Postpartum pituitary insufficiency. Report of five unusual cases with long-term follow-up. **South Med J 66**:878-882, 1973
42. Oravec D, Lichardus B: Management of diabetes insipidus in pregnancy. **Br Med J 4**:114-115, 1972 (Letter)
43. Ruiz-Velasco V, Tolis G: Pregnancy in hyperprolactinemic women. **Fertil Steril 41**:793-805, 1984
44. Sack J, Friedman E, Katznelson D, et al: Long-term treatment of diabetes insipidus with a synthetic analog of vasopressin during pregnancy. **Isr J Med Sci 16**: 406-407, 1980
45. Sheehan HL: Post-partum necrosis of the anterior pituitary. **J Pathol Bacteriol 45**:189-214, 1937
46. Shewchuk AB, Adamson GD, Lessard P, et al: The effect of pregnancy on suspected pituitary adenomas after conservative management of ovulation defects associated with galactorrhea. **Am J Obstet Gynecol 136**:659-666, 1980
47. Tyson JE, Friesen HG, Anderson MS, et al: Human lactational and ovarian response to endogenous prolactin release. **Science 177**:897-900, 1972
48. Tyson JE, Hwang P, Guyda H, et al: Studies of prolactin secretion in human pregnancy. **Am J Obstet Gynecol 113**:14-20, 1972
49. Vance ML, Evans WS, Thorner MO: Diagnosis and treatment. Drugs five years later: bromocriptine. **Ann Intern Med 100**:78-91, 1984
50. Vance ML, Thorner MO: Prolactinomas. **Endocrinol Metab Clin North Am 16**:731-753, 1987
51. Walfish PG, Chan JY: Post-partum hyperthyroidism. **Clin Endocrinol Metab 14**:417-447, 1985
52. Zárate A, Canales ES, Alger M, et al: The effect of pregnancy and lactation on pituitary prolactin-secreting tumours. **Acta Endocrinol 92**:407-412, 1979

CHAPTER 9

SPONTANEOUS SUBARACHNOID HEMORRHAGE IN PREGNANCY AND THE PUERPERIUM

PAUL D. SAWIN, MD

EPIDEMIOLOGY

Spontaneous intracranial subarachnoid hemorrhage (SAH) is an uncommon but catastrophic event which may complicate pregnancy and the puerperium. Estimates of the true incidence of SAH during pregnancy vary considerably, presumably due to differing obstetrical referral patterns and the relatively low incidence of intracranial hemorrhage in this age group in general, but range from 0.01% to 0.05% of all pregnancies.[15,18,19,25,29,60] Despite the infrequency of occurrence, however, the attendant maternal and fetal morbidity and mortality are significant. Maternal mortality from SAH has been reported in as many as 83% of cases,[64] although most published series have noted mortality figures ranging from 30% to 50%.[3,6,17,20,25] SAH has been implicated as the third leading cause of nonobstetric maternal mortality and the eighth most common cause of maternal death overall.[5] Of all maternal deaths during gestation, between 5% and 12% may be attributed to SAH.[4,5,25] Fetal mortality is also significant, occurring in 7% to 42% of pregnancies complicated by maternal SAH.[2,5,17,25,65,78]

Since Lazard reported the first verified case of SAH during pregnancy in 1899,[54] the role of pregnancy as a risk factor for SAH has remained a controversial topic. Some have estimated a five-fold increase in the incidence of intracranial hemorrhage in pregnant women when compared to age- and gender-matched nonpregnant cohorts.[95] Others have asserted that this risk may have been overestimated, as most published series to date have been based upon referred populations of pregnant women.[89] In Rochester, Minnesota, no cases of intracranial hemorrhage were reported in association with 26,099 live births spanning a 25-year period, suggesting that SAH during pregnancy may be much less common than previously surmised.[90] Unfortunately, similar studies of other well-defined populations such as this are not available to corroborate these findings, specifically in communities whose demographic characteristics are closer to the national norm.

While the true incidence remains poorly defined, SAH during pregnancy and the puerperium presents a diagnostic and therapeutic dilemma to the neurosurgeon when it occurs. Appropriate management strategies are founded upon a knowledge of the underlying pathophysiological mechanisms of intracranial hemorrhage, the influence of pregnancy on the initial and subsequent hemorrhages, the appropriate timing of surgical intervention, and the effect of diagnostic and therapeutic interventions on the developing fetus. Certainly, a multidisciplinary approach is advisable to maximize both maternal and fetal outcome.

Presentation

The clinical presentation of SAH in the pregnant patient is little different from that in the general population. Headache is the most common presenting complaint, usually of abrupt onset and severe in nature. In up to 50%, a history of "sentinel headaches" may be elicited, often occurring days to weeks prior to the definitive event.[88] Loss of consciousness at the time of the initial ictus is common but is usually short-lived, although prolonged coma is not unusual. Signs of meningeal irritation are often present, consisting of nuchal rigidity, fever, and photophobia. Occasionally, the meningitic component may be manifested by low-back pain and radicular lower extremity pain, due to irritation of the cauda equina by dependent subarachnoid blood.[30,89] Nausea and vomiting are also encountered frequently. Focal neurological dysfunction due to direct neural compression by the vascular lesion itself, concomitant intraparenchymal hemorrhage, thrombosis, embolism, vasospasm, or vascular "steal" may be evident. Global neurological dysfunction from seizure or hydrocephalus may also be present.

The principle diagnosis from which SAH must be differentiated in this setting is eclampsia. This may prove difficult when based purely upon clinical criteria, as the clinical spectra of eclampsia and SAH overlap. As in SAH, headache, mental status changes, and seizures are common manifestations of eclampsia. Two hallmark features of eclampsia, hypertension and proteinuria, have been documented in more than 10% of pregnant patients with SAH.[20] One or both of these findings was present in 34% of cases in one composite series.[25] To further complicate diagnosis, intracranial hemorrhage may result from eclampsia without a discrete vascular lesion. While the incidence of hemorrhage in nonfatal eclampsia is unknown, up to 40% of patients with fatal eclampsia exhibit SAH or intraparenchymal hemorrhage.[25,82] In this setting, bleeding is generally intraparenchymal, forming either multiple subcortical petechial hemorrhages or a single large hematoma, although isolated SAH has been observed.[19,25]

Other diagnostic considerations include intracranial arterial occlusion, venous sinus or cortical vein thrombosis, and pituitary apoplexy, all of which have been reported to occur with increased incidence during pregnancy.[7,25] In addition, demyelinating disease, meningitis, encephalitis, intra-axial lesions such as tumors or abscesses, or migraine may all present with headache and varying degrees of neurological dysfunction, and must be differentiated from SAH in this setting.

Evaluation

Definitive diagnosis of SAH often rests upon diagnostic procedures. As SAH is a potentially lethal condition for both mother and fetus, standard diagnostic procedures should not be delayed or omitted for fear of harming the fetus. However, appropriate uterine shielding should be provided to protect the fetus during radiological procedures. If SAH is suspected, cranial computed tomography (CT) should be performed at once to reveal the presence of subarachnoid blood. In addition, CT may identify concomitant intraparenchymal hemorrhage or hydrocephalus and will occasionally demonstrate the presence of a vascular lesion. This procedure will be diagnostic for SAH in over 90% of cases, obviating the need for lumbar puncture.[30] However, if CT is negative or inconclusive and suspicion of SAH remains high based upon clinical grounds, lumbar puncture should be performed to confirm the presence of subarachnoid blood or cerebrospinal fluid (CSF) xanthochromia.

Once the diagnosis of SAH has been established, four-vessel cerebral angiography should be performed expeditiously to demonstrate the presence of a causative lesion, usually an intracranial aneurysm, arteriovenous malformation (AVM), or other vascular anomaly.[25,89] Angiographic evaluation is not complete until both the carotid and vertebrobasilar systems have been imaged, as multiple structural lesions may be identified in 5% to 20% of cases.[2,65,78] Historically, angiography was often withheld from gravid patients with SAH, due to concerns of fetal compromise resulting from the procedure. However, with appropriate shielding of the uterus, radiation exposure to the fetus is minimal. Adequate maternal hydration during the procedure is mandatory to prevent fetal dehydration. Otherwise, the risk of fetal damage from administration of iodinated contrast agents is negligible, as these materials are physiologically inert.[25] This subject is also discussed in Chapter 2.

The positive yield of angiography in gravid patients with spontaneous SAH is excellent, surpassing that of the general population. Negative investigations may be obtained in up to 20% of patients with SAH in the general population; however, less than 10% of SAH associated with pregnancy will be angiographically negative.[30,74,77,78] If initial angiography fails to demonstrate the source of hemorrhage, consideration should be given to repeat angiography in a delayed fashion or to magnetic resonance imaging. The latter may demonstrate angiographically occult intracranial vascular malformations or vascular anomalies located within the spinal cord.

Physiological Changes of Pregnancy

Several cardiovascular and hemodynamic changes that accompany pregnancy and parturition may confer an increased risk of spontaneous intracranial hemorrhage. Cardiac output increases by approximately 60% during the first two trimesters of gestation, remaining relatively constant thereafter.[58,63,70] Blood volume and central venous pressure increase throughout pregnancy until term, at which time blood volume exceeds that in the nongravid state by 25% to 40%.[63,70] Due to a reduction in systemic vascular resistance, mean arterial pressure often remains constant or even decreases throughout gestation. Despite this, however, some form of hypertension occurs in 25% to 36% of all pregnancies, associated in most cases with pre-eclampsia/eclampsia.[11] Hypertension has been implicated as a causative factor in nearly 20% of patients with SAH during pregnancy.[2,6,60]

At the time of parturition, cardiac output rises by an additional 20% during uterine contractions.[48,63,70] Mean arterial pressure and central blood volume also increase significantly during each contraction.[2,48] The Valsalva maneuver induces a further increase in mean arterial pressure, in conjunction with a more transient rise in CSF pressure. This produces an acute increase in arterial transmural pressure at the end of the maneuver, potentially predisposing anomalous vasculature to hemorrhage.[2,41,78]

Hormonal changes during pregnancy may also be implicated in the pathogenesis of SAH. An increase in circulating estrogens may produce vasodilatation of anomalous vasculature, leading to increased blood flow through these lesions, enhancing their risk of hemorrhage.[56,87] Serum levels of progesterone, human chorionic gonadotropin, and relaxin are also elevated during gestation, and may influence the behavior of vascular lesions.[2,20,25] The physiology of pregnancy is also discussed in Chapter 4.

Etiology

Cranial trauma is the most common cause of SAH in all demographic groups, including gravid females. Hemorrhage from intracranial saccular aneurysms or AVMs accounts for the vast majority of nontraumatic (spontaneous) SAH. During pregnancy and the puerperium, 75% to 93% of spontaneous SAH results from the rupture of these lesions.[2,78] In most published series, aneurysms and AVMs are responsible for SAH in roughly equal proportion.[2,78,86] Others have noted a preponderance of aneurysms as the causative lesion, with an incidence approximately three-fold greater than that of AVM.[25] These reports indicate that AVMs account for a much higher percentage of SAH in gravid patients when compared to nonpregnant women of childbearing age. In the latter, only 5% to 10% of SAH episodes are produced by AVM rupture.[79]

The remaining cases of spontaneous SAH during pregnancy result from eclampsia,[19,25,82] disseminated intravascular coagulopathy,[5,37] sickle-cell anemia,[5] anticoagulation therapy,[38] cocaine abuse,[36] metastatic choriocarcinoma,[9,32] moyamoya disease,[28,66] and spinal vascular anomalies.[84] Other cerebrovascular lesions, including mycotic aneurysms, cavernous and venous angiomas, and dural AVMs, may also

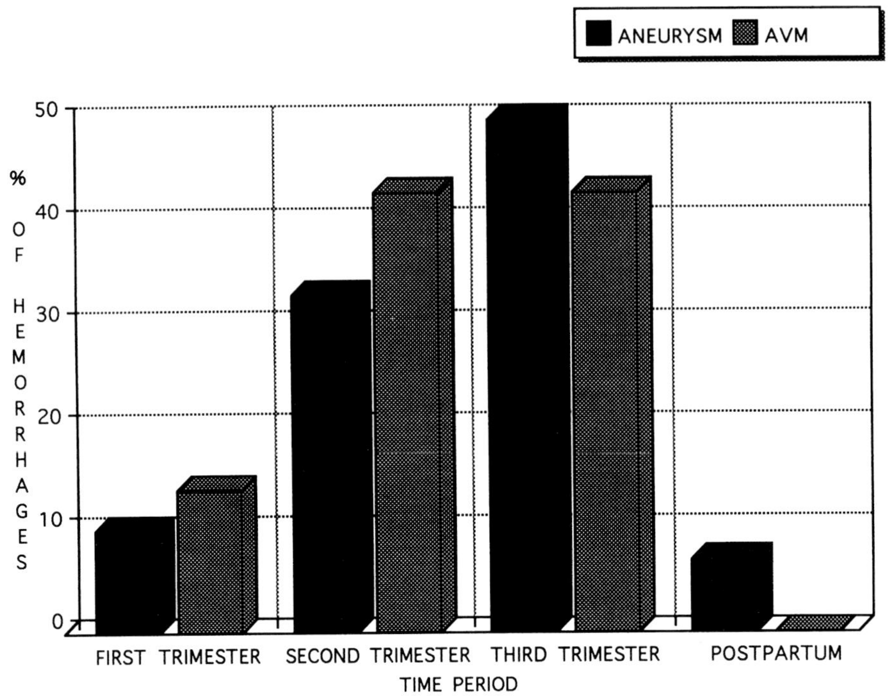

Figure 1: Distribution of SAH by gestational age. (Data derived from Dias and Sekhar[25] and Robinson et al.[78])

present with SAH, although the relationship of these lesions to pregnancy has not been studied.

Intracranial Aneurysms

Incidence and Distribution

Intracranial saccular aneurysms are found in approximately 5% of the general population at autopsy.[91] The incidence of aneurysmal SAH increases progressively with patient age, placing women of childbearing age in a relatively low-risk category. However, pregnancy appears to confer an increased risk of aneurysmal rupture on this population, up to five times that of age-matched nonpregnant women.[89] The overall incidence of aneurysmal SAH has been estimated at 0.01% to 0.03% of all pregnancies.[4,15,20,29,64] As in the general population, this incidence increases with advancing maternal age.[78,89]

The incidence of hemorrhage from an intracranial aneurysm also rises as gestation progresses (Figure 1). Fewer than 10% of initial aneurysmal ruptures are manifest within the first trimester of pregnancy. In the second trimester, the incidence increases to approximately 30%. The period of greatest risk is the third trimester, when more than 50% of all aneurysmal hemorrhages present.[41,78]

The puerperium also appears to be a period of significant risk for initial aneurysmal rupture. Approximately 5% of aneurysmal SAH occurs in the early postpartum period, generally within 6 weeks of delivery.[25,78] Despite the significant hemodynamic shifts which occur during labor and delivery, initial aneurysmal rupture is quite rare during this time.[51,89] However, rehemorrhage from a previously ruptured lesion is relatively common during parturition.[2,78,89]

Approximately 50% of women who present with aneurysmal SAH during pregnancy have had previous uncomplicated pregnancies.[89] In contrast to women with AVMs, patients with intracranial aneurysms are often multiparous, and are six times more likely to have had a prior pregnancy with a normal gestational course.[77,78,89]

The anatomical distribution of saccular aneurysms encountered during pregnancy is similar to that found in the general population. Most are located at the bifurcation of vessels constituting the circle of Willis, with 85% to 90% occurring in the anterior circulation and the remaining 10% to 15% arising posteriorly.[2,25,77,80] In 5% to 20% of cases, multiple aneurysms are identified.[2,25,65,78]

Treatment

Following aneurysmal SAH, therapeutic strategies should be focused upon minimizing maternal and fetal morbidity by reducing or eliminating the adverse sequelae of aneurysmal rupture, principally rehemorrhage and vasospasm. Rehemorrhage occurs in 33% to 50% of cases, and is associated with a maternal mortality rate of up to 70%.[15,20,25,74] In the general population, the risk of rehemorrhage from an unsecured aneurysm is greatest during the first 24 hours following SAH, as 4% will rebleed during this period.[94] Thereafter, the incidence decreases to approximately 1.5% per day, over the ensuing 13-day period. Nearly 20% of all patients with unsecured lesions will have rehemorrhaged at 2 weeks following initial rupture.[94] Whether these observations apply to the gravid patient with aneurysmal SAH is unknown.

Vasospasm is a focal or diffuse narrowing of intracranial vessels, presumably incited by blood or vasoactive by-products of hemolysis within the subarachnoid space. Arterial narrowing from vasospasm may diminish regional cerebral blood flow, producing local ischemia and neurological deficit. Symptomatic vasospasm is encountered in >30% of the general population following aneurysmal SAH, although the incidence in gravid patients is unknown. Delayed ischemic deficits from vasospasm typically occur between 5 and 12 days after SAH, although they may manifest as early as 48 hours or as late as 2 weeks after the initial hemorrhage. Neurological dysfunction may be reversible with appropriate therapy, consisting of induced arterial hypertension and intravascular volume expansion.[46] Hemodilution has also been employed with some success.

Some have postulated that the hemodynamic alterations which occur during pregnancy may be protective against the ischemic neurological dysfunction arising from vasospasm, although this concept remains purely conjecture.[30] The gravid patient is typically "hemodiluted" by the physiological anemia of pregnancy, induced by a more substantial increase in plasma volume relative to erythrocyte mass.[63,70] In addition, the intravascular volume of the pregnant patient is expanded from an increase in total blood volume, with a concomitant rise in central venous pressure.[70] The influence of these physiological changes of pregnancy on vasospasm is uncertain, as the incidence of delayed ischemic deficits following SAH has not been defined in the gravid population.

Appropriate therapy for gravid patients with aneurysmal SAH may be divided into three realms: medical, neurosurgical, and obstetric. While concern for fetal well-being is an essential element of management, it must not be allowed to compromise maternal treatment. In general, the optimal treatment for the fetus is that which maximizes maternal outcome.

Medical Management

The basic principles of medical therapy for patients with SAH are unaltered for the gravid patient. However, fetal considerations may modify specific treatment regimens somewhat. Judicious management of hypertension is critical, although care must be taken to avoid iatrogenic hypotension and uterine hypoperfusion. Uterine blood flow varies directly with maternal blood pressure, and thus any intervention that lowers mean arterial pressure precipitously may place the fetus in some jeopardy.[25] Continuous hemodynamic monitoring with arterial and central venous pressure catheters facilitates accurate blood pressure management. Continuous fetal heart rate monitoring may also be quite useful in this setting. Tachycardia and loss of normal beat-to-beat variability are early signs of fetal distress. Fetal bradycardia results from more severe maternal hypotension and uterine hypoperfusion.[93]

Routine "SAH precautions," including maintenance of a low-stimulus environment and limited visitation, are generally advocated for the pregnant patient. The cautious use of sedatives, analgesics, antiemetics, and antitussive agents is recommended. Positional modifications during bed rest are important for the gravid patient, particularly in the third trimester of pregnancy. During this time, the gravid uterus may compress the inferior vena cava and descending aorta in the supine position, producing maternal hypotension and uterine hypoperfusion.[70] The left lateral decubitus position is most conducive to minimize this effect.[70]

Several considerations unique to pregnancy may alter the selection and administration of various medications. The physiological changes of pregnancy modify the pharmacokinetics of most drugs, due to alterations in absorption, metabolism, clearance, protein binding, and volume of distribution.[16,21,45,49,50,52,53,68,69] Therefore, pharmacological therapy should be monitored closely, guided by serum drug levels whenever possible. As pregnancy is a dynamic state, serum levels must be reassessed frequently and appropriate adjustments in dosage made, in order to optimize the desired therapeutic effect while minimizing toxicity. A comprehensive overview of drug therapy in pregnancy is presented in Chapter 1.

Anticonvulsants. The potential teratogenic influence of various anticonvulsant medications has been well described. Fetal anomalies have been reported in association with virtually every anticonvulsant, including phenytoin, carbamazepine, phenobarbital, valproate, primidone, trimethadione, ethosuximide, and various benzodiazepines.[1,31,33,43,44,97] Malformations occur in 4% to 5% of the offspring of epileptics, a rate nearly twice that of the general population.[1,10,43] While this is ostensibly a multifactorial effect, anticonvulsant agents must be implicated, at least in part. Although there is a potential risk of teratogenicity, the risk of seizure (with concomitant maternal and fetal hypoxia and acidosis) justifies the use of anticonvulsants in a gravid patient with SAH.[1,25,67,79]

While many believe that the overall teratogenic potential of any one anticonvulsant is not substantially different from any other,[1,25,67] some have suggested that carbamazepine may have the most favorable teratogenicity profile, and thus should be used preferentially in this setting.[81] Although no increase in "major" fetal malformations has been noted with carbamazepine, an increase in "minor" anomalies was reported.[44] In addition, the potential for drug-induced agranulocytosis or aplastic anemia, coupled with the relative difficulty in administration of this agent to the obtunded or comatose patient (carbamazepine is supplied only in an oral form),[72] minimizes the potential advantage that carbamazepine may have over other agents, in the context of acute SAH.

The deleterious fetal effects associated with diphenylhydantoin (phenytoin) have been well characterized. The fetal hydantoin syndrome, consisting of intrauterine growth retardation, microcephaly, mental retardation, and limb defects, occurs in a minority of children born to epileptic mothers treated with phenytoin.[33] A similar syndrome has been described in association with phenobarbital and primidone.[43] Barbiturates are prone to produce fetal sedation and may precipitate fetal withdrawal symptoms when administered during the third trimester.[24,67] Maternal use of valproic acid has been associated with a 1% to 2% incidence of fetal neural tube defects, as well as craniofacial and cardiac anomalies.[43,71] Valproate also attains high levels in fetal serum following a single maternal dosing and may accumulate with repeated administration, potentially enhancing fetal toxicity.[69]

Calcium Channel Antagonists. Nimodipine is used prophylactically to ameliorate the sequelae of vasospasm associated with aneurysmal SAH. While this agent has been implicated as a teratogen in some experimental animals, its effect upon human fetuses is unknown.[25] Most advocate the use of calcium channel antagonists in gravid patients with SAH, as the potential maternal benefits are believed to justify the theoretical fetal risk.[25,27,89] Maternal hemodynamics should be monitored closely to minimize iatrogenic hypotension and uteroplacental hypoperfusion, which may result from administration of this agent.

Antifibrinolytic Agents. Epsilon-aminocaproic acid, tranexamic acid, and various other antifibrinolytic agents have been used to reduce the incidence of rehemorrhage following aneurysmal SAH, by inhibiting lysis of the clot within the aneurysmal sac. While patients receiving such therapy do enjoy a significantly lower rebleeding rate, this is accompanied by an increased incidence of ischemic deficits, vasospasm, and hydrocephalus in the general population, with no net difference in mortality.[47] Experience with the use of antifibrinolytic agents during pregnancy is limited, and studies of teratogenicity have not been performed.[73] However, the hypercoagulable state induced by pregnancy may enhance the risk of thrombotic side effects associated with the use of these agents.[89]

Diuretics. The use of osmotic diuretics such as mannitol in the gravid patient with SAH is controversial. Experimental studies in rabbits with massive doses of mannitol (≈12 g/kg body weight) demonstrated high-volume shifts of free water from fetus to mother, resulting in profound fetal dehydration.[13] Furthermore, aggressive diuresis resulted in maternal hypotension, uterine hypoperfusion, and fetal ischemia in these animals.[13] This has led to the prevailing assertion that osmotic diuretics may adversely affect the human fetus, and thus should be avoided during pregnancy.[25,34,78,89] However, more conservative doses of mannitol (≈1-2 g/kg) have been used in gravid human patients without adverse fetal sequelae.[93]

Intravascular Volume Expansion and Vasopressors. Ischemic neurological deficits from vasospasm may be reversed in nearly 75% of patients by intravascular volume expansion and induced arterial hypertension.[46] Hypervolemia is generally accomplished by the intravenous infusion of crystalloid and/or colloid fluids. Analogs of vasopressin (antidiuretic hormone) may be administered as an adjunct to fluid infusion to prevent diuresis. Arterial hypertension may be induced by a variety of vasopressor agents. These agents may diminish uteroplacental blood flow, and thus must be used with caution. A central venous or pulmonary artery catheter can simplify fluid management considerably, and should be utilized to monitor hypervolemic therapy. An arterial pressure catheter is also useful in this setting. While volume expansion and induced hypertension have become standard treatment regimens for symptomatic vasospasm in the general population, no data exist to support or refute this therapy in the gravid patient with SAH.

Corticosteroids. The efficacy of exogenous corticosteroids in the treatment of SAH in humans remains unproven. While these agents have been used extensively during pregnancy for a variety of indications without obvious adverse effects,[8] chronic use during the third trimester may result in adrenal suppression in the fetus and neonate.[25]

Surgical Management

Maternal and fetal mortality from aneurysmal SAH is significant, irrespective of therapy. Overall, maternal mortality is reported in 30% to 50% of cases.[3,6,17,20,25] With rehemorrhage, however, the maternal death rate increases significantly, up to nearly 70% in some series.[15,20,25,74] The most effective method to eliminate the risk of rehemorrhage is surgical clip ligation of the offending aneurysm, excluding it from the intracranial circulation. Other methods of operative treatment, such as internal carotid artery ligation, aneurysmal wrapping, coating, or trapping, are inferior to clip ligation in the prevention of rehemorrhage, and thus should be performed only if clipping of the aneurysmal neck is not feasible. Endovascular techniques, including balloon embolization and electrothrombosis with detachable platinum coils, have been employed as an alternative to craniotomy and aneurysmal clip ligation for the treatment of intracranial aneurysms. While the experience with these techniques is increasing, endovascular therapy remains less effective than direct surgical clipping in affording protection from rehemorrhage. The role of endovascular treatment in the gravid patient with aneurysmal SAH has yet to be defined.

Once surgical clipping has been accomplished, complete obliteration of the aneurysm must be confirmed. This may be done by direct observation, intraoperative Doppler ultrasonography, needle aspiration, or angiography. Angiography is the most definitive method currently available to ensure that the aneurysm has been eliminated.

Prompt surgical intervention may also facilitate the prevention and treatment of vasospasm. At the time of surgery, the subarachnoid

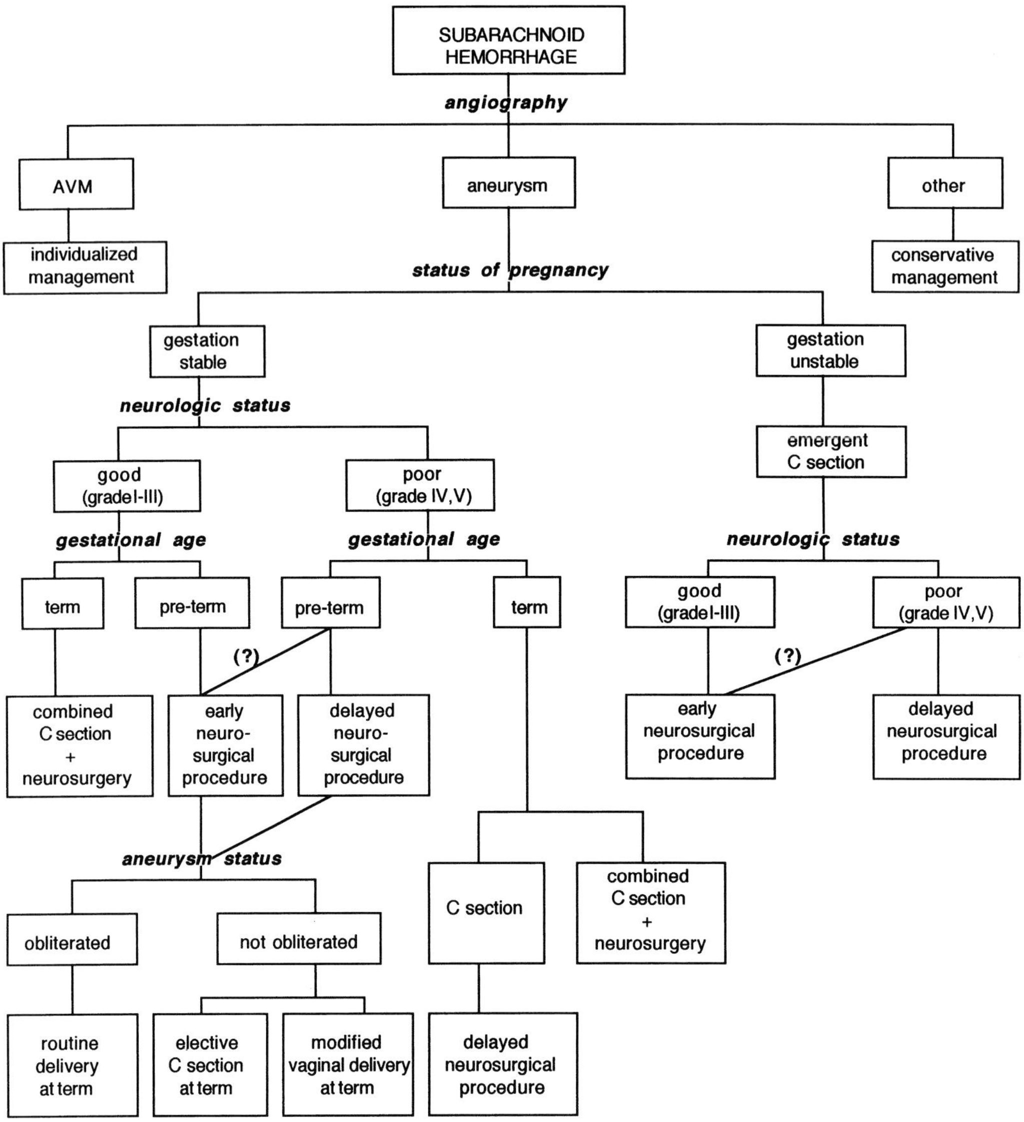

Figure 2: Treatment strategies for management of SAH during pregnancy.

clot can be partially evacuated and cisternal lavage performed, removing potentially vasoactive substances from the subarachnoid space. Once the lesion is secured, aggressive intravascular volume expansion and induced arterial hypertension are permitted, without the risk of aneurysmal rehemorrhage.

Early reports of operative intervention in gravid patients with aneurysmal SAH were fraught with high maternal and fetal mortality rates, prompting recommendations to defer surgery until after delivery, despite the high incidence of rehemorrhage.[23,75,85] With advances in operative and anesthetic techniques, however, the surgical risk has been reduced. Currently, the surgical management of intracranial aneurysms in pregnant patients is universally advocated, according to neurosurgical criteria.[2,15,17,18,20,22,25,29,30,65,78,89]

An algorithm delineating the strategy for management of the gravid patient with SAH is presented in Figure 2. In general, the timing of operative intervention is based upon neurosurgical, rather than obstetric, considerations.[2,25,41,]

[65,78,82,89] If the patient is not in active labor and there is no evidence of fetal distress, operative intervention may proceed as if the individual were not pregnant. Those with fair to excellent neurological function (i.e., grades I, II, and III, according to the classification scheme of Hunt and Hess) should undergo surgical obliteration of their aneurysms immediately. Gravid patients with unfavorable neurological conditions following SAH (i.e., Hunt and Hess grades IV and V) pose a slightly greater therapeutic dilemma. A delay in surgical intervention may facilitate the technical aspects of the procedure, by permitting dissolution of the subarachnoid clot and resolution of cerebral edema. However, the risk of rehemorrhage from the unsecured lesion during the delay is high.[94] This has encouraged some to proceed with early operative intervention in all patients, even those with poor neurological function.[26] This approach may be even more attractive in the gravid patient, if only to enhance the probability of fetal survival. In the face of neurological devastation, even maternal brain death, the pregnancy may be brought successfully to term.[35]

The only scenarios in which obstetric concerns should take precedence over neurosurgical management are active labor (which is occasionally precipitated by the hemorrhage), eclampsia, or fetal distress. In these situations, delivery should be accomplished expeditiously by cesarean section, followed immediately, or as soon as possible, by neurosurgical intervention.[27,55]

Obstetric Management

Once appropriate neurosurgical therapy has been implemented, the remainder of the gestation may proceed to term. If the aneurysm has been successfully obliterated by clip ligation at the aneurysmal neck, labor and delivery may progress normally. If, however, the offending lesion has not been surgically addressed, or has been incompletely treated with internal carotid artery sacrifice, wrapping, coating, or trapping, some modification of parturition is advisable to reduce the hemodynamic fluctuations associated with labor. Some have advocated elective cesarean section at term to avoid hemodynamic stress.[17,89] However, cesarean section appears to offer no significant advantage over a vaginal delivery with epidural anesthesia, a modified second stage of labor, and low forceps assistance.[2,15,25,29,41,63,78,83,86,96] Indeed, maternal and fetal mortality rates for vaginal and cesarean delivery are not significantly different in patients with an untreated cerebrovascular lesion following SAH.[25] With appropriate modifications, vaginal delivery can be accomplished in most instances. Cesarean section may be reserved for those situations in which obstetric concerns mandate its use.

The use of oxytocic agents in a patient with an untreated intracranial vascular lesion is controversial. Excessive administration of these agents has been associated with systemic hypertension, and should be avoided. However, judicious use appears to be well-tolerated in this context.[51,65,86]

Outcome

Maternal and fetal mortality following aneurysmal SAH is a function of neurological grade. However, independent of grade, the outcome of both mother and fetus is significantly improved by surgical intervention during pregnancy.[25] According to a composite analysis of aneurysmal SAH by Dias and Sekhar,[25] surgical management reduced maternal mortality markedly, from 63% in those managed conservatively to 11% in those treated by operative means. Fetal mortality is also reduced significantly with antepartum surgical treatment. In this series, only 5% of fetuses whose mothers were treated surgically failed to survive. Fetal mortality was 27% in cases managed nonoperatively.

Arteriovenous Malformations

Incidence and Distribution

Intracranial AVMs account for only 5% of SAH in the general population, yet they are responsible for 21% to 48% of hemorrhages

TABLE 1

GENERAL CHARACTERISTICS OF SAH FROM ANEURYSMS AND AVMS DURING PREGNANCY AND THE PUERPERIUM

Characteristic	AVM	Aneurysm
Maternal age	18 to 25 years	25 to 35 years (incidence increases with age)
Parity	Primiparous	Multiparous
Prior gestations	Complicated	Uncomplicated
Lesion location	Hemispheric (parietal most common)	Anterior circle of Willis (~85%)
Timing of hemorrhage	Second and third trimesters, labor	Third trimester, puerperium
Rehemorrhage	25% in same gestation	33% to 50%
Maternal mortality	8% to 28%	13% to 35%
Fetal mortality	9% to 18%	7% to 25%
Optimal antepartum management	?	Surgical clip ligation

during pregnancy and the puerperium.[2,25,29,77,78] This apparent predilection for rupture during pregnancy is controversial, and may be artifactual. Some have reported an 87% incidence of AVM rupture associated with pregnancy.[77] Others have disputed this strong correlation, citing a 3.5% risk of hemorrhage from AVM during gestation in patients referred for proton beam therapy, an incidence which is not significantly different from that of the general population.[40] Both study groups were based upon specialized referral populations, inviting selection bias. The true incidence of hemorrhage from AVM during pregnancy probably lies somewhere between these two estimates.

While cerebral AVM may present with seizure, headache, ischemia, bruit, or mass effect, the initial manifestation in the gravid patient is typically SAH.[79,89] Hemorrhage from AVM is more evenly distributed throughout gestation than that encountered with intracranial aneurysms (Figure 1). Most investigators have noted a predilection for angiomatous hemorrhage to arise in the second trimester of pregnancy, with the peak incidence occurring between 16 and 20 weeks' gestation.[77,78,89] This approximates the time of gestation during which cardiac output is increasing most rapidly.[48,70,89] Others contend that the rate of angiomatous hemorrhage increases with advancing gestational age, similar to that noted with saccular aneurysms.[25]

Parturition has been reported to be a high-risk period for angiomatous hemorrhage, during which time 11% of AVM ruptures occur.[60] The hemodynamic stress associated with labor and delivery has been implicated as a causative factor. This varies from the pattern of aneurysmal hemorrhage, which rarely presents initially during labor.

The incidence of rehemorrhage from an AVM is higher in gravid patients than in the general population. Following initial angiomatous hemorrhage, only 3% to 6% of nonpregnant individuals will rebleed within the first 12 months.[12,92] Approximately 25% of gravid patients will rehemorrhage during the same pregnancy.[77,79]

Comparative features of SAH from aneurysms and AVMs are presented in Table 1. Typically, women with angiomatous SAH are younger (18 to 25 years of age) than those with aneurysmal hemorrhage, in whom the incidence of rupture increases with age.[25,78,89] Hemorrhage from AVM is encountered with greater frequency in primaparous women. If an individual with angiomatous hemorrhage is multiparous, a history of previous complicated pregnancy is often obtained.[77,78,89]

The anatomical distribution of vascular malformations in pregnant patients is similar to that noted in the general population.[25] The vast majority are located within the cerebral hemispheres, often encompassing segments of more than one lobe. The parietal region is the most frequent site of involvement. This region contains at least a portion of the anomaly in 37.5% to 47% of cases.[2,25,79] Bihemispheric lesions are encountered rarely.[2,79]

Treatment

Medical Management

The fundamental medical management of the gravid patient with angiomatous SAH is not significantly different from that previously described for aneurysmal hemorrhage and does not merit comprehensive reiteration here. Strict control of hypertension and seizure activity is essential. Therapeutic strategies are again formulated to minimize maternal and fetal morbidity and mortality which may arise from rehemorrhage and vasospasm. In the patient who suffers an angiomatous hemorrhage during pregnancy, the incidence of rehemorrhage during the same gestation is approximately 25%.[25,77,79] The occurrence of vasospasm in association with angiomatous SAH is quite infrequent, although it has been reported as a devastating complication of such hemorrhage in at least one pregnant patient.[79]

Surgical Management

The role of neurosurgical intervention in the management of gravid patients with angiomatous SAH is poorly delineated. Most investigators have advocated an aggressive surgical approach to these lesions, as the incidence of rehemorrhage from an AVM during pregnancy is high and is associated with significant maternal and fetal morbidity.[78,79,89] Surgical resection of the entire anomaly affords the optimum protection against rehemorrhage. Other therapeutic modalities, including endovascular embolization and radiosurgery, do not tend to confer immediate and complete protection from rebleeding, and may actually increase the probability of hemorrhage initially. Experience with these alternative therapies in gravid patients with angiomatous SAH is minimal.

Despite the efficacy of surgical resection in reducing the incidence of rehemorrhage, a recent outcome-based metanalysis failed to demonstrate a clear benefit from antepartum excision of AVM, when defined by maternal and fetal survival as endpoints.[25] While a trend toward improved outcome of both mother and fetus was exhibited in the surgically managed group, this did not reach statistical significance. As this analysis was hampered somewhat by a small sample size, further data are required in order to define the appropriate use of surgical resection for the treatment of AVM during pregnancy. At present, the decision to proceed with surgical intervention must be individualized. As with aneurysmal SAH, this decision should be based predominantly upon neurosurgical, rather than obstetric, considerations.[2,25,78,89]

Obstetric Management

Following appropriate neurosurgical intervention, the gestation may proceed to term. Fetal well-being should be appraised frequently with serial or continuous fetal monitoring, depending upon the clinical condition of both patients. Fetal ultrasonography may also be employed to assess fetal morphology and estimate gestational age. As outlined previously, obstetric considerations should take precedence in the event of active labor, eclampsia, or fetal distress. In these instances, immediate delivery by cesarean section is recommended, followed by neurosurgical treatment.

If the AVM has been completely excised prior to parturition, labor and delivery may proceed in a routine fashion. In the event of a surgically inaccessible or subtotally resected lesion, delivery may be accomplished either by cesarean section at term, or by a modified vaginal approach, in order to minimize hemodynamic stress.[25,29,51,78,86,89]

Outcome

Irrespective of therapy, maternal and fetal mortality rates from angiomatous intracranial hemorrhage are significant.[2,25,40,78,79] Overall, maternal mortality is reported in approximately 28% of cases, with fetal death occurring in 14% of cases.[25] Antepartum operative intervention may prove to enhance both maternal and fetal survival, although at present, the influence of surgery on outcome remains unclear.

Anesthetic Considerations

Surgical anesthesia during pregnancy poses distinct hazards for mother and fetus. Anesthesia may stimulate uterine activity, precipitating premature labor. Iatrogenic maternal hypotension may result in uterine hypoperfusion and fetal hypoxia. Pharmacological agents used in the induction or maintenance of surgical anesthesia may produce teratogenic effects in the fetus.[70]

In addition to the cardiovascular and hemodynamic alterations that accompany pregnancy, changes in pulmonary function impact anesthetic management. Early in gestation, alveolar minute ventilation increases rapidly, reaching 150% to 170% of baseline by the end of the first trimester.[70] This is accomplished by a 40% increase in tidal volume, as well as a 15% increase in respiratory rate. As a result of these ventilatory changes, anesthetic induction with volatile agents is more rapid, and overall anesthetic requirements are reduced.[70] Also, this chronic hyperventilation lowers mean arterial CO_2 tension, producing a respiratory alkalosis which is accompanied by a compensatory metabolic acidosis.[70] In this setting, deliberate mechanical hyperventilation for mediation of increased intracranial pressure must be employed with caution, as this maneuver may decrease uterine blood flow, producing fetal hypoxia and acidosis.[14,57,62]

Maternal and fetal outcome may rely upon the prompt recognition of therapeutic complications. Continuous fetal heart rate monitoring is recommended during any neurosurgical procedure to detect evidence of fetal distress.[70] In the event that active labor or fetal distress is precipitated by surgery, obstetric "back-up" should be available and prepared to intercede in a timely fashion. Preoperative communication between the physicians involved in the care of both patients is essential.

Some positional modifications should be made to preserve maternal perfusion and uterine blood flow during the operative procedure. The supine position, often used for craniotomy, may produce maternal and fetal hypotension secondary to compression of the inferior vena cava and aorta by the gravid uterus. Over 90% of pregnant women at term have complete obstruction of the inferior vena cava when lying supine.[69] This concern may be eliminated by placing the patient in a lateral decubitus position for the procedure.

Induced Hypotension

Induced hypotension is occasionally desirable for neurovascular procedures, both to minimize the risk of intraoperative rupture, and, if rupture occurs, to reduce hemorrhage into the operative field. The use of induced hypotension in the gravid patient with an intracranial vascular lesion is controversial. As a rule, any intervention which lowers maternal blood pressure may lower uterine blood flow, and should be employed with extreme caution. However, with appropriate fetal monitoring, induced hypotension has been used safely in this setting.[30,65,93]

The choice of agents used to induce hypotension in the gravid patient is also a matter of considerable debate. Sodium nitroprusside may provide a small degree of uterine blood flow protection in the face of systemic maternal hypotension,[93] and has been used for this application without incident on several occasions.[39,76,93] However, cyanide levels may accumulate within the fetus, leading to fetal cyanide toxicity.[61,93] Volatile agents, such as halothane and isoflurane, are capable of decreasing maternal mean arterial pressure up to 25%, while maintaining uteroplacental blood flow.[93] Beta-adrenergic antagonists may induce uterine irritability, fetal bradycardia, hypotension, and hypoglycemia, although judicious use of labetalol and metoprolol appears to be well-tolerated.[93] Hydralazine is transferred across the placenta in significant amounts and may accumulate in the fetus, although it has been used in obstetric procedures without apparent adverse sequelae.[93] Trimetaphan camsylate has been utilized successfully to induce hypotension in gravid patients with cerebrovascular lesions, and has minimal placental transfer due to its high molecular weight.[65,93]

Hypothermia

The cerebral protection afforded by hypothermia is often desirable when manipulating complex cerebrovascular lesions. This technique has been used frequently in gravid patients, and appears to be well-tolerated by both mother and fetus.[34,39,59,78]

Unruptured Aneurysms and Arteriovenous Malformations

Unruptured intracranial aneurysms may be discovered incidentally through cranial imaging for evaluation of trauma or atypical headaches, or may manifest symptoms related to embolic episodes or direct neural compression. Most neurological surgeons now advocate elective clip ligation of any unruptured aneurysm with a maximum diameter that exceeds 9 mm, as these lesions have a significantly higher propensity for subsequent rupture.[91] The management of smaller intracranial aneurysms is more controversial and may vary with patient age and general medical status. The discovery of an unruptured aneurysm during pregnancy is an exceedingly unusual event, and the natural history of such a lesion has not been studied. Consequently, no standard therapeutic recommendations regarding antepartum surgery for an unruptured aneurysm can be made.

Unruptured AVMs may present with seizures, headaches, an audible bruit, ischemic deficits from vascular steal phenomena, or mass effect. Asymptomatic lesions may also be encountered as incidental findings on cranial imaging. Again, the discovery of such a lesion during pregnancy is extremely rare. At present, it may be difficult to justify elective excision of an unruptured AVM during pregnancy, as the benefits of antepartum surgery for a ruptured anomaly have yet to be established. Further investigation is required to determine the natural history of these lesions during pregnancy, as well as to define the role of surgical intervention in their management.

References

1. American Academy of Pediatrics Committee on Drugs: Anticonvulsants and pregnancy. **Pediatrics 63:**331-333, 1979
2. Amias AG: Cerebral vascular disease in pregnancy. I: Haemorrhage. **J Obstet Gynaecol Br Comm 77:**100-120, 1970
3. Andersen SB, Lamkee MJ, De Alvaraz RR: Subarachnoid hemorrhage and pregnancy. Report of a case. **Obstet Gynecol 18:**116-119, 1961
4. Barnes JE, Abbott KH: Cerebral complications incurred during pregnancy and the puerperium. **Am J Obstet Gynecol 82:**192-207, 1961
5. Barno A, Freeman DW: Maternal deaths due to spontaneous subarachnoid hemorrhage. **Am J Obstet Gynecol 125:**384-392, 1976
6. Barrett JM, Van Hooydonk JE, Boehm FH: Pregnancy-related rupture of arterial aneurysms. **Obstet Gynecol Surv 37:**557-566, 1982
7. Beal MF, Wechsler LR, Davis KR: Cerebral vein thrombosis and multiple intracranial hemorrhages by computed tomograpy. **Arch Neurol 39:**437-438, 1982
8. Biggs JSG, Allan JA: Medication and pregnancy. **Drugs 21:**69-75, 1981
9. Biller J, Adams HP: Cerebrovascular disorders associated with pregnancy. **Am Fam Phys 33(6):**125-132, 1986
10. Bjerkedal T, Bahna SL: The course and outcome of pregnancy in women with epilepsy. **Acta Obstet Gynecol Scand 52:**245-248, 1973
11. Brinkman CR III: Hypertensive disorders of pregnancy, in Hacker NF, Moore JG (eds): **Essentials of Obstetrics and Gynecology.** Philadelphia, PA: WB Saunders, 1986, pp 125-133
12. Brown RD Jr, Weibers DO, Forbes G, et al: The natural history of unruptured intracranial arteriovenous malformations. **J Neurosurg 68:**352-357, 1988
13. Bruns PD, Linder RO, Drose VE, et al: The placental transfer of water from fetus to mother following intravenous infusion of hypertonic mannitol to the maternal rabbit. **Am J Obstet Gynecol 86:**160-166, 1963
14. Buckley TA, Yau GHM, Poon WS, et al: Caesarean section and ablation of a cerebral arteriovenous malformation. **Anaesth Intensive Care 18:**248-251, 1990
15. Cannell DE, Botterell EH: Subarachnoid hemorrhage and pregnancy. **Am J Obstet Gynecol 72:**844-855, 1956
16. Chen S, Perucca E, Lee JN, et al: Serum protein binding and free concentration of phenytoin and phenobarbitone in pregnancy. **Br J Clin Pharmacol 13:**547-552, 1982
17. Conley JW, Rand CW: Spontaneous subarachnoid hemorrhage occurring in noneclamptic pregnancy. **Arch Neurol Psychiatry 66:**443-463, 1951

18. Copeland EL, Mabon RF: Spontaneous intracranial bleeding in pregnancy. **Obstet Gynecol 20:**373-378, 1967
19. Crawford S, Varner MW, Digre KB, et al: Cranial magnetic resonance imaging in eclampsia. **Obstet Gynecol 70:**474-477, 1987
20. Daane TA, Tandy RW Sr: Rupture of congenital intracranial aneurysms in pregnancy. **Obstet Gynecol 15:**305-314, 1960
21. Dam M, Christiansen J, Munck O, et al: Antiepileptic drugs: metabolism in pregnancy. **Clin Pharmacokinet 4:**53-62, 1979
22. Davey LM, Fiorito JA, Hehre FW: Intracranial aneurysms in late pregnancy. Report of a successful operation utilizing hypothermia. **J Neurosurg 23:** 542-546, 1965
23. De Carle DW: Pregnancy and cerebrovascular complications. **West J Surg Obstet Gynecol 57:**181-189, 1949
24. Desmond MM, Schwanecke RP, Wilson GS, et al: Maternal barbiturate utilization and neonatal withdrawal symptomatology. **J Pediatr 80:**190-197, 1972
25. Dias MS, Sekhar LN: Intracranial hemorrhage from aneurysms and arteriovenous malformations during pregnancy and the puerperium. **Neurosurgery 27:**855-866, 1990
26. Disney L, Weir B, Grace M, et al: Factors influencing the outcome of aneurysm rupture in poor grade patients: a prospective series. **Neurosurgery 23:**1-9, 1988
27. Donaldson JO: Neurologic emergencies in pregnancy. **Obstet Gynecol Clin North Am 18:**199-212, 1991
28. Enomoto H, Goto H: Moyamoya disease presenting as intracerebral hemorrhage during pregnancy: case report and review of the literature. **Neurosurgery 20:**33-35, 1987
29. Fliegner JRH, Hooper RS, Kloss M: Subarachnoid haemorrhage and pregnancy. **J Obstet Gynaecol Br Comm 76:**912-917, 1969
30. Giannona SL, Daniels J, Goide SH, et al: Ruptured intracranial aneurysms during pregnancy: a report of four cases. **J Reprod Med 31:**139-147, 1986
31. Goldman AS, Yaffe SJ: Fetal trimethadione syndrome. **Teratology 17:**103-106, 1978
32. Gurwitt LJ, Long JM, Clark RE: Cerebral metastatic choriocarcinoma. A postpartum cause of "stroke." **Obstet Gynecol 45:**583-588, 1975
33. Hanson JW, Smith DW: The fetal hydantoin syndrome. **J Pediatr 87:**285-290, 1975
34. Hehre FW: Hypothermia for operations during pregnancy. **Anesth Analg 44:**424-428, 1965
35. Heikkinen JE, Rinne Ri, Alahuhta SM, et al: Life support for 10 weeks with successful fetal outcome after fatal maternal brain damage. **Br Med J 290:** 1237-1238, 1985
36. Henderson CE, Torbey M: Rupture of intracranial aneurysm associated with cocaine use during pregnancy. **Am J Perinatol 5:**142-143, 1988
37. Heron JR, Hutchinson EC, Boyd WN, et al: Pregnancy, subarachnoid haemorrhage, and the intravascular coagulation syndrome. **J Neurol Neurosurg Psychiatry 37:**521-525, 1974
38. Hirsh J, Cade JF, Gallus AS: Anticoagulants in pregnancy: a review of indications and complications. **Am Heart J 83:**301-305, 1972
39. Holcomb WL Jr, Petrie RH: Cerebrovascular emergencies in pregnancy. **Clin Obstet Gynecol 33:** 467-471, 1990
40. Horton JC, Chambers WA, Lyons SL, et al: Pregnancy and the risk of hemorrhage from cerebral arteriovenous malformations. **Neurosurgery 27:** 867-872, 1990
41. Hunt HB, Schifrin BS, Suzuki K: Ruptured berry aneurysms and pregnancy. **Obstet Gynecol 43:** 827-837, 1973
42. Hunt WE, Hess RM: Surgical risk as related to time of intervention in the repair of intracranial aneurysms. **J Neurosurg 28:**14-20, 1968
43. Janz D: The teratogenic risk of antiepileptic drugs. **Epilepsia 16:**159-169, 1975
44. Jones KL, Lacro RV, Johnson KA, et al: Patterns of malformations in the children of women treated with carbamazepine during pregnancy. **N Engl J Med 30:**1661-1666, 1989
45. Kanto JH: Use of benzodiazepines during pregnancy, labour, and lactation, with particular reference to pharmacokinetic considerations. **Drugs 23:**354-380, 1982
46. Kassell NF, Peerless SJ, Durward QJ, et al: Treatment of ischemic deficits from vasospasm with intravascular volume expansion and induced arterial hypertension. **Neurosurgery 11:**337-342, 1982
47. Kassell NF, Torner JC, Adams HP Jr: Antifibrinolytic therapy in the acute period following aneurysmal subarachnoid hemorrhage. Preliminary observations from the Cooperative Aneurysm Study. **J Neurosurg 61:**225-230, 1984
48. Kerr MG: Cardiovascular dynamics in pregnancy and labour. **Br Med Bull 24:**19-24, 1968
49. Kochenour NK, Emery MG, Sawchuk RJ: Phenytoin metabolism in pregnancy. **Obstet Gynecol 56:** 577-582, 1980
50. Kriel RL, Cloyd J: Clonazepam and pregnancy. **Ann Neurol 11:**544, 1982
51. Laidler JA, Jackson IJ, Redfern N: The management of caesarean section in a patient with an intracranial arteriovenous malformation. **Anaesthesia 44:** 490-491, 1989
52. Lander CM, Edwards VE, Eadie MJ, et al: Plasma anticonvulsant concentrations during pregnancy. **Neurology 27:**125-131, 1977
53. Landon MJ, Kirkley M: Metabolism of diphenylhydantoin (phenytoin) during pregnancy. **Br J Obstet Gynecol 86:**125-132, 1979
54. Lazard EM: A case of cerebral hemorrhage following labor. **Philadelphia Med J 4:**1091-1092, 1899
55. Lennon RL, Sundt TM Jr, Gronert GA: Combined cesarean section and clipping of intracerebral aneurysm. **Anesthesiology 60:**240-242, 1984
56. Letterman G, Schurter M, Barter RH, et al: Hemangiomas of pregnancy. **South Med J 50:**594-599, 1957
57. Levinson G, Shnider SM, deLorimier AA, et al: Effects of maternal hyperventilation on uterine blood flow and fetal oxygenation and acid-base status. **Anesthesiology 40:**340-347, 1974
58. Mashini IS, Albazzaz SJ, Fadel HE, et al: Serial noninvasive evaluation of cardiovascular hemodynamics

during pregnancy. **Am J Obstet Gynecol 156:** 1208-1213, 1987
59. Matsuki A, Oyama T: Operation under hypothermia in a pregnant woman with an intracranial arteriovenous malformation. **Can Anaesth Soc J 19:**184-191, 1972
60. Maymon R, Fejgin M: Intracranial hemorrhage during pregnancy and puerperium. **Obstet Gynecol Surg 45:**157-159, 1990
61. McDowall DG, Keaney NP, Turner JM, et al: The toxicity of sodium nitroprusside. **Br J Anaesth 46:** 327-332, 1974
62. Meschia G: Placental respiratory gas exchange and fetal oxygenation, in Creasy RK, Resnik R (eds): **Maternal-Fetal Medicine: Principles and Practice.** Philadelphia, PA: WB Saunders, 1984, pp 274-285
63. Metcalfe J, McAnulty JH, Ueland K: Cardiovascular physiology. **Clin Obstet Gynecol 24:**693-710, 1981
64. Miller HJ, Hinckley CM: Berry aneurysms in pregnancy: a 10 year report. **South Med J 63:**279-285, 1970
65. Minielly R, Yuzpe AA, Drake CG: Subarachnoid hemorrhage secondary to ruptured cerebral aneurysm in pregnancy. **Obstet Gynecol 53:**64-70, 1978
66. Miyakawa I, Lee HC, Haruyama Y, et al: Occlusive disease of the internal carotid arteries with vascular collaterals (Moyamoya disease) in pregnancy. **Arch Gynecol 237:**175-180, 1986
67. Montouris GD, Fenichel GM, McLain LW Jr: The pregnant epileptic: a review and recommendations. **Arch Neurol 36:**601-603, 1979
68. Mygind KI, Dam M, Christiansen J: Phenytoin and phenobarbitone clearance during pregnancy. **Acta Neurol Scand 54:**160-166, 1976
69. Nau H, Rating D, Koch S, et al: Valproic acid and its metabolites: placental transfer, neonatal pharmacokinetics, transfer via mother's milk, and clinical status in neonates of epileptic mothers. **J Pharmacol Exp Ther 219:**768-777, 1981
70. Pedersen H, Finster M: Anesthetic risk in the pregnant surgical patient. **Anesthesiology 151:**439-451, 1979
71. **Physicians' Desk Reference, 48th ed.** Montvale, NJ: Medical Economics, 1994, pp 411-413
72. **Physicians' Desk Reference, 48th ed.** Montvale, NJ: Medical Economics, 1994, pp 585-587
73. **Physicians' Desk Reference, 48th ed.** Montvale, NJ: Medical Economics, 1994, pp 1063-1064
74. Pool JL: Treatment of intracranial aneurysms during pregnancy. **JAMA 192:**209-214, 1963
75. Rhoads EE: Congenital aneurysms of the circle of Willis associated with pregnancy. **Am J Obstet Gynecol 54:**533-536, 1947
76. Rigg D, McDonagh A: Use of sodium nitroprusside for deliberate hypotension during pregnancy. **Br J Anaesth 53:**985-987, 1981
77. Robinson JL, Hall CS, Sedzimir CB: Arteriovenous malformations, aneurysms, and pregnancy. **J Neurosurg 41:**63-70, 1974
78. Robinson JL, Hall CJ, Sedzimir CB: Subarachnoid hemorrhage in pregnancy. **J Neurosurg 36:**27-33, 1972
79. Sadasivan B, Malik GM, Lee C, et al: Vascular malformations and pregnancy. **Surg Neurol 33:**305-313, 1990
80. Sahs AH, Perrot GE, Locksley HB, et al: **Intracranial Aneurysms and Subarachnoid Hemorrhage: A Cooperative Study.** Philadelphia, PA: JB Lippincott, 1969
81. Saunders M: Epilepsy in women of childbearing age. If anticonvulsants cannot be avoided use carbamazepine. **Br Med J 299:**581, 1989
82. Schwartz J: Pregnancy complicated by subarachnoid hemorrhage. **Am J Obstet Gynecol 62:**539-547, 1951
83. Sencer W: The management of spontaneous intracranial hemorrhage in non-eclamptic pregnancy. **J Mt Sinai Hosp 31:**487-539, 1964
84. Shephard RH: Spinal arteriovenous malformations and subarachnoid haemorrhage. **Br J Neurosurg 6:** 5-12, 1992
85. Strohschein DF, Suzuki M: Ruptured intracranial aneurysm and pregnancy. **Grace Hosp Bull 25:**71-78, 1947
86. Tuttelman RM, Gleicher N: Central nervous system hemorrhage complicating pregnancy. **Obstet Gynecol 58:**651-656, 1981
87. Ueland K, Paver JT: Effects of estrogens of the cardiovascular system of the ewe. **Am J Obstet Gynecol 96:**400-406, 1966
88. Verweij R, Wijdicks EFM, van Gijn J: Warning headache in aneurysmal subarachnoid hemorrhage. A case-control study. **Arch Neurol 45:**1019-1020, 1988
89. Wiebers DO: Subarachnoid hemorrhage in pregnancy. **Semin Neurol 8:**226-229, 1988
90. Wiebers DO, Whisnant JP: The incidence of stroke among pregnant women in Rochester, Minn, 1955 through 1979. **JAMA 254:**3055-3057, 1985
91. Wiebers DO, Whisnant JP, Sundt TM Jr, et al: The significance of unruptured intracranial saccular aneurysms. **J Neurosurg 66:**23-29, 1987
92. Wilkins RH: Natural history of intracranial vascular maltormations: a review. **Neurosurgery 16:**421-430, 1985
93. Willoughby JS: Sodium nitroprusside, pregnancy and multiple intracranial aneurysms. **Anaesth Intensive Care 12:**351-357, 1984
94. Winn HR, Richardson AE, Jane JA: The long-term prognosis in untreated cerebral aneurysms, I. The incidence of late hemorrhage in cerebral aneurysm: a 10-year evaluation of 364 patients. **Ann Neurol 1:** 358-370, 1977
95. Wong MC, Giuliani MJ, Haley E Jr: Cerebrovascular disease and stroke in women. **Cardiology 77(Suppl 2):**80-90, 1990
96. Young DC, Leveno KJ, Whalley PJ: Induced delivery prior to surgery for ruptured cerebral aneurysm. **Obstet Gynecol 61:**749-752, 1983
97. Zackai EH, Mellman WJ, Neiderer B, et al: The fetal trimethadione syndrome. **J Pediatr 87:**280-284, 1975

CHAPTER 10

VENOUS THROMBOTIC DISORDERS IN PREGNANCY

MARK G. HAMILTON, MDCM, FRCS(C), WENDY ZIAI, MD,
RUSSELL D. HULL, MB,BS, MSc, FCCP, GRAHAM F. PINEO, MD, FRCP(C), AND
KAREN A. VALENTINE, MD, PHD, FRCP(C)

Venous thrombotic disease, both extracranial and intracranial, is an important cause of obstetric morbidity and mortality.[11,16,49,59,65,72,83,90,91,267,287,288,313] Extracranial thromboembolic disease, which includes deep vein thrombosis (DVT) and pulmonary embolism (PE), is the leading cause of death after a live birth in the United States[11] and is an important source of morbidity and mortality in patients with neurological disease.[132,133] Pregnancy increases the risk of venous thrombosis five-fold.[11] Many neurosurgical disorders also significantly increase the risk of venous thrombosis.[133] A variety of neurological disorders, including brain tumors,[132] spinal cord injury, head injury, and stroke (embolic ischemic stroke, subarachnoid hemorrhage, intracerebral hemorrhage), substantially increase the risk of extracranial thrombotic disease.[133] Thromboembolic disease, therefore, represents a significant management issue when treating neurological disorders that occur during pregnancy or during the puerperium (first 6 weeks after delivery). Those caring for these patients must, therefore, recognize the risk factors for the development of DVT and PE to be able to effectively and quickly make a diagnosis and initiate treatment, frequently within the confines of caring for both mother and fetus. To adequately manage patients with DVT and PE, the physician requires a thorough understanding of the pharmacokinetics of heparin and warfarin and knowledge of their role in the treatment strategies for which there is proven efficacy and safety during pregnancy. More importantly, an awareness of the risk associated with the development of thromboembolic disease during pregnancy in patients with neurological disorders enhances the ability to initiate adequate prophylactic measures.[57,115,132,133,251] There are prophylactic strategies which can be applied to dramatically reduce the incidence of thromboembolism and these should be applied on a routine basis. The standard prophylactic methods for thromboembolic prophylaxis include mechanical devices (e.g., graduated leg stockings, and intermittent external pneumatic calf compression) and pharmacological agents (e.g., low-dose heparin). In addition, a knowledge base concerning low-molecular weight heparins and heparinoids is essential because these new agents have a promising role in both the prophylaxis and treatment of pregnant patients with neurological disease. The principles concerning the prophylaxis and management of venous thromboembolic disease in pregnant patients with neurosurgical disorders are dealt with in this review. In addition, intracranial thrombotic disease (intracranial venous thrombosis), with an estimated incidence ranging from one in 2,500 to one in 10,000 deliveries,[288] can be a significant problem during pregnancy. The authors have, therefore, briefly reviewed current epidemiological, clinical, diagnostic, and therapeutic information to allow for management of cerebral venous thrombosis during pregnancy and the puerperium.

Extracranial Thrombotic Disorders

Pregnancy poses a significant risk for thromboembolism. When a pregnant patient experiences a neurosurgical condition such as a brain tumor, spinal cord injury, stroke, or subarachnoid hemorrhage, the associated thromboembolic risk potential is enhanced. Those caring for pregnant patients must therefore be capable of recognizing the risk factors for the development of venous thrombosis, be able to effectively and quickly make a diagnosis and initiate proper treatment, and in particular be aware of the special considerations associated with the management of DVT and PE. In addition, awareness of the risk factors for the development of thromboembolic disease in this patient population allows for the initiation of adequate prophylactic measures.[57,115,133,251] In this section we review current epidemiological, clinical, diagnostic, and therapeutic information to allow state-of-the-art prophylaxis and treatment of thromboembolic disease in pregnant patients with neurosurgical disorders.

Epidemiology

Overview

A number of epidemiological reports have identified specific patient risk factors for DVT: older age, obesity, varicose veins, immobility, pregnancy, puerperium, estrogen therapy, previous DVT or PE, deficiency of antithrombin III or protein C or protein S, trauma, surgery, malignancy, heart failure, and infection.[11,32,46,69,123,181,186,209,212,237,243,254,278,313] The risk factors for a patient with neurological disease generally fall into one of these categories.[132,133,277]

Many reports have documented the scope of the problem created by DVT and PE.[23,69,115] Dalen and Alpert[78] estimated the incidence of PE in the United States to range as high as 630,000 cases per year, resulting in 200,000 (32%) deaths. Coon[69] estimated the incidence of clinically recognized DVT in the United States at over 250,000 cases per year; the actual total incidence of DVT is estimated to be three- to five-fold greater than the incidence of PE: 1.8 million to 3.2 million cases per year. With DVT comes a substantial risk both for PE and for the postphlebitic syndrome.[80,203] The postphlebitic syndrome occurs as a result of venous hypertension produced in the lower extremities by incompetence of the venous valves. It produces significant morbidity, including venous ulceration of the lower extremities. The prevalence of the postphlebitic syndrome has been estimated at between 1% and 2% of the general population: potentially over 5 million patients in the United States. In addition, approximately 500,000 Americans have or have had venous ulceration.[80]

To best appreciate the epidemiological data concerning DVT and PE, it is important to determine how these data were collected. A clinical study that utilized a diagnostic test for DVT or PE that has high sensitivity and high predictive value should not be compared with a study that utilized low-sensitivity tests because of the potential differences in DVT or PE incidence. It is therefore necessary to understand the different methods by which DVT and PE can be diagnosed.

Clinical Diagnosis of DVT and PE

The clinical diagnosis of DVT is at best extremely unreliable. When the physician is faced with the so-called classic clinical features such as a swollen, tender, hot calf with venous dilatation or a positive Homan's sign, DVT will actually be found only 20% to 50% of the time.[70,139,223] More importantly, about 50% to 60% of patients with DVT will not have these clinical symptoms, as documented in screening studies using ^{125}I fibrinogen, impedance plethysmography, or venography, and by the substantial number of patients presenting with PE without any clinical evidence of DVT.[80,310] The clinical diagnosis of PE is also extremely nonspecific.[116,171] When presented with the so-called cardinal clinical features such as dyspnea, hemoptysis, pleuritic chest pain, pleural friction rub, fever, right heart failure, or cardiovascular collapse, the physician is faced with substantial differential diagnoses which may range from atelectasis to cardiac tamponade.[171] However, to deal with this clinical uncertainty, a host of techniques are available to either confirm or exclude the diagnosis of DVT or PE.

Levels of Evidence for Diagnosis of Venous Thromboembolism and Use of Antithrombotic Agents

To adequately judge the value of a clinical trial evaluating a particular method of prophylaxis, diagnosis, or treatment requires a set of guidelines to determine the quality of the evidence presented. The American College of Chest Physicians developed rules of evidence to allow clinical recommendations on the use of antithrombotic agents for prophylaxis (Table 1).[68,268,269] From the rules of evidence, a definition of the "level of evidence" was constructed from which a "grading of recommendation" could then be stated. Level I studies are appropriately sized randomized trials with clear-cut results which have low risk of error and are classified as Grade A. Level II studies are small randomized trials with uncertain results because of low power and are designated as Grade B. Level III studies are nonrandomized trials with contemporaneous controls. Level IV studies are nonrandomized trials with historical controls, while Level V studies are case series reports without controls. Level III, IV, and V studies warrant only a Grade C recommendation.

TABLE 1

RULES OF EVIDENCE AND CLINICAL RECOMMENDATIONS ON THE USE OF ANTITHROMBOTIC AGENTS*

Levels of Evidence	
I	Randomized trials with low false-positive (alpha) and low false-negative (beta) errors
II	Randomized trials with high false-positive (alpha) and high false-negative (beta) errors
III	Nonrandomized concurrent cohort studies
IV	Nonrandomized historical cohort studies
V	Case series
Grading of Recommendation	
A	Supported by Level I evidence
B	Supported by Level II evidence
C	Supported by Level III, IV, or V evidence

*From Cook et al.[68]

Guidelines for levels of evidence regarding methods used to diagnose DVT and PE have been established according to criteria similar to those described for the use of antithrombotic agents. These rules are modified because randomized trials are not always required to meet the criteria for Level I evidence. In fact, three different types of studies provide Level I evidence for diagnostic testing: 1) a large prospective study evaluating sensitivity, specificity, and predictive value of an experimental diagnostic test compared with a gold standard; 2) a rigorous randomized clinical trial comparing the clinical outcome of interest against the outcomes observed using a gold standard; and 3) a prospective clinical trial determining the safety of withholding therapy after negative findings of the experimental diagnostic test. These basic principles can also be equally applied to the evaluation of treatment modalities.

Laboratory Diagnosis of DVT: General Principles

When faced with the clinical symptoms that suggest DVT, there are a number of valid ways to approach making a rapid and accurate diagnosis in the pregnant patient.[108,139,173] The accepted reference gold standard for diagnosis remains contrast venography.[320] However, while venography is the most definitive method to confirm or exclude thrombosis of the lower extremities or pelvic veins, it is also moderately invasive, and other noninvasive diagnostic techniques have been developed.

Calf vein thrombi have less clinical significance than thrombi in the proximal thigh veins. There is considerable evidence to suggest that calf vein thrombi are relatively benign unless they extend into the popliteal vein or the proximal veins, which occurs about 30% to 50% of the time. While isolated calf vein thrombi result in PE in <1% of cases,[156,164,173,230] approximately 40% to 50% of thrombi in the proximal veins of the lower extremities will produce clinically important pulmonary emboli, thereby making the identification of thrombus extension extremely important. Careful serial objective testing is required to exclude propagation of calf thrombus into the proximal veins since all proximal thrombi require treatment to prevent PE.

There is a vast body of Level I evidence to support the use of serial impedance plethysmography to exclude or confirm the diagnosis of significant proximal vein thrombi.[64,157,164,173,326] This technique monitors the decreasing electrical impedance that blood produces as it leaves the calf veins through the proximal leg veins, after relaxation of a pneumatic tourniquet. With obstruction of the proximal veins by thrombus, the egress of blood from the calf is abnormal. Impedance plethysmography is not sensitive for the detection of isolated calf thrombi. However, when used in a serial fashion for about 2 weeks after an initial negative test (e.g., Days 1, 2, 5, and 10) impedance plethysmography is effective in its ability to predict which patients will require treatment: the risk of PE with negative serial evaluations is <1%. This principle holds true for impedance plethysmography even when calf thrombi are documented by ^{125}I fibrinogen.[164] One advantage is that it is relatively easy to perform and there is very little inter- or intraobserver variation.[28] False-positive results can occur with a number of disorders which interfere with venous outflow or arterial inflow: severe congestive heart failure, constrictive pericarditis, hypotension, external venous compression (e.g., late pregnancy), or severe arterial insufficiency. A false-negative result can occur in cases of nonocclusive proximal DVT and in cases of proximal DVT with well-developed collateral vessels. Immobilization of the limb by a cast or other brace or the inability to properly position the patient because of pain or other medical reasons are the only other conditions which preclude the use of impedance plethysmography. In summary, a positive result is indicative of proximal DVT; while a negative result does not exclude the diagnosis of DVT, impedance plethysmography must be repeated in a serial fashion for at least a 2-week period. This test is extremely cost-effective and can replace venography as the primary diagnostic tool in most situations.[156,162,173,230] When impedance plethysmography is not available or is contraindicated, venography remains an acceptable alternative.

Two other diagnostic methods are commonly described: Doppler ultrasound[28,71,139,173,327] and radioisotopes.[28,139,173,279,283] Doppler ultrasound, now frequently combined with real-time B-mode ultrasound imaging, utilizes the same basic principle as impedance plethysmography in that, using the Doppler principle, it seeks to detect abnormal egress of blood from the calf when thrombus is present within the deep veins of the leg. B-mode imaging has been added to allow visualization of the affected vein thrombus and to image the compressibility of the vein. There have been a number of Level I evidence studies evaluating the efficacy of Doppler with B-mode ultrasound in symptomatic patients.[138,202,327] These combined Level I studies report the sensitivity of Doppler ultrasound with B-mode imaging to be about 95% and the specificity 99%.[138,202,327] An advantage, compared with impedance plethysmography, includes the ability to perform the investigation in patients who are immobilized or who have lower-leg casts or amputations. In addition, ultrasound is more readily available in most treatment centers. Some of the conditions which limit the effectiveness of impedance plethysmography are also encountered with Doppler ultrasound. However, the major limitation concerns the actual performance of the test: data interpretation can be highly subjective and requires a high level of user skill, which is not required with impedance plethysmography. Doppler ultrasound with B-mode imaging is an acceptable alternative to either venography or impedance plethysmography if performed by a skilled and experienced technician. The principle of serial examination must also apply to patients with an initial negative Doppler/B-mode ultrasound examination.

A number of different radioisotopes can be used to assist in the diagnosis of DVT. The high sensitivity of ^{125}I fibrinogen has been well described.[28,283] The radiolabeled fibrinogen is incorporated into developing thrombus and a positive signal is recorded over these regions. This technique is overly sensitive and expensive. The sensitivity of ^{125}I fibrinogen, although impractical for daily clinical use, has been very effective for the assessment of new prophylactic or treatment strategies, and ^{125}I fibrinogen has made major contributions to our understanding of the natural history of DVT and the clinical efficacy of prophylactic and treatment strategies. However, it has been withdrawn from use because of concerns about the potential risk of human immunodeficiency virus or hepatitis contamination. The other commonly used nuclear medicine technique is a form of radioisotope venography and blood pool scanning method using ^{99}Tc-labeled red blood cells. This method identifies thrombus by the presence of changes in the pattern of venous blood flow, but only has a sensitivity of about 75% for proximal extension of calf thrombi.[285] It has not been evaluated in a fashion to satisfy Level I evidence criteria, and its routine use to exclude DVT cannot be justified. Other radioisotopes being developed and assessed include ^{111}In-labeled platelets, ^{99}Tc plasmin, and ^{111}In-labeled antifibrin monoclonal antibodies,[279] and can only be considered experimental.

Laboratory Diagnosis of PE: General Principles

The diagnosis of PE can also be difficult.[171] A significant number of patients will die within the first hour or will be critically ill because of cardiopulmonary dysfunction. Establishing a diagnosis in these patients is usually not difficult. Problems arise with the patient who has survived an initial PE and a diagnosis is essential to ensure that recurrent embolism is prevented. Arterial blood gas measurements, chest x-ray, and electrocardiography (ECG) are all insensitive and nonspecific methods. Normal arterial blood gases do not rule out PE. Chest x-ray and ECG may be useful if they demonstrate another cause for the patients' symptoms such as pneumothorax, pneumonia, or myocardial infarction.

The gold standard for diagnosis of PE has been pulmonary angiography, with or without superselective technique, looking for evidence of filling defects within the pulmonary vessels.[100,165,166,171,230] However, pulmonary angiography is invasive, with a minimum 3% to 4% risk of significant complications including tachyarrhythmias, cardiac injury or perforation, cardiac arrest, or allergic reactions to contrast media.[166,171] In addition to these important risks, about 20% of patients will be too critically ill to undergo this investigation and difficulty interpreting the angiogram may be encountered for technical reasons or if other pulmonary pathology is present. As in DVT diagnosis, less invasive alternatives have been developed for diagnosing PE.

A significant volume of Level I evidence has been obtained using ventilation-perfusion lung scanning as a method for the noninvasive diagnosis of PE.[100,165,171,185,250] A chest x-ray is required to interpret this study. The perfusion lung scan is performed with ^{99}Tc-labeled macroaggregated albumin and detects abnormalities of pulmonary blood flow associated with PE. Ventilation lung scanning is performed at the time of the perfusion scan and typically uses a gas such as ^{133}Xe- or ^{99}Tc-labeled aerosols, such as sulfur colloid or diethylene triamine penta-acetic acid. With PE one would expect a perfusion defect without an associated ventilation defect. A perfusion defect associated with a ventilation defect may represent another underlying pathology such as atelectasis or pneumonia. A normal ventilation-perfusion lung scan effectively rules out PE. When perfusion defects are present, an abnormal scan is graded as high, intermediate, or low probability for PE based on the number and degree of ventilation-perfusion segmental mismatches present. In a patient with clinically suspected embolism, the chances with high-, intermediate-, and low-probability ventilation-perfusion scanning are 88%, 33%, and 12% respectively.[250] High-probability scans therefore warrant a positive diagnosis of PE, while intermediate- and low-probability scans do not rule out the possibility and require pulmonary angiography to determine the proper diagnosis. Finally, in the presence of intermediate- or low-probability ventilation-perfusion scanning, establishing the presence of DVT with any of the accepted methods described above is sufficient (given that the anticoagulant treatment for DVT and PE is identical) and eliminates the need for pulmonary angiography.

Thromboembolic Risk During Pregnancy

PE remains the leading cause of maternal death in the United States.[11] Untreated DVT in pregnancy results in a 15% risk of PE with a 13% mortality rate. In addition to the risk of PE, the late sequelae of DVT (postphlebitic syndrome) causes significant long-term morbidity in this relatively young patient population.[208]

Pregnancy increases the risk of thromboembolic disease five- to six-fold as compared to nonpregnant, nonpuerperal women.[11,34,194,266] If pregnancy is complicated by an underlying thrombophilia, the risk of thrombosis may be increased to 15% to 30%.[66,85] However, because the absolute risk for thrombosis during pregnancy is low, very few prospective studies have been published, and the true incidence of DVT is unknown. The best estimate of the incidence of DVT and PE in pregnant women without a prior history of thromboembolism comes from a few retrospective studies based on objective diagnostic criteria for DVT or PE in symptomatic patients: 0.06% to 0.09%.[194,261,266] The risk of recurrent thrombosis in pregnant women with a history of DVT has been estimated to be as high as 4% to 12%.[13,295] Again, however, these estimates are based on retrospective reports and no prospective studies are available.

Thromboembolic complications may present at any time during pregnancy or the puerperium. While it has been suggested that PE may occur more frequently in the postpartum period, particularly in a patient undergoing a cesarean section, two recent prospective studies have indicated that the risk for DVT is evenly distributed throughout pregnancy.[106,169] Peculiar to pregnancy is the striking predilection for pregnancy-associated DVT to develop in the left leg.[106]

Factors that have been suggested to increase the risk of pregnancy-associated DVT or PE include: history of venous thrombosis or PE, age and parity, obesity, prolonged hospitalization (immobilization), operative procedures (i.e., mode of delivery cesarean section), and underlying hypercoagulable states. It becomes immediately apparent that many of these risk factors are shared with nonpregnant patients. More importantly, it is essential to recognize that thromboembolic risk factors are undoubtedly additive: pregnant patients have a potential spectrum of DVT/PE risk that increases according to the risk associated with their neurosurgical disorder.

General Neurosurgical Population

There are numerous reports available concerning patients in a neurosurgical population[133] describing a risk for PE ranging between 0% and 5%, with a mortality rate of 9% to 50%.[54,183,284,305,306,311,324,335] Puls et al[256] reported a 24.8% incidence of PE in a consecutive autopsy series of 101 patients, with PE the primary cause of death in almost one-half of these patients. The risk of developing clinically evident DVT in a general neurosurgical population was reported by Joffe to be 4.3%[183] but has been more effectively established using sensitive investigative techniques such as ^{125}I-labeled fibrinogen.[203] With this technique, the incidence ranges between 19% and 50%.

While this information regarding the general neurosurgical population is important, it would be even more useful to know the risk of DVT and PE in specific subpopulations of neurosurgery patients. This knowledge would allow certain high-risk patients to be targeted for prophylaxis. Limited details are available regarding patients with head injury[190] or subarachnoid hemorrhage[31] and patients undergoing lumbar discectomy.[257] Ramirez and Thisted[257] reported an incidence of PE in only 0.1% of 28,395 patients undergoing lumbar discectomy. Much more information is available concerning patients with brain tumor, stroke, and spinal cord injury. These patients, in particular, have a high risk for thromboembolic events.

Brain Tumor. The incidence of DVT and PE in the patient with a brain tumor is considered to be quite dramatic.[4-6,47,67,191,219,264,274,275,294,300,324] However, in comparison to certain other neurological disorders (e.g., spinal cord injury), this conclusion is actually based upon only a small number of clinical and investigative reports. In many of the reports reviewed here, information about brain tumor patients has been extracted from a general neurosurgical population.

Kayser-Gatchalian and Kayser[191] reported a 27.5% incidence of DVT in 334 autopsies of patients with brain tumors. Tomita and Raimondi[300] described a 2.5% clinical incidence of DVT in 80 patients undergoing craniotomy for brain tumor. Choucair et al[56] described a 1% incidence and Constantini et al[67] a 5% incidence of clinical DVT in retrospective reviews of, respectively, 915 and 492 patients undergoing treatment for glioma and metastatic brain tumors. Levi et al[204] described a clinical thromboembolic incidence (failing to distinguish between DVT and PE) of only 1.7% in a retrospective review of 1,703 patients undergoing craniotomy for cerebral tumor.

The risk of developing DVT has been more effectively established using sensitive investigative techniques such as ^{125}I-labeled fibrinogen uptake. Turpie et al,[306] Sawaya et al,[276] Bynke et al,[52] Valladares,[310] and Skillman et al[284] determined the incidence of DVT to range between 22% and 45% in patients with brain tumor. The incidence determined by sensitive techniques, while potentially overrepresenting the clinical impact of DVT, is important to clarify the true pathophysiology in these patients. Finally, given that the clinical diagnosis of DVT is so highly unreliable, these sensitive techniques are essential to allow for objective assessment of any prophylactic strategy.

In 1960, Wetzel et al[324] retrospectively reviewed a series of 6,065 neurosurgical patients and found a 3% incidence of fatal pulmonary emboli among 599 autopsies, with 14 of the 18 deaths occurring in patients with brain tumors. Brisman and Mendell[47] documented a 6.7% incidence of PE in autopsies of 223 patients with supratentorial brain tumors, while 33.3% of patients with suprasellar brain tumors had autopsy evidence of thromboembolic disease. Tomita and Raimondi[300] described a 3.8% clinical incidence of PE in 80 patients undergoing craniotomy for brain tumor. Choucair et al[56] described a 3% incidence (37% mortality) and Constantini et al[67] a 4% incidence (37% mortality) of PE in retrospective reviews of, respectively, 915 and 492 patients undergoing treatment for glioma and metastatic brain tumors. Muchmore et al[232] reported a 22% incidence (20% mortality) in 23 patients with malignant gliomas. Sawaya et al[276] reported one death from PE in a group of 46 brain tumor patients (2.2%) screened for DVT with ^{125}I fibrinogen, although 40% of patients with positive scans received treatment for venous thrombosis (thereby potentially decreasing the true incidence of PE in this population). The clinical incidence of PE has been reported to range from 2% to 39% in four different patient series describing the surgical treatment of cerebral meningioma, with mortality ranging from 0% to 100% in affected patients.[4,5,219,294]

In addition, there are also specific data concerning how the risk for DVT and PE is dependent upon the tumor location and tumor histology. Brisman and Mendell[47] in an autopsy series reported that patients with tumors in the suprasellar location had a risk of PE that was almost five times that for tumors in other locations. In a case report and review of the literature, Sawaya et al[274] also suggested that the suprasellar location was a significant risk factor. However, this has not been substantiated by any other reports. Constantini et al[67] identified significant risk factors for clinical DVT and PE in a series of 633 patients with brain tumor that included supratentorial (not suprasellar) location of the tumor, malignant glioma, and the presence of para- or hemiparesis. Levi et al[204] in a retrospective series of 1,703 brain tumor patients found a combined clinical diagnosis of DVT and PE in 3.1% of meningioma patients and 1% of both glioma and metastasis patients. Valladares,[310] using ^{125}I fibrinogen, found that the incidence of DVT was 40% in patients with benign tumors and 25% in those with malignant tumors. In a review of 46 patients with brain tumor, using ^{125}I fibrinogen, Sawaya et al[276] reported the incidence of DVT in patients with meningioma, malignant glioma, and metastasis to be, respectively, 72%, 60%, and 20%. There may be some intrinsic feature of specific tumors, such as malignant glioma and meningioma, that contributes to the development of DVT, while other features such as leg paralysis may also play a significant role.

Stroke. The risk of death from PE after stroke is sizable.[36,40,84,104,200,220,221,229,280,308,316-318] In a review of 1,538 patients in a Stroke Registry in the Union of Soviet Socialist Republics (USSR), reported in 1988 by Scmidt et al,[280] PE was the cause in 13.6% of 573 patient deaths occurring within 3 weeks of stroke and in an additional 5.2% of 596 deaths occurring between 3 weeks and 7 years. Other reports are compatible with this high incidence: 2% to 19.8% incidence of PE with mortality ranging from 25% to 100%. The study by Scmidt et al did not examine the incidence of DVT. Using investigational techniques, the incidence of DVT ranges from 28% to 75%, with the paralyzed leg the typical site of the DVT.[104,200,316-318] Warlow et al,[316] using ^{125}I fibrinogen, documented DVT in the paralyzed leg of 53% of patients with stroke, but in only an additional 7% of nonparalyzed legs.

Spinal Cord Injury. The volume of literature concerning the risk for DVT and PE in the patient with spinal cord injury is the largest of any subpopulation in neurosurgery or neurology.[37,42,86,98,227,233,234,245,246,248,256,263,299,303,334] This is a reflection of the enormous risk present in this patient group: the incidence of DVT ranges as high as 100% when documented by ^{125}I fibrinogen[233,299] and as high as 21.4% in autopsy studies.[127,256,303] In a review of 5,131 patients with spinal cord injury over a 7-year period at seven centers in the United States, DeVivo et al[86] reported a 9% overall mortality (459 deaths) with 28 deaths occurring secondary to PE. The incidence of PE exceeded the age-adjusted expected value by 45.2 times. This substantial risk of death secondary to thromboembolism is apparently dependent not just on the immobilization that typically occurs after spinal injury, but more specifically on the presence of spinal cord injury: in two studies looking at spinal fracture without spinal cord injury, the risk of DVT, using sensitive ^{125}I fibrinogen techniques, was low (0%-8.3%).[233,246]

Mechanisms and Risk Factors for Thrombosis

The general thromboembolic clinical features of the neurosurgery population and pregnancy have already been reviewed. The risk for DVT appears highest in patients with spinal cord injury, brain tumor, and stroke, while a less specific increased risk is present in the general neurosurgical population. These patients typically have one or more of the previously described common risk factors such as immobility, malignancy, trauma, surgery, or older age. However, it appears that there is more involved in the increased risk for thrombosis in the patient with neurological disease than the nonspecific risk factors such as trauma, immobility, or malignancy. While more common in a paretic leg, differences in the incidence of DVT exist depending upon such things as the type of brain tumor present, or whether spinal cord injury occurs with the spinal fracture. Abnormalities of coagulation which may represent predisposition to thrombosis include: 1) elevations of fibrinopeptide A and fibrinogen fragment B(β)15-42 in neurosurgical patients;[38] 2) decreased activated partial thromboplastin time (APTT) and increased fibrinopeptide A levels,[199,200] increased platelet count and plasma fibrinogen level with lowered platelet adhesiveness and plasminogen levels,[318] and decreased fibrinolysis in the superficial veins of the paralyzed limbs of stroke patients;[225] 3) subclinical disseminated intravascular coagulation[273,275] in brain tumor patients; and 4) increases in factor VIII and platelet aggregation in patients with spinal cord injury.[263] Hypotheses regarding the mechanisms for these changes are less definite. While the brain contains the highest concentration of thromboplastin in the human body and it is speculated that trauma, infarction, or surgery to the brain results in release of tissue thromboplastin and activation of the coagulation cascade,[251,277,297] there is no direct evidence to support this hypothesis.

Pregnancy is also probably associated with a hypercoagulable state.[59,66,83,85,267] Levels of factors XII, IX, X, VIII, VIII:Ag, VII, V, and fibrinogen increase and factors XIII and XI decrease during pregnancy. In addition, levels of protein C remain normal, whereas levels of both total and free protein S decrease during pregnancy.[66,85] Levels of plasminogen increase during pregnancy, while reports conflict about the levels of plasminogen activator activity and antigen.[14,112,198,332] Thus, there appears to be an overall increase in the activation of coagulation during pregnancy that is compensated for by an increase in fibrinolytic activity.[35,331] A decrease in the altered fibrinolytic potential could greatly enhance the hypercoagulable state, thereby potentiating venous thrombosis. However, the exact mechanisms whereby this imbalance in the altered coagulation state of pregnancy tilts toward a hypercoagulable state remain undetermined.

Thromboembolic Prophylaxis

Overview

It is more cost-effective to prevent than to treat DVT and subsequent PE (with risk of death) and the postphlebitic syndrome.[9,57,115,137,167,188,271] With a well-structured program for prophylaxis of thrombosis in place as the accepted standard of care for each neurosurgical and neurological center, the incidence of DVT and PE is dramatically reduced and considerable human life, health-care energy, and health-care dollars are saved.[236] However, even with the advances that have occurred in the prophylaxis of venous thromboembolism, there are three axioms which must be constantly remembered: 1) patients who receive thrombosis prophylaxis can and do develop DVT and PE; 2) both DVT and PE have protean clinical manifestations ranging from minimal symptoms to sudden death; therefore, a high index of suspicion is required as the possibility of thromboembolism must be constantly evaluated and re-evaluated as a potential diagnosis ("the diagnosis must be thought of before it can be made"); and 3) the physician must be aware of the limitations of the diagnostic methods to ensure that the conclusions resulting from these investigations lead to proper clinical decisions. With these basic principles in mind, an approach to thromboembolic prophylaxis can be developed.

Risk Stratification of Thromboembolism in Pregnancy

An approach to prophylaxis of venous thromboembolism begins with identifying the relevant risk factors and using this to construct a classification of the risk pattern.[172,177,236] Patients are generally rated as low risk (calf vein thrombosis risk <10%), moderate risk (calf vein thrombosis risk 10%-40%), or high risk (calf vein thrombosis risk 40%-80%) for development of thromboembolism.[172] While pregnancy increases the risk for DVT and PE, most uncomplicated pregnancies without other significant risk factors are considered low risk for thromboembolic events. However, the risk level is greatly enhanced for a pregnant patient with a neurological condition associated with an increased risk for thromboembolic events. Patients suffering stroke with hemiparesis,[316-318] subarachnoid hemorrhage,[31] brain tumor (especially meningioma and malignant glioma),[132] head injury,[190] or spinal cord injury with paraplegia or quadriplegia[233,256,334] conform to the definition for the moderate- or high-risk groups, while patients undergoing surgeries such as laminectomy or discectomy of the lumbar and cervical regions are typically associated with low thromboembolic risk. Patients with spinal fracture but no spinal cord injury[233,246] or patients undergoing lumbar discectomy[257] appear to have a low risk of DVT and PE.

It is often difficult, from the finite information available, to sort out the specific risk for individual patients when no specific risk data are available. At this point, a reasonable approach for defining risk is to apply basic principles.[172] Low-risk patients are defined as being <40 years old, with minimal general risk factors, and (if undergoing operation) will have anesthesia of <30 minutes' duration (e.g., carpal tunnel release). Moderate-risk patients are defined as those >40 years old, patients with malignancy, prolonged bed rest, extensive surgical dissection, varicose veins and obesity, or those undergoing an operation >30 minutes' duration (e.g., most spinal operations and most craniotomies). Patients with high risk have the previous features plus a prior history of DVT or PE, or associated abdominal surgery for advanced malignant disease or major orthopedic surgery of the lower limbs. It is important to remember that the thromboembolic risk profile for an individual patient may be represented by the summation of the neurological and pregnancy-associated risks.

Methods of Prophylaxis

Thromboembolic prophylaxis is undertaken using two basic methods which can be used either alone or in combination: mechanical or pharmacological.

Mechanical DVT Prophylaxis. Mechanical techniques attempt to reduce or eliminate venous stasis, while also typically increasing local and systemic fibrinolysis.[177,321] The mechanical procedures include graduated compression stockings, electrical stimulation of the calf muscles, intermittent external pneumatic calf compression, and rotating tables. All of these techniques have proven efficacy in reducing the incidence of DVT in patients.[22,58,158,177] External intermittent pneumatic compression (IPC) of the calf and electrical stimulation of the calf muscles are the two most effective techniques in this category. Static compression stockings should not be used because they do not provide any proven benefit against development of DVT.[282] The commonly used graduated stockings (TED Anti-Embolism Stockings, Kendall Company, Mansfield, MA) are efficacious because they apply graduated pressure to the leg which progressively decreases between the ankle and the thigh, thereby promoting venous emptying. The main advantages of these mechanical techniques are that there is minimal risk associated with their use and they are relatively inexpensive and simple to use. They can be used safely by neurosurgery patients in whom the risk of bleeding complications associated with pharmacological agents such as heparin might be deemed excessive, or used in conjunction with pharmacological agents to augment their efficacy.[97,226,328] Mechanical techniques offer adequate prophylaxis for low-risk patients and many moderate-risk patients. The disadvantage is the suboptimal efficacy with higher-risk patients.

Pharmacological DVT Prophylaxis. The pharmacological agents used for thrombotic prophylaxis are typically targeted at altering the coagulation system (e.g., aspirin, dextran, unfractionated heparin, low-molecular weight heparins (LMWHs) and heparinoids, or warfarin).[57,92,115,172,177] Aspirin has a very limited role in the prevention of venous thrombosis, mostly because its main action is platelet inhibition and platelets seem to play only a minor role in venous thrombosis. Dextran is a polysaccharide originally introduced as a blood volume expansion agent and has multiple antithrombotic properties.[177] It has modest antithrombotic effectiveness in different surgical populations.[126] There are three main pharmacological agents that have proven efficacy to prevent DVT in various patient populations: low-dose and adjusted-dose unfractionated heparin, warfarin, and the more recently described group of LMWHs and heparinoids.[26,27,33,53,58,62,128,129,143,163,168,172,177,228,238,309]

The efficacy of low-dose heparin for prevention of DVT and PE has been documented in many well-designed clinical trials.[58,62] The typical protocol delivers 5,000 IU subcutaneously starting 2 hours before elective surgery or immediately upon presentation at hospital (e.g., trauma and myocardial infarction) and continuing doses of 5,000 IU two to three times daily until the risk of thrombosis has been eliminated. Heparin does not cross the placenta and is considered safe for use during pregnancy. The primary concern about using this agent lies in its bleeding potential. In most general surgical populations, the risk of hemorrhagic complications is quite small. However, there has been a reluctance to use this agent in neurosurgery patients because of the possible catastrophic consequences of hemorrhage.[54,56]

More intense prophylactic approaches have been recommended in high-risk patients, where low-dose heparin is not as effective. These include adjusted-dose heparin and adjusted-dose warfarin.[172,188,207] With heparin, varying doses are given to maintain an APTT value at the upper end of the normal range, while with warfarin, the target range is a prothrombin time (PT) which is 1.3-1.5 times control using rabbit brain thromboplastin (international normalized ratio (INR) 2.0-3.0). However, while these approaches are effective, there is an associated increased risk of bleeding.[119,172] With this increase, there is even more reluctance to use these in neurosurgical patients. Additional specific concerns exist concerning the use of warfarin during pregnancy.

Warfarin is contraindicated for use during pregnancy because of the risk of warfarin embryopathy (e.g., stippled epiphyses and nasal and limb hypoplasia) following exposure prior to 12 weeks' gestation and the increased risk of central nervous system (CNS) abnormalities (e.g., agenesis of the corpus callosum, Dandy-Walker malformation, midline cerebellar atrophy, and ventral midline dysplasia manifested by optic atrophy and hemorrhage) throughout the second trimester.[109,131] Rates of spontaneous abortions and stillbirths are elevated in the third trimester, likely as a result of fetal hemorrhage. A review of 1,325 pregnancies from 186 studies reported a 16.9% incidence of adverse outcomes with the use of warfarin during pregnancy, after excluding pregnancies with maternal co-morbid conditions and prematurity with normal outcomes. Warfarin is not secreted in breast milk and therefore may be used with reasonable safety in the postpartum period.[222]

The latest class of agents shown to have efficacy for thromboembolic prophylaxis are the LMWHs and heparinoids.[26,27,53,92,128,129,143,163,168,177,188,228,238,301,309] Nonfractionated heparin is a mixture of a number of heparin fragments of different molecular weights with varying antithrombotic and anticoagulant properties. LMWHs are derived from standard unfractionated heparin by enzymatic or chemical cleavage. This process results in compounds of molecular weight 4000-5000 Da as compared to 12,000-16,000 Da for standard heparin. LMWHs possess a number of advantages over standard heparin. Pharmacokinetic studies[17,29,45,99,136,217] and small clinical trials in selected patients with venous thrombosis[44,152] indicate that the bioavailability of LMWH fractions following subcutaneous injection is on the order of 80% to 90%. For example, Bratt et al[45] reported that the bioavailability of LMWH after a subcutaneous injection of 120 factor Xa U/kg to healthy volunteers was approximately 90% of an equivalent intravenous dose. The plasma half-life (antifactor Xa activity) is also prolonged compared to unfractionated heparin.[2,17,217] The anticoagulant response (factor Xa U/ml) observed with a given dose of LMWH is highly correlated with body weight.[217] All of these features suggest that LMWH can be effective when given in standard doses (factor Xa U/kg) once daily, without laboratory monitoring. The differential effects of these compounds on thrombin and factor Xa inhibition result in maintenance of anticoagulant effect without prolongation of the APTT at equivalent factor Xa levels.[148] It is the potential for an LMWH to possess a high ratio of antithrombotic effect to bleeding risk that makes some of the LMWH agents more attractive to physicians.[177,301] In general, when compared to unfractionated heparin, these drugs may possess a higher antithrombotic potency. However, a recent clinical trial reported by Hull et al,[163] comparing the efficacy of the LMWH Logiparin with warfarin for prophylaxis against DVT after hip or knee implantation, found similar efficacy but with the major bleeding rate for warfarin of 1.2% compared to 2.8% for Logiparin (p=0.04). Therefore, it appears that while the antithrombotic properties of many LMWHs are significant, the anticoagulant properties of LMWHs have not yet been satisfactorily evaluated to allow for a blanket recommendation for the use of LMWHs or heparinoids in the prophylaxis of neurosurgery patients.

In addition, when scrutinizing the literature, the physician must be aware that there are a potentially large number of different LMWH agents and there is currently no justification for considering all LMWH agents to have equivalent efficacy or safety.[128,142] Each individual LMWH found to be effective in a randomized clinical trial is only appropriate for the conditions established by that particular trial. For example, using venography to evaluate DVT as an endpoint, there is convincing evidence that several LMWHs are safe and effective in patients undergoing elective hip surgery[163,249] and elective general surgical procedures.[187,238]

Other classes of pharmacological agents are being developed and evaluated: pentasaccharides, dermatan sulfate, heparan sulfate, synthetic lactobionic acid amides, depolymerized heparinoids, polydeoxyribonucleotide derivatives, synthetic peptides and related drugs, and recombinant hirudin and related anticoagulants.[92] Information regarding these agents is still preliminary and judgment concerning efficacy and safety must await the results of properly designed clinical trials.

TABLE 2

THROMBOEMBOLIC PROPHYLAXIS IN PATIENTS WITH NEUROLOGICAL DISEASE*

Author	Level	No.	Assessment	Method	Deep Vein Thrombosis (%)	Pulmonary Embolism (%)
General Population						
Turpie et al, 1977[306]	I	63	^{125}I	Control	19.3	0
		65		IPC	1.5	0
Cerrato et al, 1978[54]	I	50	^{125}I	Control	34	–
		50		Heparin	6	–
Skillman et al, 1978[284]	I	48	^{125}I	Control	25	4.2
		47		IPC	8.5	0
Turpie et al, 1979[305]	I	96	^{125}I	Control	20.8	0
		103		IPC	7.8	0
Zelikovski et al, 1981[335]	I	20	^{125}I	Control	50	5
		23		IPC	4.3	0
Turpie et al, 1989[307]	I	81	IPG	Control	19.8	0
		80		Grad stockings	8.8	0
		78		Grad stockings/IPC	9	1.3
Bucci et al, 1989[48]	I	38	IPG	IPC	2.6	0
		32		Grad stockings	3.1	0
Boström et al, 1986[39]	II	49	^{125}I	Heparin	10	–
		40		Electric/dextran	13	–
Black et al, 1986[30]	V	523	Doppler ultrasound/clinical	IPC	2.3	1.8
Flinn et al, 1989[95]	V	361	Doppler ultrasound	IPC & Grad stockings	4.7	0.6
Brain Tumor						
Turpie et al, 1977[306]	I	27	^{125}I	Control	22.2	0
		28		IPC	4.0	0
Cerrato et al, 1978[54]	I	36/50	^{125}I	Control	34‡	–
		42/50		Heparin	6‡	–
Skillman et al, 1978[284]	I	20	^{125}I	Control	35	0
		11		IPC	9.1	0
Bynke et al, 1987[52]	I	31†	^{125}I	Control	19.3	–
		31†		IPC	0	–
Boström et al, 1986[39]	II	16/49	^{125}I	Heparin	4.5**	–
		14/40		Electric/dextran		
Black et al, 1986[30]	V	59	Doppler ultrasound/clinical	IPC	3.4	5.1
Flinn et al, 1989[95]	V	78	Doppler ultrasound	IPC & Grad stockings	14	0
Stroke						
McCarthy et al, 1977[221]	I	16	^{125}I	Control	75	–
		16		Heparin	12.5	–
Gelmers, 1980[102]	I	49	^{99}Tc	Control	23	4
		52		Heparin	2	0
McCarthy & Turner, 1986[220]	I	161	^{125}I	Control	72.2	20.5
		144		Heparin	22.2	4.9
Turpie et al, 1987[308]	I	25	^{125}I	Control	28	8
		50		LMWH	4	0

TABLE 2 (continued)

THROMBOEMBOLIC PROPHYLAXIS IN PATIENTS WITH NEUROLOGICAL DISEASE*

Author	Level	No.	Assessment	Method	Deep Vein Thrombosis (%)	Pulmonary Embolism (%)
Subarachnoid Hemorrhage						
Black et al, 1986[31]	III	56	Doppler ultrasound	Control	17.9	0
		90		IPC	5.6	0
Spinal Cord Injury						
Green et al, 1988[119]	I	29	IPG/Doppler ultrasound	Heparin	31	10.3
		29		Adjusted heparin	7	0
Merli et al, 1988[227]	I	17	^{125}I	Control	47	0
		16		Heparin	50	0
		15		Heparin/Electric	6.7	0
Green et al, 1990[120]	I	21	IPG/Doppler ultrasound	Heparin	23.8	9.5
		20		LMWH	0	0
Frisbie & Sasahara, 1981[98]	II	17	IPG	Control	5.9	–
		15		Heparin	6.7	–
Becker et al, 1987[22]	II	5	^{125}I/IPG	Control	80	–
		10		Rotating table	10	–
Green et al, 1982[121]	III	18	^{125}I	Control	72	–
		15		IPC	60	–
		12		IPC/aspirin/ dipyridamole	25	–
Merli et al, 1992[226]	IV	19	^{125}I	Control	35.3	–
				Grad stockings/ IPC/heparin	5.3	–
Jarrell et al, 1983[182]	V	209	^{125}I	Heparin	62††	–

* Level = level value of study;[68] ^{125}I = ^{125}I fibrinogen; IPG = impedance plethysmography; IPC = intermittent pneumatic calf compression; ^{99}Tc = technetium 99 albumin; Grad stockings = graduated stockings; Electric = electrical calf stimulation; heparin = fixed dose of 5,000 IU 2-3 times per day. PE was diagnosed clinically except when screened for by autopsy.

† In this study there were 31 patients with one leg assigned to be the control and the other leg receiving treatment.

‡ Incidence of total population (majority had brain tumors).

** Combined incidence for both treatment groups.

††In this portion of the study all patients with evidence of DVT were anticoagulated to prevent PE.

Thromboembolic Prophylaxis in Pregnant Neurosurgical Patients

Overview. A summary of well-designed clinical trials evaluating prophylaxis of thromboembolism in neurosurgery patients that have been published in the English language is presented in Table 2. The reports have been ranked according to the level of evidence to which they correspond and grouped according to type of patient population.[22,30,31,39,48,52,54,95,98,102,119-121,182,220,221,227,284,305-308,335] While reviewing Table 2, it should become immediately apparent that with adequate prophylaxis a significant impact can be made on the incidence of DVT and PE.[252,292]

Mechanical Prophylaxis. There is enough evidence to encourage certain conservative but effective techniques in all patients at risk: early ambulation and graduated compression stockings.[48,95,307] The clinical trial reported by Bucci et al,[48] comparing graduated stockings with IPC of the lower extremity, demonstrated similar efficacy for both methods using impedance plethysmography surveillance. The efficacy of IPC has also been documented in several Level I trials completed in the general neurosurgical population.[52,284,305,306,335] IPC should not be used in any patient with suspected or confirmed DVT. When used, it should be continued until the patient is either ambulating for more than 3 to 4 hours per day or until the major risk period has passed or an effective alternative agent has been started. The advantages of IPC are the ease with which it is used and its safety, particularly in patients with intracranial hemorrhage. It is less effective in high-risk patients (patients with stroke, spinal cord injury, or brain tumor). To balance these two issues, some advocate the use of IPC during the first 10 to 14 days after a high-risk DVT event, such as spinal cord or head injury, followed by low-dose heparin. To date there are no studies of IPC in the pregnant patient at risk for development of DVT. In addition, since most pregnant patients are ambulatory, IPC would be expected to be of limited utility. However, IPC remains a valuable, practical option for DVT prophylaxis. Finally, while there is evidence to substantiate an effective role for electric calf muscle stimulation[39,227] and rotating tables[22] in neurosurgical patients, these methods are not accepted for general use.

Pharmacological Prophylaxis. The bulk of pharmacological clinical trials evaluate low-dose nonfractionated heparin, adjusted-dose heparin, or some of the new LMWH agents. Warfarin will not be reviewed here because of the contraindications to its use during pregnancy. The prime concern with the use of these agents in patients harboring pathology in the CNS has been the risk of intracranial or intraspinal hemorrhage. There is substantial evidence to suggest that low-dose nonfractionated heparin can be used safely in neurosurgical patients and during pregnancy with minimal risk of significant hemorrhage. Experiences with low-dose heparin have been reported by Barnett et al[19] in 150 patients undergoing a neurosurgical operation (two wound hematomas) and by van Dulken and Thomeer[312] on 983 general neurosurgical patients (one wound hematoma). Cerrato et al[54] reported a randomized trial comparing low-dose heparin with no prophylaxis in 100 neurosurgery patients undergoing craniotomy, with no postoperative bleeding complications in the 50 patients receiving heparin. Gelmers[102] and McCarthy and Turner[220] reported similar randomized studies in, respectively, 101 and 305 patients suffering acute stroke. In Gelmers' study there were minor bleeding episodes in two of the 52 patients on low-dose heparin. There was no increase in the risk for hemorrhagic cerebral infarction in the 144 patients receiving low-dose heparin in McCarthy and Turner's report. In a report by Green et al[119] of patients with spinal cord injury, there were no bleeding events in the 29 patients receiving low-dose heparin; however, seven of the 29 patients receiving adjusted-dose heparin suffered bleeding complications. Clinical experience using low-dose heparin in high-risk pregnant patients has substantiated safety for both the fetus and mother.[34,76,131,140, 141,295] Heparin does not cross the placenta and is not associated with any increased risk of fetal morbidity and mortality, even when used in therapeutic doses,[107,109,111,131] although there is potential concern regarding hemorrhage at the time of delivery.[7] The pregnant patient is also at risk for developing several of the side effects for heparin therapy, including heparin-induced osteoporosis (exact risk unknown)[18,75,125, 154,286,330] and thrombocytopenia (1%-5% risk).[124,315] Heparin-induced osteoporosis will be reviewed in the treatment section.

Low-dose heparin appears most efficacious in patients in the general neurosurgical population,[39,54] with less effectiveness in high-risk disorders such as stroke and spinal cord injury. The incidence of DVT in patients with stroke ranges from 2% to 22% and in patients with spinal cord injury as high as 50%. Green et al[119] showed that adjusted-dose heparin offered better protection from DVT than low-dose heparin (7% vs. 31%), with no incidence of PE in the adjusted-dose heparin group. However, the increased efficacy came at the cost of bleeding complications in 24% of the patients.

It is well known that heparin requirements fluctuate throughout pregnancy with wide individual variation.[76] The efficacy of low-dose heparin in pregnant patients at high risk for DVT or PE has been variable, possibly related to dosing problems. Tengborn et al[295] failed to demonstrate efficacy with low-dose heparin prophylaxis in high-risk pregnant patients, but this may have been due to underdosing. Hellgren et al[140] produced a significant reduction in DVT recurrence in pregnant patients by adjusting heparin dosage using plasma heparin concentrations. A Level I study examining low-dose heparin prophylaxis has not yet been performed.

The LMWHs and heparinoids are promising agents for the prevention of DVT. In a Level I study, Turpie et al[308] assessed the heparinoid Org 10172 in 75 patients with acute stroke: in 50 patients receiving treatment evaluated by ^{125}I fibrinogen, DVT occurred in 4% and none had PE, while in control patients DVT occurred in 28% and 8% experienced PE. There were no episodes of hemorrhage related to Org 10172. In another Level I trial, Green et al[120] evaluated the LMWH Logiparin in the prophylaxis of thrombosis in 41 spinal cord-injured patients. Compared with low-dose unfractionated heparin, the incidence of DVT evaluated by impedance plethysmography and Doppler ultrasound was 23.8%, with 9.5% experiencing fatal PE in the regular heparin group; there were no episodes of DVT or PE in the LMWH group. Again, there were no episodes of significant bleeding in the LMWH group, while in the low-dose heparin group use of the drug was halted in 10% of the patients because of severe bleeding. These two well-designed clinical trials, using different LMWH agents, demonstrated efficacy that appears superior to low-dose heparin[120] while offering significantly greater safety than adjusted-dose heparin.[119] Very limited experience is available concerning utilization of LMWH agents therapeutically[82,96,224,240] and prophylactically[105,291] in pregnant patients. Reports from Sturridge et al[291] and Gillis et al[105] have suggested a promising role for LMWH agents in prophylaxis of DVT in pregnant patients but this is, at best, Level IV evidence.

It should become immediately apparent that with adequate prophylaxis a significant impact can be made on the incidence of DVT, and hopefully, PE.[52,54,284,306] However, it is also obvious that only a limited assessment of the problem of venous thrombotic prophylaxis has been undertaken in neurosurgical patients and even less investigation has been performed in pregnant patients, let alone pregnant neurosurgical patients. The need for comprehensive, well-designed clinical trials to establish the true natural history of venous thromboembolism in neurosurgical patients is essential.

Prophylaxis Recommendations in the Pregnant Neurosurgical Patient

The current recommendations for pregnant neurosurgical patients can therefore be summarized: 1) earliest possible ambulation; 2) where ambulation is inhibited, graduated stockings should be worn except when IPC is being used; and 3a) IPC in all patients prior to surgical treatment or in patients with hemiplegia or paraplegia, as a minimum mode of prophylaxis (Grade A recommendation), or 3b) low-dose heparin given subcutaneously (5,000 IU q12 hourly until 36 weeks' gestation; 7,500 IU q12 hourly or 5,000 IU q8 hourly until delivery and in the postpartum period for 4 to 6 weeks[34,59]) in combination with IPC for all patients prior to surgical therapy or in hemiplegic/paraplegic patients (Grade B recommendation). Ideally, low-dose heparin should be started before a neurosurgical procedure; however, a number of clinicians prefer to start heparin prophylaxis in the postoperative period. A distinction between recommendations 3a and 3b is made to attempt to deal with the reservations that many clinicians have about using heparin in these patients. While the authors feel that a significant volume of data has been published demonstrating the relative safety of low-dose heparin in this patient population and that the addition of heparin adds significantly to venous thromboembolic prophylaxis (Grade B recommendation), they are willing to accept IPC as a minimum standard of surgical prophylaxis until efficacy and safety of low-dose heparin have been clearly defined in a well-designed prospective clinical trial involving neurosurgical patients. Finally, the dosing recommendations that have been provided are based only on Grade B and C studies and further information is required to better define these important details.

The recommendation for combining low-dose heparin with IPC has not been assessed with a Level I clinical trial. Given the lack of complete efficacy of either heparin or IPC alone for certain high-risk patients, the rationale seems reasonable and there does not appear to be any contraindication to this combination (Grade B recommendation). In addition, one may speculate that the different mechanisms of action of the two modalities may achieve a cumulative effect in DVT prophylaxis. One trial evaluated low-dose heparin and electric calf muscle stimulation,[227] and another, the mechanical means of prophylaxis. This Level I trial documented a dramatic increase in the efficacy of prophylaxis when heparin was combined with electric stimulation. The incidence of DVT, as evaluated with ^{125}I fibrinogen, was 50% in 16 patients treated with low-dose heparin compared with only 6.7% in 15 patients using both methods. Frim et al[97] compared IPC alone against IPC and heparin in a Level II trial in neurosurgical patients and noted a decrease in the clinical incidence of DVT to 0% from 3.2%. Merli et al[226] assessed a combination of graduated compression stockings, IPC, and low-dose unfractionated heparin in a Level IV trial. Using ^{125}I fibrinogen, they identified DVT in 5.5% of treated spinal cord-injured patients compared with 35.3% of patients without prophylaxis.

While adjusted-dose heparin appears to be efficacious, it carries a significant risk of bleeding complications and cannot be recommended at this time in pregnant neurosurgical patients. Furthermore, as previously noted, warfarin is contraindicated during pregnancy.

We speculate that various LMWH agents will supplant the role that low-dose heparin now has in the prophylaxis of thrombosis in neurosurgical and neurological patients. The LMWH Logiparin has proven efficacy for patients with spinal cord injury, as does the LMWH Org 10172 for patients with acute stroke. LMWH agents have been successfully utilized in pregnant patients in Level IV studies. However, more experience scrutinizing the efficacy and safety of this class of drugs in a variety of larger subpopulations of patients with neurological disorders, including pregnant patients, will be required before their definitive role can be established.

Management of Thromboembolic Disease in Pregnant Patients

Laboratory Diagnosis of DVT and PE During Pregnancy

The accepted reference gold standard for diagnosis of DVT remains contrast venography.[320] However, while venography is the most definitive method to confirm or exclude thrombosis of the lower extremities, it is also moderately invasive and may produce pain or, less commonly, phlebitis. Furthermore, the risk of exposing the fetus to ionizing radiation must be considered. Impedance plethysmography is the only noninvasive method of diagnosing DVT to be validated in pregnant patients.[81,169] The safety of withholding anticoagulant therapy in pregnant patients with clinically suspected DVT and serially negative plethysmography testing was demonstrated in a prospective Level I trial.[172] Serial impedance plethysmography testing in 152 patients (Days 1, 3, 5 or 7, 10, and 14) was negative in 139 patients studied and none of these developed thromboembolism during long-term follow-up. Additional studies have determined that late in pregnancy, impedance plethysmography should be performed with the patient in the lateral decubitus position.[60,81] While a number of careful studies have evaluated B-mode compression ultrasonography in the general population,[138,202] this technique has not been validated in pregnant patients.

The gold standard for diagnosis of PE is pulmonary angiography.[165,250] Because of potential complications and technical difficulties performing pulmonary angiography in critically ill patients, ventilation-perfusion scanning has displaced pulmonary angiography for PE diagnosis in most patients.[165,250] Neither method has been evaluated in pregnant patients in a Level I study. However, ventilation-perfusion scanning is utilized in pregnant patients because of strong evidence supporting its role in the general population. Furthermore, the risk of exposure of the fetus to ionizing radiation during pulmonary angiography, in comparison to ventilation-perfusion scanning, must also be considered.

Ginsberg et al[108] conducted a review of the literature concerning the risks of in utero exposure to low-dose (<5,000 mrad) radiation coupled with estimates of fetal radiation exposure during investigation of DVT or PE: 1) contrast venography diagnosis of DVT can be performed with <500 mrad exposure to the fetus, which can be further reduced to <50 mrad with limited venography and abdominal shielding; 2) pulmonary angiography exposes the fetus to 405 mrad when performed by the femoral technique or <50 mrad if a brachial route is utilized with abdominal shielding; and 3) ventilation-perfusion scanning exposes the fetus to <55 mrad. Ginsberg's review also suggested that there was a statistically significant increase in the risk of childhood cancers (relative risk 1.2 to 2.4 increase) following in utero radiation exposure, although the absolute risk increase would be likely very small given incidence of childhood cancer in the general population is estimated at only 0.1%.

Therefore, venography or ventilation-perfusion scanning can be performed with techniques that expose the fetus to very low doses of ionizing radiation, such that the risks of the slight increase in oncogenicity are more than outweighed by the benefits of establishing a correct diagnosis of DVT or PE and instituting appropriate therapy. Impedance plethysmography can safely replace venography for the investigation of most pregnant patients and pulmonary angiography must be decided on an individual basis, weighing the risks and benefits. The recommendations for investigation of suspected DVT or PE in a pregnant patient, therefore, are very similar to those for the general population: 1) impedance plethysmography for diagnosis of DVT with the understanding that false-positive results can occur during the third trimester due to extrinsic compression by the gravid uterus; 2) serial impedance plethysmography if the initial test is negative; 3) impedance plethysmography diagnosis confirmation when venography is positive during the third trimester; 4) ventilation-perfusion scanning for diagnosis or exclusion of PE; 5) impedance plethysmography or venography to confirm DVT diagnosis with intermediate probability ventilation-perfusion scanning; and 6) pulmonary angiography when impedance plethysmography or venography is negative with intermediate probability ventilation-perfusion scanning.

Treatment of DVT and PE: General Principles

After confirming a diagnosis of either DVT or PE, an established protocol for treatment should immediately be initiated. The main objectives of treatment are: 1) prevent death from PE; 2) prevent the postphlebitic syndrome; 3) reduce morbidity from the acute event; and 4) achieve the previous objectives with minimum side effects and cost.[79,146] The therapeutic approaches used to accomplish these objectives include: 1) preventing extension of the thrombus by inhibiting blood coagulation;[25,51,79,101,144,150,153,160,161,170,174,175,178,193,230,247,262,270,272,323] 2) preventing PE from DVT by interrupting the inferior vena cava;[122,211] and 3) in rare circumstances, removing the thrombus by mechanical or enzymatic means.[8,113,114,151,211,296] It is not the intent to review specific details of therapy, but rather to discuss principles of treatment and to point out some of the difficulties commonly encountered during management of neurosurgical patients and to focus on specific features associated with pregnancy.

Overview of Anticoagulant Therapy. It would be useful to review some key points and discuss some of the recognized problems that exist before addressing issues of specific relevance to patients with neurological disease. The efficacy of therapeutic anticoagulation as treatment for DVT and PE is well established, yet if improperly used, anticoagulation will either inadequately treat the thrombotic state or will result in excessive anticoagulation with potential bleeding complications. Anticoagulant therapy is highly efficacious and prevents death from PE in >95% of patients. Wheeler et al[325] documented inadequate anticoagulation with heparin in 60% of 65 patients during the first 24 hours after diagnosis was established. They identified five common practices that led to the problem of nontherapeutic anticoagulation in the majority of these patients: 1) failure to start heparin therapy at the time of initial clinical suspicion; 2) choice of unfractionated heparin bolus and continuous infusion dosage insufficient to elevate APTT to >1.5 times control; 3) delay in obtaining the first APTT after starting heparin therapy beyond the recommended 4 to 6 hours (average 11.7 hours); 4) insufficient heparin therapy in response to a low APTT; and 5) excessive and prolonged reductions in heparin therapy in response to an APTT level in excess of 3 times control. All of these problems have their basis in a poor understanding of heparin kinetics and can be avoided. Some of these problems can be alleviated by using a heparin protocol which ensures that patients are quickly brought into the therapeutic range early in treatment.[73,176]

Recent Level I evidence has substantiated the efficacy and safety for starting warfarin on the same day as the heparin therapy is started.[175] Warfarin should always be overlapped with heparin for 4 to 5 days;[178] with this approach, heparin therapy can usually be discontinued in 5 to 7 days rather than the typical 10- to 14-day period with the earlier approach which started warfarin on Day 5 to Day 10.[101,174,175,262] No benefit is gained by postponing the start of warfarin therapy beyond this suggested time period. In addition, there is substantial Level I evidence supporting the recommended therapeutic INR range of 2.0 to 3.0 for anticoagulation with warfarin.[145,147,149,150,161] This recommended INR range is much lower than historical levels but is equally efficacious with a dramatically reduced risk of bleeding complications. A thorough understanding of the pharmacokinetics of warfarin,[323] all of the possible deleterious drug interactions, and the testing procedures done to evaluate its anticoagulant effect are required to allow for its safe use in patients. Warfarin is contraindicated in pregnancy, although not in the puerperium, unless hemorrhage risk is a concern.[109,111,131,222]

Finally, a growing experience with LMWH agents to treat DVT or PE has demonstrated their effectiveness and safety. The advantages of LMWH agents include a long half-life and the elimination of laboratory monitoring.[3,43-45,61,118,135,148,155,174,210,255]

Alternative Treatment Strategies. The major dilemma in treatment strategy, therefore, concerns this latter group of patients with absolute or relative contraindications for anticoagulant therapy. Future evaluation of LMWHs and heparinoids may provide further evidence of their efficacy and safety and better define their role in thromboembolism management in patients with neurological disorders. In addition, there is evidence supporting the efficacy of filters in the inferior vena cava to interrupt venous return to the right atrium and therefore prevent either primary or recurrent PE in the patient with DVT.[122,182,192,211,232,239] Inferior vena cava filters provide a temporary alternative to full anticoagulation in those patients at highest risk for catastrophic hemorrhagic complications. However, the role for inferior vena cava filters is limited and full anticoagulation should be reconsidered after a patient has passed out of the high-risk period for bleeding complications (e.g., beyond securement of aneurysm or beyond 1 to 2 weeks after intracranial surgery).

The role of thrombolytic therapy has not been clearly defined for patients with DVT and PE[8,296] and is associated with a substantial risk of hemorrhagic complications[117] in most patients with neurological disease. Therefore, the routine use of thrombolytic therapy cannot be recommended.

General Recommendations for DVT and PE Treatment. The current Grade A recommendation for care of patients with DVT and PE is based on Level I evidence: 1) in the acute stage, anticoagulation can be accomplished with an intravenous bolus followed by continuous intravenous infusion of nonfractionated heparin or with adjusted-dose subcutaneous nonfractionated heparin, both aiming to prolong the APTT from 1.5 to 2.0 times control value,[178] or using a fixed-dose of the LMWH Logiparin (175 International factor Xa inhibitory U/kg of body weight every 24 hours);[174] 2) when heparin therapy is initiated, treatment with the oral agent warfarin[178] can begin with a dose of 10 mg per day, adjusted to maintain the INR between 2.0 and 3.0 (1.3 to 1.5 times control using North American thromboplastin); 3) an acceptable alternative when oral anticoagulants are either contraindicated or inconvenient is to use adjusted-dose heparin to prolong the APTT to 1.5 times the control at the mid-dosing interval[160,178] or fixed-dose LMWH;[174,231] 4) treatment should continue for a minimum of 3 to 6 months (Grade A recommendation)[178] or indefinitely in patients with recurrent venous thrombosis or continuing risk factors such as antithrombin III deficiency, protein C or S deficiency, or malignancy (Grade C recommendation).

Anticoagulants in the Pregnant Neurosurgical Patient

The principle concern about using anticoagulants to treat DVT and PE in the pregnant neurosurgical patient relates to the bleeding potential[79,205] and the catastrophic consequences that would be expected if an intracranial or intraspinal hemorrhage occurred.[117,285] However, there is sufficient evidence to support the relative safety of heparin and warfarin (although contraindicated during pregnancy) in most patients with neurological disease.[6,56,67,88,130,239,244,245,264,293,319] Although the outcome of any intracranial hemorrhage while on anticoagulant therapy might be fatal, there is no doubt about the very high mortality associated with PE. Furthermore, there is ample evidence documenting the safety of anticoagulant treatment utilizing therapeutic levels of unfractionated heparin or LMWH agents in pregnant patients.[63,82,96,107,215,224,240] Simple observation of a patient with DVT or PE is not acceptable management.

The only current absolute contraindications for anticoagulation are patients with an unsecured aneurysm after a subarachnoid hemorrhage or patients with an acute intracerebral hemorrhage or hematomyelia. There is no information available to define the magnitude or duration of the risk for hemorrhage associated with the use of anticoagulants after any of these events, or during the first 6 weeks after intracranial surgery.[329] There is weaker evidence to suggest the safety of therapeutic anticoagulation between postoperative Week 1 and Week 6.[6,56,239,264]

Treatment of DVT or PE in the pregnant patient requires consideration of a few unique issues. As previously discussed, heparin can be safely utilized during pregnancy because it does not cross the placenta.[63,107,215] Warfarin is contraindicated during pregnancy but can be used during the puerperium. Therefore, after initial treatment with intravenous heparin to achieve therapeutic anticoagulation, long-term treatment of DVT and PE during pregnancy is accomplished with subcutaneous heparin administration. Heparin requirements fluctuate throughout pregnancy with wide individual variation;[76] changes in these requirements are likely a reflection of dilutional effects, changes in glomerular filtration rate, increases in heparin binding proteins and platelet factor IV, and placental catabolism. These physiological changes generally produce increased heparin requirements during the second trimester, followed by marked decreases in requirements as the pregnancy comes to term and immediately postpartum. The short half-life of unfractionated heparin and fluctuating heparin requirements throughout pregnancy necessitate twice daily subcutaneous injections, frequent laboratory monitoring, and dose adjustments to maintain therapeutic levels of heparin. An additional special concern arising from the prolonged use of therapeutic doses of heparin is osteoporosis.[18,75,125,154,286,330]

Heparin-induced osteoporosis in pregnancy is poorly documented. The literature contains scattered case reports of women with clinically relevant vertebral fractures associated with heparin therapy.[125,286,330] A small randomized controlled trial reported by Howell et al[154] demonstrated that one of 20 women randomized to receive heparin prophylaxis (10,000 U subcutaneously twice daily) developed osteoporotic spinal fractures as compared to none of the control patients. The patient numbers in this study are too small for the results to be used as a reliable estimate of heparin-associated osteoporosis. More recently, two prospective case-controlled studies, using bone density as the outcome measure, demonstrated statistically significant decreases in bone density in the heparin-treated groups with variable degrees of resolution after discontinuation of heparin treatment.[18,77] However, the relationship between heparin dose, duration of exposure, and the risk of development of osteoporosis is unclear as no prospective trials addressing this issue have been reported: osteoporotic fractures have been reported in patients using <15,000 U of heparin daily for 7 weeks,[75,125] while studies of bone density have failed to establish a clear dose response of heparin.[18,74,110]

Randomized controlled prospective trials using LMWH for the treatment of thromboembolism in pregnancy have not been published to date. Several LMWH preparations have been used in pregnant patients which have not been shown to cross the placenta[82,96,224,240] and, therefore, are unlikely to harm the fetus. Additionally, one study suggested a lower risk of osteoporosis when used in the long-term management of nonpregnant individuals,[231] although animal studies have conflicted with this observation.[218] There are several case reports and small series describing the use of LMWH agents in pregnant women for treatment of thromboembolic disease.[105,224,231] The limited evidence from this Level IV and V data suggests that LMWHs may be effective in treatment of DVT in pregnancy and as of yet have not been associated with an increased adverse outcome. Of interest, Sturridge et al[291] reported Level IV data in which the length of gestation had no significant effect on the dose of Enoxaparine needed to obtain anti-factor Xa levels (in contrast to regular heparin). This latter result must be interpreted with caution as there is very little published data on the pharmacokinetics of LMWHs in pregnancy. However, it does suggest that dose adjustment throughout pregnancy may not be required with this agent and possibly other LMWH agents.

Treatment Recommendations in the Pregnant Neurosurgical Patient

In summary, clinical trials have established the need for initial treatment of DVT and PE with heparin or with LMWH followed by outpatient treatment with heparin or LMWH (warfarin can be used during the puerperium). In addition, these trials have demonstrated that an adequate intensity of treatment with these anticoagulant agents is required to prevent recurrent thromboembolism. A comprehensive knowledge of the pharmacokinetics of these treatment agents is therefore essential for efficacious and safe usage.

Full anticoagulation is relatively safe in most pregnant patients with neurological disease, except in those patients with unsecured, recently ruptured intracranial aneurysms, in the presence of recent intracerebral hemorrhage or hematomyelia, or in the first week after intracranial surgery. The risk for hemorrhagic complications is not well defined for these situations and each patient must be evaluated on an individual basis. Recommended treatment is based upon Level IV data[24,63,107,111,215] (Grade C recommendation), extrapolating from Level I data in nonpregnant patients:[160] intravenous heparin for 6 days followed by adjusted-dose subcutaneous heparin for the remainder of the pregnancy and for 4 to 6 weeks postpartum. Subcutaneous heparin therapy is administered every 12 hours and is monitored by measurement and adjustment of the mid-interval APTT to the therapeutic range (1.5 to 2.5 times control). The major support for this recommendation is from Level I data comparing the efficacy of prolonged adjusted-dose subcutaneous heparin versus warfarin after initial treatment with intravenous heparin for documented proximal DVT in nonpregnant patients.[160] There is a risk of life-threatening bleeding at parturition in patients receiving adjusted-dose heparin and precautions to prevent this must be taken (i.e., discontinuation of heparin 12 hours prior to induction or with the onset of labor).[7]

The role for LMWHs and heparinoids in pregnant neurosurgery patients is not clearly defined at this time, but appears promising. The long half-life of some LMWH agents and the ability to predict dosing requirements based upon body weight, potentially without the concern about fluctuations of LMWH dosing requirements during different phases of pregnancy, offers the possibility of a once daily subcutaneous treatment protocol, potentially in an outpatient setting without the need for laboratory monitoring. In addition, there may be less risk of bleeding with LMWH agents at parturition and in the high-risk setting associated with many neurosurgical conditions (if one extrapolates from the observed 91% risk reduction in the rate of clinically important bleeding observed during a Level I assessment of the therapeutic role of an LMWH as compared with therapeutic doses of unfractionated heparin in nonpregnant, non-neurosurgical patients[253]). The limited data available concerning the use of LMWH agents during pregnancy or in neurosurgical patients preclude their recommendation at this time as first-line anticoagulants for treatment of DVT or PE in these patients.

Insertion of an inferior vena cava filter is an alternative to anticoagulation in these high-risk patients or in patients experiencing hemorrhagic complications from anticoagulant therapy (Grade C recommendation). Limited clinical experience has been published concerning the use of filters in pregnant patients, either alone[1] or in combination with anticoagulants.[235] If an inferior vena cava filter is used alone for PE prevention in a patient with DVT, anticoagulation should be reconsidered when the risk of hemorrhagic complications diminishes, both to increase the efficacy of PE prevention and to reduce the risk of lower extremity complications. There is no role for thrombolytic therapy in neurosurgical patients or during pregnancy.

Finally, the need for well-designed clinical studies to evaluate the important questions that have been addressed here cannot be understated. A cooperative effort will be required to accomplish this goal.

Intracranial Thrombotic Disorders

Intracranial thrombotic disease (intracranial venous thrombosis) occurs with an estimated incidence of one in 2,500 to one in 10,000 deliveries.[16,72,288] While the neurosurgeon is only infrequently actively involved in the care of these patients, a basic understanding of the disease and treatment is required. In this section we briefly review current epidemiological, clinical, diagnostic, and therapeutic information to allow for management of cerebral venous thrombosis during pregnancy and the puerperium.

Epidemiology

Overview

Intracranial venous thrombotic disease remains a diagnostic challenge, mainly because of the protean, nonspecific initial symptoms such as headache with nausea and vomiting that rarely alert physicians to this specific diagnosis. Venous occlusion may involve one or more sinuses and/or the cerebral veins, either cortical or deep: typically, cerebral venous thrombosis is rarely limited to one sinus (<30% of cases[41]) and involves cortical veins more commonly than internal cerebral and cerebellar veins. The incidence of intracranial venous thrombosis is at best uncertain.[189] Autopsy studies have reported an incidence of superior sagittal sinus thrombosis ranging from 0.03% to a high of 9%.[20,90,302] Undoubtedly, the true clinical incidence is higher than identified by autopsy studies, and given the nonspecific clinical manifestations, intracranial venous thrombosis is probably significantly underdiagnosed in certain populations such as adolescents and young adults.[12]

Pregnancy, and more significantly the puerperium, is associated with an increased risk for intracranial venous thrombosis. The vast majority occur 3 days to 4 weeks after delivery, with 80% occurring in the second or third week postpartum.[16,91,179,287] A minority of patients actually present with cerebral venous thrombosis during pregnancy.[16,93,201]

Pathophysiology

The majority of patients with intracranial venous thrombosis are categorized as idiopathic after excluding trauma, infection (decreased substantially in North America and Europe during the modern "antibiotic era"), polycythemia vera, leukemia, dehydration, and sickle cell anemia.[20,41,103] The etiology during pregnancy and the puerperium in patients with idiopathic intracranial venous thrombosis is undoubtedly related to an ill-defined hypercagulable state.[14,35,59,65,66,83,85,91,112,198,267,290,331,332] Furthermore, up to about 12% of patients who present with intracranial thrombosis may have an underlying DVT or PE, further illustrating the systemic hypercoagulable state that exists in many of these patients.[87,288] Any additional factors that may predispose to a hypercoagulable state, such as the neurosurgical conditions previously discussed with reference to risk for DVT (e.g., stroke, brain tumors, and spinal cord injury), may enhance the risk potential.

Clinical Presentation

The symptoms of intracranial venous thrombosis are protean and nonspecific and may include headache and vomiting (almost 100%), seizures (50%-80%), focal neurological deficit (50%-60%), fever, and decreased level of consciousness ranging from slight alteration in mental status to coma (50%-60%).[16,41,103,179,288,298] Symptoms are caused by ischemic or hemorrhagic infarction, increased intracranial pressure secondary to cerebral edema, cerebral hemorrhage, or hydrocephalus.[196]

Diagnosis

The antemortem diagnosis of intracranial venous thrombosis is based upon a combination of clinical findings with radiographic confirmation of venous occlusion. Meningitis, tumors, arterial ischemic events, subarachnoid hemorrhage, or nonvenous occlusive intracerebral hemorrhage must be excluded. This is a diagnosis for which the clinician must have a high index of suspicion. Historically, the diagnosis was established with cerebral angiography;[10,195,197,333] however, the diagnosis can now be noninvasively confirmed with computed tomography (CT) scanning[50,55,242,258,314,322] and magnetic resonance imaging (MRI).[159,180,184,213,304] MRI technology, and now more specifically MR angiography (MRA) and MR venography (MRV), have effectively replaced cerebral angiography for the diagnosis of intracranial venous thrombosis, especially when thrombosis has occurred in a dural sinus.[184,216,241,260,265] CT is the most commonly utilized diagnostic modality during investigation of a patient with suspected intracranial venous thrombosis,[50,55,242,258,314,322] and can effectively rule out many potential etiologies. CT findings include hemorrhagic or nonhemorrhagic infarcts (Figure 1), cerebral edema, mass effect associated with small ventricles, enlarged ventricles, or subarachnoid space. In addition, a contrast-enhanced CT study may identify fresh thrombus in a thrombosed vein ("cord sign")[15] or in a dural sinus ("empty delta sign").[41,50,314] The "empty delta sign" (empty triangle or negative delta sign) represents dural leaf enhancement with central nonopacified thrombus in superior sinus thrombosis. This sign is relatively specific but only observed in about 10% to 30% of patients with intracranial venous thrombosis.[41,50,314]

MRI is undoubtedly the most sensitive noninvasive diagnostic modality available to identify intracranial venous thrombosis.[159,180,184,213,216,241,260,265,304] (Figures 1 and 2). Thrombus within the dural sinuses can be directly visualized because of the characteristic imaging signals produced by hemoglobin degradation products within the thrombosed sinuses.[184,213] Subacute thrombus has a characteristic hyperintense signal on T1-weighted images due to methemoglobin (Figure 2). Phase-contrast MRA techniques produce high signal from protons within flowing blood and can provide high-resolution venograms (Figure 1). In addition, MRI can identify intracerebral hematomas and cerebral infarction (hemorrhagic or nonhemorrhagic) and can rule out other diagnostic possibilities.

Angiographic evaluation includes the direct imaging and identification of the thrombosed part of the vessel (vein or dural sinus), including identification of the adjacent collateral venous drainage.[195,197,333] (Figure 1). In most situations angiography is not required to establish the diagnosis. However, cerebral angiography may be needed in highly suspect patients for whom the diagnosis cannot be confirmed by either CT or MRI (MRA/MRV) or in situations where MRI is not available. In addition, cerebral angiography may be necessary if endovascular treatment is required.[21,281] Previously discussed issues concerning exposure of the fetus to ionizing radiation also apply during the investigation of thrombosis. However, the relatively infrequent occurrence of this disorder during pregnancy limits this concern to a small subpopulation of patients.

Other diagnostic procedures including lumbar puncture and electroencephalography, radionucleotide imaging, and ultrasound imaging have a limited role in the diagnosis, although in certain situations one of these investigations may establish another diagnosis.

Management

Overview

Many patients with intracranial venous thrombosis will have mild to moderate symptoms and have a good prognosis. Although the general prognosis for this disease is believed to be quite good, patients who are very ill with this

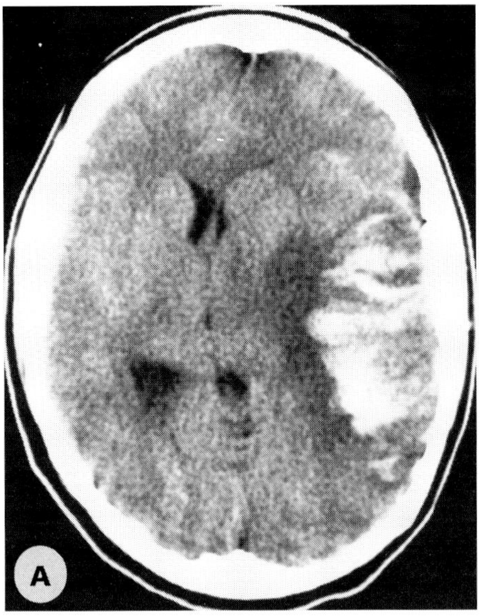

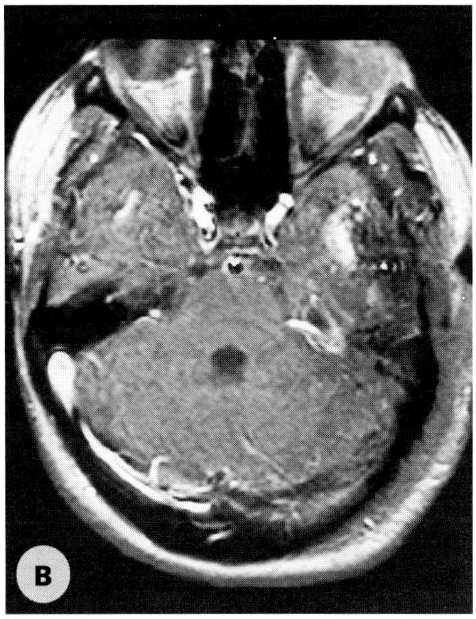

Figure 1: A) This 32-year-old female with a history of smoking presented with sudden loss of consciousness and right hemiparesis with a dilated fixed left pupil 4 days after a cesarean section. Axial CT scan demonstrates a hemorrhage in the left temporal and parietal lobes. Urgent surgery was performed to evacuate the hematoma. **B**) Postoperative MRI (TR 40, TE 5.0 Fr) scan demonstrates post-hemorrhage and surgical effects in the left temporal lobe and absent flow in the left transverse and sigmoid sinuses. Normal flow in the right transverse and sigmoid sinuses is hyperintense (white) with this imaging technique. The diagnosis was established as transverse and sigmoid sinus thrombosis. **C**) Venous phase angiogram after left vertebral injection. The right transverse sinus, sigmoid sinus, and jugular vein can be clearly seen, whereas flow through the left transverse and sigmoid sinuses is absent because of intraluminal thrombus. This patient made an uncomplicated early recovery and 6 months postoperatively had residual dysphasia but no hemiparesis.

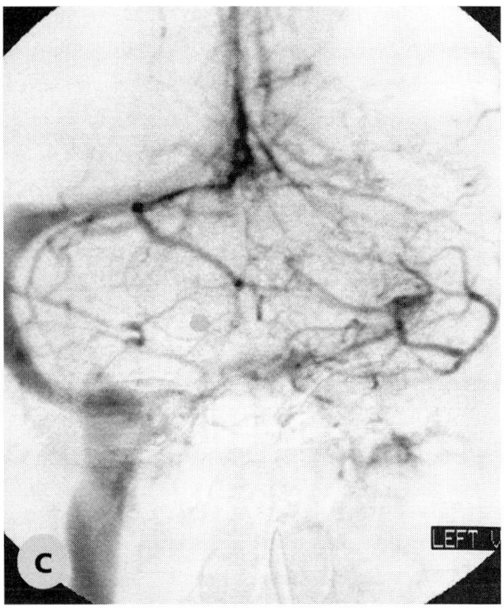

condition have a more unpredictable outcome. A major problem with establishing what comprises optimal management for these patients is the poor understanding about what constitutes the natural history for the various subgroups of patients with this disorder. Although favorable results have been reported for treatment with anticoagulants and/or fibrinolysis,[21,41,89,196,206] this is not universally accepted as standard of care.[103] Thus far, management recommendations for patients with this condition are based upon minimal Level II and maximal Level IV and V data (Grade C) or on experimental studies. With this understanding, the therapeutic goals for management of these patients can be organized into three subsets: 1) alleviation of the secondary effects associated with the venous thrombosis, such as seizures, cerebral edema, and raised intracranial pressure; 2) treatment of the intracranial venous thrombosis directly with anticoagulants, thrombolysis, or surgery; and 3) treatment of the underlying disease

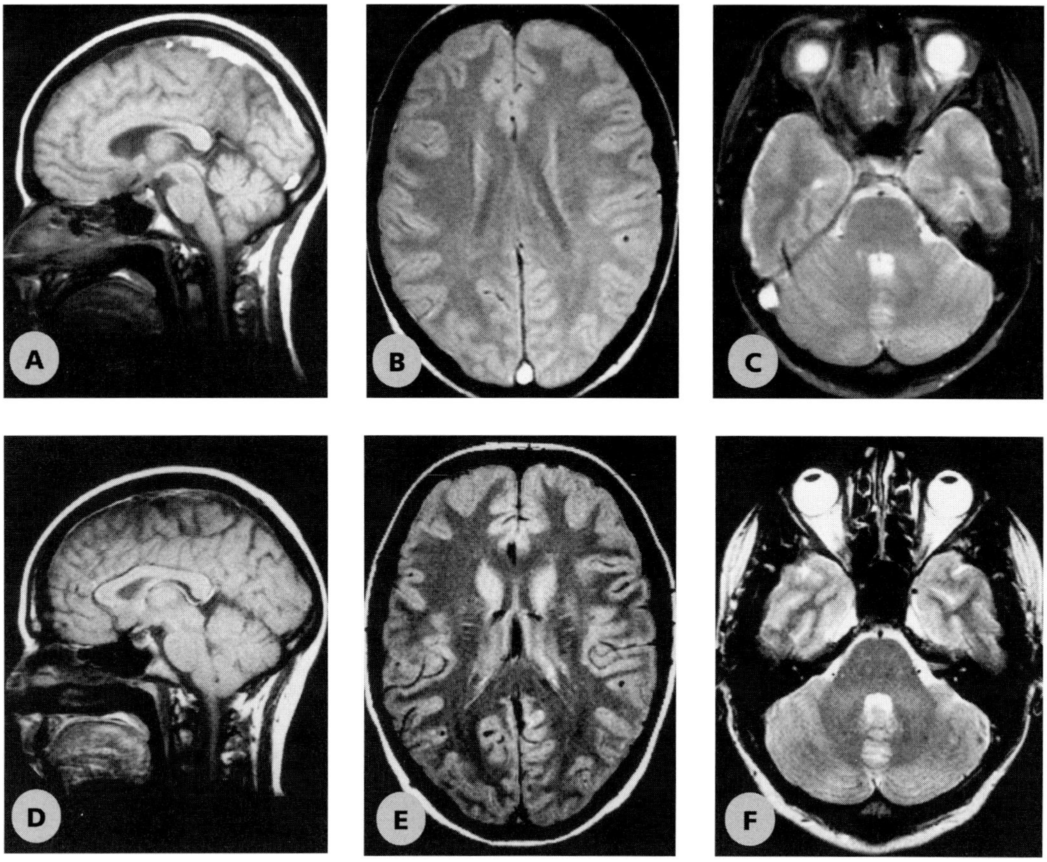

Figure 2: A) This 28-year-old female presented with severe headaches 3 weeks after a routine pregnancy and delivery. She had no neurological complaints and a normal neurological examination. Sagittal T1-weighted MRI (TR 600, TE 25) demonstrates hyperintense (white) subacute clot within the sagittal sinus and torcula. **B**) Axial T2-weighted MRI (TR 2000, TE 30) demonstrates hyperintense (white) clot within the sagittal sinus. **C**) Axial T2-weighted MRI (TR 2000, TE 25) demonstrates hyperintense (white) clot within the right sigmoid sinus. **D**) This patient was treated acutely with intravenous heparin followed by warfarin for 6 months. This follow-up sagittal T1-weighted MRI (TR 600, TE 27) demonstrates resolution of the sagittal sinus thrombus. **E**) Follow-up axial T2-weighted MRI (TR 2000, TE 18) demonstrates resolution of the sagittal sinus thrombus. **F**) Follow-up axial T2-weighted MRI (TR 3200, TE 90) demonstrates resolution of the sigmoid sinus thrombus.

process, such as infection or trauma (Table 3).

Treatment of symptoms is directed at alleviation of cerebral edema, hydrocephalus, and seizures. The methods for dealing with these neurosurgical problems include diuretics, mannitol, hyperventilation, ± barbiturates, ventriculostomy, and anticonvulsants.[41,91,103,134,214] The specifics of dealing with these problems are not reviewed in this section.

Treatment aimed directly at the thrombosis is more controversial and can be subdivided into three frequently overlapping categories: anticoagulation, fibrinolysis, and surgery.[21,41,69,91,196,206,259] Interestingly, the role of straightforward anticoagulation is less clear (Level II evidence; Grade B recommendation) than for fibrinolytic therapy or surgery, both of which are typically utilized in critically ill patients in an effort to salvage poor clinical situations (Level IV and V evidence; Grade C recommendation).

Anticoagulants have been used since the early 1940s[289] to treat patients with intracranial venous thrombosis. Most published information concerning the use of anticoagulants has at best been only Level IV or V evidence. Again, a failure to understand the natural history of this disease, reinforced by a lack of well-designed randomized controlled clinical trials, has

TABLE 3

Therapeutic Approaches to the Management of Intracranial Venous Thrombosis

Symptomatic Treatment

- Treat intracranial hypertension/edema (fluid restriction, diuretics, mannitol, barbiturates, hyperventilation)
- Ventricular drainage for hydrocephalus
- Anticonvulsants for seizures
- Surgical decompression for large hematomas
- General medical care of patient (stress ulcer prophylaxis, DVT/PE prophylaxis, blood pressure control, protect airway with intubation if necessary)

Intracranial Venous Thrombosis Treatment

- Heparin (high dose: 1,000 IU/hr to start; APTT >1.5-2 times control)
- Local (endovascular) or intravenous fibrinolysis (urokinase, streptokinase, tissue-type plasminogen activator) followed by heparinization
- Surgical thrombectomy or combined surgical/endovascular thrombectomy

Specific Treatment of Underlying Disease

- Antibiotics for infection
- Surgical drainage of infected sinuses or mastoidectomy for infection
- Treat dehydration if present

allowed the controversy concerning the anticoagulant management to continue for over 50 years. Concerns about using anticoagulation include increased risk of spontaneous bleeding, such as hemorrhagic transformation of infarcted areas, and the risk of precipitating disseminated intravascular coagulation. More recently, Einhäupl et al[89] in 1991 reported a small (20 patients), randomized, blinded placebo-controlled evaluation of heparin for treating patients with venous sinus thrombosis. These authors suggested that patients treated with dose-adjusted intravenous heparin had significantly better neurological outcome compared to placebo and recommended heparin anticoagulation (Level II evidence; Grade B recommendation). Furthermore, these authors also retrospectively evaluated 102 additional patients (Level IV evidence), suggesting no significant risk for intracerebral hemorrhage during treatment with heparin in the presence of a prior intracerebral hematoma and significantly lower mortality in those treated with heparin (15%) compared to those treated without heparin (69%). Data for the utilization of LMWHs are extremely limited (Level V evidence).[94] The role for long-term anticoagulation has not been adequately investigated.

The philosophy behind both fibrinolysis (streptokinase, urokinase, and tissue-type plasminogen activator) and surgery is that reestablishment of venous flow will significantly reduce cerebral venous hypertension.[21,41,89,91,196,206,259] Thrombolytic therapy can be administered systemically or directly into the jugular venous system or dural sinus at the site of thrombosis (via the transfemoral or transjugular approach). Thrombolysis is usually followed by standard anticoagulation. Although promising Level IV and V evidence suggests that these treatment methodologies may be quite effective, clinical experience is very limited and both should be considered only in the context of a controlled clinical study. Furthermore, systemic administration of thrombolytic agents is contraindicated in pregnant patients because of the risk of fetal and maternal hemorrhage, although local application of fibrinolytic agents may be considered, given the substantially lower doses that are required.

Treatment Recommendations

The prognosis for patients with intracranial venous thrombosis is not well-defined and the general impression is that most recover without serious sequelae. However, the average mortality rate for these patients is approximately 25%.[50,189,196,197,289] Undoubtedly, this disease has a spectrum of severity that extends from the minor clinical symptoms to coma and death. The ability to establish a clinical grading scale, define the natural history for the different clinical grades, and compare treatment for the different grades of patients would allow for confident treatment recommendations. At this time only Grade B and (mostly) Grade C recommendations can be offered (Table 3). All patients should be symptomatically treated. There is currently only limited evidence to support acute anticoagulation with intravenous heparin (Grade B recommendation). Long-term anticoagulant treatment is typically continued using warfarin for several months to several years[43] (Grade C recommendation). Fibrinolysis (systemically or locally administered) and surgery should be considered only in the context of a controlled clinical study with systemic fibrinolysis contraindicated during pregnancy.

REFERENCES

1. Aburahma AF, Bastug DF, Tiley EH III, et al: Management of deep vein thrombosis of the lower extremity in pregnancy. **W Va Med J 89:**445-447, 1993
2. Aiach M, Michaud A, Balian JL, et al: A new low molecular weight heparin derivative. *In vitro* and *in vivo* studies. **Thromb Res 31:**611-621, 1983
3. Albada J, Nieuwenhuis HK, Sixma JJ: Treatment of acute venous thromboembolism with low molecular weight heparin (Fragmin). Results of a double-blind randomized study. **Circulation 80:**935-940, 1989
4. Al-Mefty O, Fox JL, Smith RR: Petrosal approach for petroclival meningiomas. **Neurosurgery 22:**510-517, 1988
5. Al-Mefty O, Holoubi A, Rifai A, et al: Microsurgical removal of suprasellar meningiomas. **Neurosurgery 16:**364-372, 1985
6. Altschuler E, Moosa H, Selker RG, et al: The risk and efficacy of anticoagulant therapy in the treatment of thromboembolic complications in patients with primary malignant brain tumors. **Neurosurgery 27:** 74-77, 1990
7. Anderson DR, Ginsberg JS, Burrows R, et al: Subcutaneous heparin therapy during pregnancy: a need for concern at the time of delivery. **Thromb Haemost 65:**248-250, 1991
8. Anderson DR, Levine MN: Thrombolytic therapy for the treatment of acute pulmonary embolism. **Can Med Assoc J 146:**1317-1324, 1992
9. Arcelus JI, Caprini JA, Traverso CI: International perspective on venous thromboembolism prophylaxis in surgery. **Semin Thromb Hemost 17:**322-325, 1991
10. Askenasy HM, Kosary IZ, Braham J: Thrombosis of the longitudinal sinus. Diagnosis by carotid angiography. **Neurology 12:**288-292, 1962
11. Atrash HK, Koonin LM, Lawson HW, et al: Maternal mortality in the United States, 1979-1986. **Obstet Gynecol 76:**1055-1060, 1990
12. Averback P: Primary cerebral venous thrombosis in young adults: the diverse manifestations of an underrecognized disease. **Ann Neurol 3:**81-86, 1979
13. Badaracco MA, Vessey MP: Recurrence of venous thromboembolic disease and use of oral contraceptives. **Br Med J 1:**215-217, 1974
14. Ballegeer V, Mombaerts P, Declerck PJ, et al: Fibrinolytic response to venous occlusion and fibrin fragment D-Dimer levels in normal and complicated pregnancy. **Thromb Haemost 58:**1030-1032, 1987
15. Banna M, Groves JT: Deep vascular congestion in dural venous thrombosis on computed tomography. **J Comput Assist Tomogr 3:**539-541, 1979
16. Bansal BC, Gupta RR, Prakash C: Stroke during pregnancy and puerperium in young females below the age of 40 years as a result of cerebral venous/venous sinus thrombosis. **Jpn Heart J 21:** 171-183, 1980
17. Bara L, Billaud E, Gramond G, et al: Comparative pharmacokinetics of a low molecular weight heparin (PK 10 169) and unfractionated heparin after intravenous and subcutaneous administration. **Thromb Res 39:**631-636, 1985
18. Barbour LA, Kick SD, Steiner JF, et al: A prospective study of heparin-induced osteoporosis in pregnancy using bone densitometry. **Am J Obstet Gynecol 170:** 862-869, 1994
19. Barnett HG, Clifford JR, Llewellyn RC: Safety of mini-dose heparin administration for neurosurgical patients. **J Neurosurg 47:**27-30, 1977
20. Barnett HJM, Hyland HH: Non-infective intracranial venous thrombosis. **Brain 76:**36-49, 1953
21. Barnwell SL, Higashida RT, Halbach VV, et al: Direct endovascular thrombolytic therapy for dural sinus thrombosis. **Neurosurgery 28:**135-142, 1991
22. Becker DM, Gonzalez M, Gentili A, et al: Prevention of deep venous thrombosis in patients with acute spinal cord injuries: use of rotating treatment tables. **Neurosurgery 20:**675-677, 1987
23. Benotti JR, Dalen JE: The natural history of pulmonary embolism. **Clin Chest Med 5:**403-410, 1984
24. Bergqvist A, Bergqvist D, Hallböök T: Deep vein thrombosis during pregnancy: a prospective study. **Acta Obstet Gynecol Scand 62:**443-448, 1983
25. Bergqvist D: Current trends in the management of postsurgical thromboembolism: the role of low molecular weight heparin. **Semin Thromb Hemost 17:** 332-335, 1991
26. Bergqvist D: Perioperative hemorrhagic complications in patients on low molecular weight heparins. **Semin Thromb Hemost 19 (Suppl 1):**128-130, 1993
27. Bergqvist D: Principal view on dose adjustment of low molecular weight heparins. **Semin Thromb Hemost 19 (Suppl 1):**107-110, 1993
28. Bergqvist D, Bergentz SE: Diagnosis of deep vein thrombosis. **World J Surg 14:**679-687, 1990
29. Bergqvist D, Hedner U, Sjörin E, et al: Anticoagulant effects of two types of low molecular weight heparin administered subcutaneously. **Thromb Res 32:** 381-391, 1983
30. Black PM, Baker MF, Snook CP: Experience with external pneumatic calf compression in neurology and neurosurgery. **Neurosurgery 18:**440-444, 1986
31. Black PM, Crowell RM, Abbott WM: External pneumatic calf compression reduces DVT in patients with ruptured intracranial aneurysms. **Neurosurgery 18:** 25-28, 1986
32. Blaisdell FW: Acquired and congenital clotting syndromes. **World J Surg 14:**664-669, 1990
33. Blaisdell FW: Preventing postoperative thromboembolism. **West J Med 151:**188-189, 1989 (Editorial)
34. Bonnar J: Venous thromboembolism and pregnancy. **Clin Obstet Gynecol 8:**455-473, 1981
35. Bonnar J, McNichol GP, Douglas AS: Fibrinolytic enzyme system and pregnancy. **Br Med J 3:**387-389, 1969
36. Bornstein NM, Norris JW: Deep vein thrombosis after ischemic stroke: rationale for a therapeutic trial. **Arch Phys Med Rehabil 69:**955-958, 1988

37. Bors E, Conrad CA, Massell TB: Venous occlusion of lower extremities in paraplegic patients. **Surg Gynecol Obstet 99**:451-454, 1954
38. Boström S, Holmgren E, Jonsson O, et al: Fibrinopeptide A and fibrinogen fragment B(β)15-42 and their relation to the operative trauma and postoperative thromboembolism in neurosurgical patients. **Acta Neurochir 88**:49-55, 1987
39. Boström S, Holmgren E, Jonsson O, et al: Post-operative thromboembolism in neurosurgery. A study on the prophylactic effect of calf muscle stimulation plus dextran compared to low-dose heparin. **Acta Neurochir 80**:83-89, 1986
40. Bounds JV, Wiebers DO, Whisnant JP, et al: Mechanisms and timing of deaths from cerebral infarction. **Stroke 12**:474-477, 1981
41. Bousser MG, Chiras J, Bories J, et al: Cerebral venous thrombosis—a review of 38 cases. **Stroke 16**:199-213, 1985
42. Brach BB, Moser KM, Cedar L, et al: Venous thrombosis in acute spinal cord paralysis. **J Trauma 17**: 289-292, 1977
43. Bratt G, Åberg W, Johansson M, et al: Two daily subcutaneous injections of Fragmin as compared with intravenous standard heparin in the treatment of deep vein thrombosis (DVT). **Thromb Haemost 64**: 506-510, 1990
44. Bratt G, Törnebohm E, Granqvist S, et al: A comparison between low molecular weight heparin (Kabi 2165) and standard heparin in the intravenous treatment of deep venous thrombosis. **Thromb Haemost 54**:813-817, 1985
45. Bratt G, Törnebohm E, Widlund L, et al: Low molecular weight heparin (Kabi 2165, Fragmin): pharmacokinetics after intravenous and subcutaneous administration in human volunteers. **Thromb Res 42**:613-620, 1986
46. Breddin HK: Thrombosis and Virchow's triad: what is established? **Semin Thromb Hemost 15**:237-239, 1991
47. Brisman R, Mendell J: Thromboembolism and brain tumors. **J Neurosurg 38**:337-338, 1973
48. Bucci MN, Papadopoulos SM, Chen JC, et al: Mechanical prophylaxis of venous thromboembolism in patients undergoing craniotomy: a randomized trial. **Surg Neurol 32**:285-288, 1989
49. Buchanan DS, Brazinsky JH: Dural sinus and cerebral venous thrombosis. Incidence in young women receiving oral contraceptives. **Arch Neurol 22**:440, 1970
50. Buonanno FS, Moody DM, Ball MR, et al: Computed cranial tomographic findings in cerebral sinovenous occlusion. **J Comput Assist Tomogr 2**: 281, 1978
51. Bussey HI, Force RW, Bianco TM, et al: Reliance on prothrombin time ratios causes significant errors in anticoagulation therapy. **Arch Intern Med 152**: 278-282, 1992
52. Bynke O, Hillman J, Lassvik C: Does peroperative external pneumatic leg muscle compression prevent post-operative venous thrombosis in neurosurgery? **Acta Neurochir 88**:46-48, 1987
53. Caprini JA, Arcelus JI, Traverso CI, et al: Low molecular weight heparins and external pneumatic compression as options for venous thromboembolism prophylaxis: a surgeon's perspective. **Semin Thromb Hemost 17**:356-366, 1991
54. Cerrato D, Ariano C, Fiacchino F: Deep vein thrombosis and low-dose heparin prophylaxis in neurosurgical patients. **J Neurosurg 49**:378-381, 1978
55. Chiras J, Bousser MG, Meder JF, et al: CT in cerebral thrombophlebitis. **Neuroradiology 27**:145-154, 1985
56. Choucair AK, Silver P, Levin VA: Risk of intracranial hemorrhage in glioma patients receiving anticoagulant therapy for venous thromboembolism. **J Neurosurg 66**:357-358, 1987
57. Clagett GP, Anderson FA Jr, Levine MN, et al: Prevention of venous thromboembolism. **Chest 102 (Suppl)**:391S-407S, 1992
58. Clagett GP, Reisch JS: Prevention of venous thromboembolism in general surgical patients. Results of meta-analysis. **Ann Surg 208**:227-240, 1988
59. Clarke-Pearson DL, Hume RF Jr: Venous thromboembolic disease in obstetrics and gynecology: prevention, diagnosis, and treatment. **Curr Probl Obstet Gynecol Fertil 12**:38-63, 1989
60. Clarke-Pearson DL, Jelovsek FR: Alterations of occlusive cuff impedance plethysmography results in the obstetric patient. **Surgery 89**:594-598, 1981
61. A Collaborative European Multicentre Study: A randomized trial of subcutaneous low molecular weight heparin (CY 216) compared with intravenous unfractionated heparin in the treatment of deep vein thrombosis. **Thromb Haemost 65**:251-256, 1991
62. Collins R, Scrimgeour A, Yusuf S, et al: Reduction in fatal pulmonary embolism and venous thrombosis by perioperative administration of subcutaneous heparin. Overview of results of randomized trials in general, orthopedic and urologic surgery. **N Engl J Med 318**:1162-1172, 1988
63. Colvin BT, Barrowcliffe TW: The British Society for Haematology guidelines on the use and monitoring of heparin 1992: second revision. **J Clin Pathol 46**: 97-103, 1993
64. Comerota AJ, White JV, Katz ML: Diagnostic methods for deep vein thrombosis: venous Doppler examination, phleborheography, iodine-125 fibrinogen uptake, and phlebography. **Am J Surg 150(4A)**: 14-24, 1985
65. Comp PC, Thurnau GR, Welsh J, et al: Functional and immunologic protein S levels are decreased during pregnancy. **Blood 68**:881-885, 1986
66. Conard J, Horellou MH, Van Dreden P, et al: Thrombosis and pregnancy in congenital deficiencies in AT III, protein C or protein S: study of 78 women. **Thromb Haemost 63**:319-320, 1990 (Letter)
67. Constantini S, Kornowski R, Pomeranz S, et al: Thromboembolic phenomena in neurosurgical patients operated upon for primary and metastatic brain tumours. **Acta Neurochir 109**:93-97, 1991
68. Cook DJ, Guyatt GH, Laupacis A, et al: Rules of evidence and clinical recommendations on the use of antithrombotic agents. **Chest 102 (Suppl)**: 305S-311S, 1992
69. Coon WW: Venous thromboembolism. Prevalance, risk factors, and prevention. **Clin Chest Med 5**: 391-401, 1984
70. Cranley JJ, Canos AJ, Sull WJ: The diagnosis of deep venous thrombosis. Fallibility of clinical symptoms and signs. **Arch Surg 111**:34-36, 1976
71. Cronan JJ, Dorfman GS: Advances in ultrasound imaging of venous thrombosis. **Semin Nucl Med 21**:

297-312, 1991
72. Cross JN, Castro PO, Jennett WB: Cerebral strokes associated with pregnancy and the puerperium. **Br Med J 3:**214-218, 1968
73. Cruickshank MK, Levine MN, Hirsh J, et al: A standard heparin nomogram for the management of heparin therapy. **Arch Intern Med 151:**333-337, 1991
74. Dahlman T, Lindvall N, Hellgren M: Osteopenia in pregnancy during long-term heparin treatment: a radiological study post partum. **Br J Obstet Gynaecol 97:**221-228, 1990
75. Dahlman TC: Osteoporotic fractures and the recurrence of thromboembolism during pregnancy and the puerperium in 184 women undergoing thromboprophylaxis with heparin. **Am J Obstet Gynecol 168:**1265-1270, 1993
76. Dahlman TC, Hellgren MSE, Blombäck M: Thrombosis prophylaxis in pregnancy with use of subcutaneous heparin adjusted by monitoring heparin concentration in plasma. **Am J Obstet Gynecol 161:** 420-425, 1989
77. Dahlman TC, Sjöberg HE, Ringertz H: Bone mineral density during long-term prophylaxis with heparin in pregnancy. **Am J Obstet Gynecol 170:**1315-1320, 1994
78. Dalen JE, Alpert JS: Natural history of pulmonary embolism. **Prog Cardiovasc Dis 17:**259-270, 1975
79. Dalen JE, Hirsh J: American College of Chest Physicians and the National Heart, Lung, and Blood Institute National Conference on Antithrombic Therapy. **Arch Intern Med 146:**462-472, 1986
80. Dalen JE, Paraskos JA, Ockene IS, et al: Venous thromboembolism. Scope of the problem. **Chest 89 (Suppl):**370S-373S, 1986
81. de Boer K, Büller HR, ten Cate JW, et al: Deep vein thrombosis in obstetric patients: diagnosis and risk factors. **Thromb Haemost 67:**4-7, 1992
82. de Boer K, Heyboer H, ten Cate JW, et al: Low molecular weight heparin treatment in a pregnant woman with allergy to standard heparins and heparinoid. **Thromb Haemost 61:**1481, 989 (Letter)
83. Demers C, Ginsberg JS: Deep venous thrombosis and pulmonary embolism in pregnancy. **Clin Chest Med 13:**645-656, 1992
84. Denham MJ, Farran H, James G: The value of ^{125}I fibrinogen in the diagnosis of deep venous thrombosis in hemiplegia. **Age Ageing 2:**207-210, 1973
85. De Stefano V, Leone G, Mastrangelo A, et al: Thrombosis during pregnancy and surgery in patients with congenital deficiency of antithrombin III, protein C, protein S. **Thromb Haemost 71:**799-780, 1994
86. DeVivo MJ, Kartus PL, Stover SL, et al: Cause of death for patients with spinal cord injuries. **Arch Intern Med 149:**1761-1766, 1989
87. Diaz JM, Schiffman JS, Urban ES, et al: Superior sagittal sinus thrombosis and pulmonary embolism: a syndrome rediscovered. **Acta Neurol Scand 86:** 390-396, 1992
88. Di Ricco G, Marini C, Rindi M, et al: Pulmonary embolism in neurosurgical patients: diagnosis and treatment. **J Neurosurg 60:**972-975,1984
89. Einhäupl KM, Villringer A, Meister W, et al: Heparin treatment in sinus venous thrombosis. **Lancet 338:**597-600, 1991
90. Erez N, Babuna C, Uner A: Low incidence of thromboembolic disease. An evaluation of obstetric and gynecologic patients in Istanbul. **Obstet Gynecol 27:**833-837, 1966
91. Estanol B, Rodriguez A, Conte G, et al: Intracranial venous thrombosis in young women. **Stroke 10:** 680-684, 1979
92. Fareed J: Venous thromboembolism in the 1990s: a perspective. **Semin Thromb Hemost 17:**317-321, 1991
93. Fehr PE: Sagittal sinus thrombosis in early pregnancy. **Obstet Gynecol 59 (Suppl):**7-9, 1982
94. Février MJ, Nguyen JP, Brugières P, et al: Thrombophlébe du sinus longitudinal supérieur au stade chirurgical. A propos d'un cas. Intérêt de l'héparine de bas poids moléculaire. **Neurochirurgie 33:** 490-493, 1987
95. Flinn WR, Sandager GP, Cerullo LJ, et al: Duplex venous scanning for the prospective surveillance of perioperative venous thrombosis. **Arch Surg 124:** 901-905, 1989
96. Forestier F, Sole Y, Aiach M, et al: Absence of transplacental passage of Fragmin (Kabi) during the second and the third trimesters of pregnancy. **Thromb Haemost 67:**180-181, 1992 (Letter)
97. Frim DM, Barker FG II, Poletti CE, et al: Postoperative low-dose heparin decreases thromboembolic complications in neurosurgical patients. **Neurosurgery 30:**830-833, 1992
98. Frisbie JH, Sasahara AA: Low dose heparin prophylaxis for deep venous thrombosis in acute spinal cord injury patients: a controlled study. **Paraplegia 19:** 343-346, 1981
99. Frydman AM, Bara L, Le Roux Y, et al: The antithrombotic activity and pharmacokinetics of enoxaparine, a low molecular weight heparin, in humans given single subcutaneous doses of 20 to 80 mg. **J Clin Pharmacol 28:**609-618, 1988
100. Fulkerson WJ, Coleman RE, Ravin CE, et al: Diagnosis of pulmonary embolism. **Arch Intern Med 146:** 961-967, 1986
101. Gallus A, Jackaman J, Tillett J, et al: Safety and efficacy of warfarin started early after submassive venous thrombosis or pulmonary embolism. **Lancet 2:**1293-1296, 1986
102. Gelmers HJ: Effects of low-dose subcutaneous heparin on the occurrence of deep vein thrombosis in patients with ischemic stroke. **Acta Neurol Scand 61:**313-318, 1980
103. Gettelfinger DM, Kokmen E: Superior sagittal sinus thrombosis. **Arch Neurol 34:**2-6, 1977
104. Gibberd FB, Gould SR, Marks P: Incidence of deep vein thrombosis and leg oedema in patients with strokes. **J Neurol Neurosurg Psychiatry 39:** 1222-1225, 1976
105. Gillis S, Shushan A, Eldor A: Use of low molecular weight heparin for prophylaxis and treatment of thromboembolism in pregnancy. **Int J Gynaecol Obstet 39:**297-301, 1992
106. Ginsberg JS, Brill-Edwards P, Burrows RF, et al: Venous thrombosis during pregnancy. Leg and trimester of presentation. **Thromb Haemost 67:** 519-520, 1992
107. Ginsberg JS, Hirsh J: Use of antithrombotic agents during pregnancy. **Chest 102 (Suppl):**385S-390S, 1992
108. Ginsberg JS, Hirsh J, Rainbow AJ, et al: Risks to the fetus of radiologic procedures used in the diagnosis

of maternal venous thromboembolic disease. **Thromb Haemost 61**:189-196, 1989
109. Ginsberg JS, Hirsh J, Turner DC, et al: Risks to the fetus of anticoagulant therapy during pregnancy. **Thromb Haemost 61**:197-203, 1989
110. Ginsberg JS, Kowalchuk G, Hirsh J, et al: Heparin effect on bone density. **Thromb Haemost 64**: 286-289, 1990
111. Ginsberg JS, Kowalchuk G, Hirsh J, et al: Heparin therapy during pregnancy. Risks to the fetus and mother. **Arch Intern Med 149**:2233-2236, 1989
112. Gjønnaess H, Fagerhol MK: Studies on coagulation and fibrinolysis in pregnancy. With special reference to cold activation of Factor VII. **Acta Obstet Gynecol Scand 54**:363-367, 1975
113. Goldhaber SZ: Evolving concepts in thrombolytic therapy for pulmonary embolism. **Chest 101 (Suppl)**:183S-185S, 1992
114. Goldhaber SZ: Tissue plasminogen activator in acute pulmonary embolism. **Chest 95 (Suppl)**:282S-289S, 1989
115. Goldhaber SZ, Morpurgo M: Diagnosis, treatment, and prevention of pulmonary embolism. Report of the WHO/International Society and Federation of Cardiology Task Force. **JAMA 268**:1727-1733, 1992
116. Goodall RJR, Greenfield LJ: Clinical correlations in the diagnosis of pulmonary embolism. **Ann Surg 191**:219-223, 1980
117. Gore JM: Prevention of severe neurologic events in the thrombolytic era. **Chest 101 (Suppl)**:124S-130S, 1992
118. Green D, Hirsh J, Heit J, et al: Low molecular weight heparin: a critical analysis of clinical trials. **Pharmacol Rev 46**:89-109, 1994
119. Green D, Lee MY, Ito VY, et al: Fixed- vs adjusted-dose heparin in the prophylaxis of thromboembolism in spinal cord injury. **JAMA 260**:1255-1258, 1988
120. Green D, Lee MY, Lim AC, et al: Prevention of thromboembolism after spinal cord injury using low-molecular-weight heparin. **Ann Intern Med 113**:571-574, 1990
121. Green D, Rossi EC, Yao JST, et al: Deep vein thrombosis in spinal cord injury: effect of prophylaxis with calf compression, aspirin, and dipyridamole. **Paraplegia 20**:227-234, 1982
122. Greenfield LJ, Michna BA: Twelve-year clinical experience with the Greenfield vena caval filter. **Surgery 104**:706-712, 1988
123. Greengard JS, Eichinger S, Griffin JH, et al: Brief report: variability of thrombosis among homozygous siblings with resistance to activated protein C due to an Arg to Gln mutation in the gene for factor V. **N Engl J Med 331**:1559-1562, 1994
124. Greinacher A, Michels I, Mueller-Eckhardt C: Heparin-associated thrombocytopenia: the antibody is not heparin specific. **Thromb Haemost 67**: 545-551, 1992
125. Griffiths HT, Liu DTY: Severe heparin osteoporosis in pregnancy. **Postgrad Med J 60**:424-425, 1984
126. Gruber UF, Saldeen T, Brokop T, et al: Incidences of fatal postoperative pulmonary embolism after prophylaxis with dextran 70 and low-dose heparin: an international multicentre study. **Br Med J 280**:69-72, 1980
127. Gruber UF, Thöni F: Prevention of thromboembolic complications in paraplegics. **Paraplegia 23**:124, 1985
128. Haas S, Blümel G: An objective evaluation of the clinical potential of low molecular weight heparins in the prevention of thromboembolism. **Semin Thromb Hemost 15**:424-434, 1989
129. Haas S, Haas P: Efficacy of low molecular weight heparins: an overview. **Semin Thromb Hemost 19 (Suppl 1)**:101-106, 1993
130. Hachen HJ: Anticoagulant therapy in patients with spinal cord injury. **Paraplegia 12**:176-187, 1974
131. Hall JG, Pauli RM, Wilson KM: Maternal and fetal sequelae of anticoagulation during pregnancy. **Am J Med 68**:122-140, 1978
132. Hamilton MG, Hull RD, Pineo GF: Prophylaxis of venous thromboembolism in brain tumor patients. **J Neurooncol 22**:111-126, 1994
133. Hamilton MG, Hull RD, Pineo GF: Venous thromboembolism in neurosurgery and neurology patients: a review. **Neurosurgery 34**:280-296, 1994
134. Hanley DF, Feldman E, Borel CO, et al: Treatment of sagittal sinus thrombosis associated with cerebral hemorrhage and intracranial hypertension. **Stroke 19**:903-909, 1988
135. Harenberg J, Huck K, Bratsch H, et al: Therapeutic application of subcutaneous low-molecular-weight heparin in acute venous thrombosis. **Haemostasis 20 (Suppl 1)**:205-219, 1990
136. Harenberg J, Würzner B, Zimmermann R, et al: Bioavailability and antagonization of the low molecular weight heparin CY 216 in man. **Thromb Res 44**: 549-554, 1986
137. Hauch O, Khattar SC, Jørgensen LN: Cost-benefit analysis of prophylaxis against deep vein thrombosis in surgery. **Semin Thromb Hemost 17 (Suppl)**: 280-283, 1991
138. Heijboer H, Büller HR, Lensing A-WA, et al: A comparison of real-time compression ultrasonography with impedance plethysmography for the diagnosis of deep-vein thrombosis in symptomatic outpatients. **N Engl J Med 329**:1365-1369, 1993
139. Heijboer H, ten Cate JW, Buller HR: Diagnosis of venous thrombosis. **Semin Thromb Hemost 17 (Suppl)**:259-268, 1991
140. Hellgren M, Hahn L, Dahlman T: Thromboprophylaxis during pregnancy. **Am J Obstet Gynecol 162**: 1338, 1990 (Letter)
141. Hellgren M, Nygårds EB: Long-term therapy with subcutaneous heparin during pregnancy. **Gynecol Obstet Invest 13**:76-89, 1982
142. Hemker HC: A standard for low molecular weight heparins? **Haemostasis 19**:1-4, 1989 (Editorial)
143. Hirsh J: Low molecular weight heparin. **Thromb Haemost 70**:204-207, 1993
144. Hirsh J: Substandard monitoring of warfarin therapy in North America. Time for change. **Arch Intern Med 152**:257-258, 1992 (Editorial)
145. Hirsh J, Deykin D, Poller L: "Therapeutic range" for oral anticoagulant therapy. **Chest 89 (Suppl)**: 11S-15S, 1986
146. Hirsh J, Hull RD: Treatment of venous thromboembolism. **Chest 89 (Suppl)**:426S-433S, 1986
147. Hirsh J, Levine M: Therapeutic range for the control of oral anticoagulant therapy. **Arch Neurol 43**: 1162-1164, 1986
148. Hirsh J, Levine MN: Low molecular weight heparin.

Blood 79:1-17, 1992
149. Hirsh J, Levine MN: The optimal intensity of oral anticoagulant therapy. **JAMA 258:**2723-2726, 1987
150. Hirsh J, Poller L, Deykin D, et al: Optimal therapeutic range for oral anticoagulants. **Chest 95 (Suppl):** 5S-11S, 1989
151. Hirsh J, Turpie AGG: Use of plasminogen activators in venous thrombosis. **World J Surg 14:**688-693, 1990
152. Holm HA, Ly B, Handeland GF, et al: Subcutaneous heparin treatment of deep vein thrombosis: a comparison of unfractionated and low molecular weight heparin. **Haemostasis 16 (Suppl 2):**30-37, 1986
153. Hommes DW, Bura A, Mazzolai L, et al: Subcutaneous heparin compared with continuous intravenous heparin administration in the initial treatment of deep vein thrombosis. A meta-analysis. **Ann Intern Med 116:**279-284, 1992
154. Howell R, Fidler J, Letsky E, et al: The risks of antenatal subcutaneous heparin prophylaxis: a controlled trial. **Br J Obstet Gynaecol 90:**1124-1128, 1983
155. Huet Y, Janvier G, Bendriss PH, et al: Treatment of established venous thromboembolism with Enoxaparin: preliminary report. **Acta Chir Scand 556 (Suppl):**116-120, 1990
156. Huisman MV, Büller HR, Ten Cate JW, et al: Management of clinically suspected acute venous thrombosis in outpatients with serial impedance plethysmography in a community hospital setting. **Arch Intern Med 149:**511-513, 1989
157. Huisman MV, Büller HR, ten Cate JW, et al: Serial impedance plethysmography for suspected deep venous thrombosis in outpatients. The Amsterdam general practitioner study. **N Engl J Med 314:** 823-828, 1986
158. Huisman MV, Nurmohamed M, ten Cate JW: Mechanical prophylaxis of deep vein thrombosis. **Semin Thromb Hemost 17 (Suppl):**269-271, 1991
159. Hulcelle PJ, Dooms GC, Mathurin P, et al: MRI assessment of unsuspected dural sinus thrombosis. **Neuroradiology 31:**217-221, 1989
160. Hull R, Delmore T, Carter C, et al: Adjusted subcutaneous heparin versus warfarin sodium in the long-term treatment of venous thrombosis. **N Engl J Med 306:**189-194, 1982
161. Hull R, Hirsh J, Jay R, et al: Different intensities of oral anticoagulant therapy in the treatment of proximal-vein thrombosis. **N Engl J Med 307:**1676-1681, 1982
162. Hull R, Hirsh J, Sackett DL, et al: Cost effectiveness of clinical diagnosis, venography, and noninvasive testing in patients with symptomatic deep-vein thrombosis. **N Engl J Med 304:**1561-1567, 1981
163. Hull R, Raskob G, Pineo G, et al: A comparison of subcutaneous low-molecular-weight heparin with warfarin sodium for prophylaxis against deep-vein thrombosis after hip or knee implantation. **N Engl J Med 329:**1370-1376, 1993
164. Hull RD, Hirsh J, Carter CJ, et al: Diagnostic efficacy of impedance plethysmography for clinically suspected deep-vein thrombosis. A randomized trial. **Ann Intern Med 102:**21-28, 1985
165. Hull RD, Hirsh J, Carter CJ, et al: Diagnostic value of ventilation-perfusion lung scanning in patients with suspected pulmonary embolism. **Chest 88:**819-828, 1985
166. Hull RD, Hirsh J, Carter CJ, et al: Pulmonary angiography, ventilation lung scanning, and venography for clinically suspected pulmonary embolism with abnormal perfusion lung scan. **Ann Intern Med 98:** 891-899, 1983
167. Hull RD, Hirsh J, Sackett DL, et al: Cost-effectiveness of primary and secondary prevention of fatal pulmonary embolism in high-risk surgical patients. **Can Med Assoc J 127:**990-995, 1982
168. Hull RD, Pineo GF: Therapeutic use of low molecular weight heparins: The knowledge to date as applied to therapy. **Semin Thromb Hemost 19 (Suppl 1):**111-115, 1993
169. Hull RD, Raskob GE, Carter CJ: Serial impedance plethysmography in pregnant patients with clinically suspected deep-vein thrombosis. Clinical validity of negative findings. **Ann Intern Med 112:**663-667, 1990
170. Hull RD, Raskob GE, Hirsh J, et al: Continuous intravenous heparin compared with intermittent subcutaneous heparin in the initial treatment of proximal-vein thrombosis. **N Engl J Med 315:** 1109-1114, 1986
171. Hull RD, Raskob GE, Hirsh J: The diagnosis of clinically suspected pulmonary embolism. Practical approaches. **Chest 89 (Suppl):**417S-425S, 1986
172. Hull RD, Raskob GE, Hirsh J: Prophylaxis of venous thromboembolism. An overview. **Chest 89 (Suppl):**374S-383S, 1986
173. Hull RD, Raskob GE, LeClerc JR, et al: The diagnosis of clinically suspected venous thrombosis. **Clin Chest Med 5:**439-456, 1984
174. Hull RD, Raskob GE, Pineo GF, et al: Subcutaneous low-molecular-weight heparin compared with continuous intravenous heparin in the treatment of proximal-vein thrombosis. **N Engl J Med 326:** 975-982, 1992
175. Hull RD, Raskob GE, Rosenbloom D, et al: Heparin for 5 days as compared with 10 days in the initial treatment of proximal venous thrombosis. **N Engl J Med 322:**1260-1264, 1990
176. Hull RD, Raskob GE, Rosenbloom D, et al: Optimal therapeutic level of heparin therapy in patients with venous thrombosis. **Arch Intern Med 152:** 1589-1595, 1992
177. Husted SE: Principles of thromboprophylaxis in surgical patients. **Semin Thromb Hemost 17 (Suppl):**254-258, 1991
178. Hyers TM, Hull RD, Weg JG: Antithrombotic therapy for venous thromboembolic disease. **Chest 95:** 37-51, 1989
179. Imai WK, Everhart FR Jr, Sanders JM Jr: Cerebral venous sinus thrombosis: report of a case and review of the literature. **Pediatrics 70:**965-970, 1982
180. Irving RM, Jones NS, Hall-Craggs MA, et al: View from within: radiology in focus. CT and MR imaging in lateral sinus thrombosis. **J Laryngol Otol 105:** 693-695, 1991
181. Janssen HF, Schachner J, Hubbard J, et al: The risk of deep venous thrombosis: a computerized epidemiologic approach. **Surgery 101:**205-212, 1987
182. Jarrell BE, Posuniak E, Roberts J, et al: A new method of management using the Kim-Ray Greenfield filter for deep venous thrombosis and pulmonary embolism in spinal cord injury. **Surg Gynecol Obstet 157:** 316-320, 1983
183. Joffe SN: Incidence of postoperative deep vein thrombosis in neurosurgical patients. **J Neurosurg**

42:201-203, 1975
184. Johnson BA, Fram EK: Cerebral venous occlusive disease: pathophysiology, clinical manifestations, and imaging. **Neuroimaging Clin North Am 2**:769, 1991
185. Juni JE, Alavi A: Lung scanning in the diagnosis of pulmonary embolism: the emperor redressed. **Semin Nucl Med 21**:281-296, 1991
186. Kakkar VV: Pathophysiologic characteristics of venous thrombosis. **Am J Surg 150(4A)**:1-6, 1985
187. Kakkar VV, Murray WJG: Efficacy and safety of low-molecular-weight heparin (CY216) in preventing postoperative thrombo-embolism: a co-operative study. **Br J Surg 72**:786-791, 1985
188. Kakkar VV, Stringer MD: Prophylaxis of venous thromboembolism. **World J Surg 14**:670-678, 1990
189. Kalbag RM, Woolf AL: **Cerebral Venous Thrombosis.** London: Oxford University, 1967
190. Kaufman HH, Satterwhite T, McConnell BJ, et al: Deep vein thrombosis and pulmonary embolism in head injured patients. **Angiology 34**:627-638, 1983
191. Kayser-Gatchalian MC, Kayser K: Thrombosis and intracranial tumors. **J Neurol 209**:217-224, 1975
192. Kempczinski RF: Surgical prophylaxis of pulmonary embolism. **Chest 89 (Suppl)**:384S-388S, 1986
193. Kessler CM: Anticoagulation and thrombolytic therapy. Practical considerations. **Chest 95 (Suppl)**: 245S-256S, 1989
194. Kierkegaard A: Incidence and diagnosis of deep vein thrombosis associated with pregnancy. **Acta Obstet Gynecol Scand 62**:239-243, 1983
195. Kim KS, Walczak TS: Computed tomography of deep cerebral venous thrombosis. **J Comput Assist Tomogr 10**:386-390, 1986
196. Krayenbühl H: Cerebral venous and sinus thrombosis. **Clin Neurosurg 14**:1-24, 1967
197. Krayenbühl H: Cerebral venous thrombosis: the diagnostic value of cerebral angiography. **Schweiz Arch Neurol Psychiatr 74**:261-287, 1954
198. Kruithof EKO, Tran-Thang C, Gudinchet A, et al: Fibrinolysis in pregnancy: a study of plasminogen activator inhibitors. **Blood 69**:460-466, 1987
199. Landi G, D'Angelo A, Boccardi E, et al: Hypercoagulability in acute stroke: prognostic significance. **Neurology 37**:1667-1671, 1987
200. Landi G, D'Angelo A, Boccardi E, et al: Venous thromboembolism in acute stroke. Prognostic importance of hypercoagulability. **Arch Neurol 49**: 279-283, 1992
201. Lavin PJM, Bone I, Lamb JT, et al: Intracranial venous thrombosis in the first trimester of pregnancy. **J Neurol Neurosurg Psychiatry 41**:726-729, 1978
202. Lensing AWA, Prandoni P, Brandjes D, et al: Detection of deep-vein thrombosis by real-time B-mode ultrasonography. **N Engl J Med 320**:342-345, 1989
203. Le Quesne LP: Relation between deep vein thrombosis and pulmonary embolism in surgical patients. **N Engl J Med 291**:1292-1294, 1974
204. Levi ADO, Wallace MC, Bernstein M, et al: Venous thromboembolism after brain tumor surgery: a retrospective review. **Neurosurgery 28**:859-863, 1991
205. Levine MN, Raskob G, Hirsh J: Hemorrhagic complications of long-term anticoagulant therapy. **Chest 95 (Suppl)**:26S-36S, 1989
206. Levine SR, Twyman RE, Gilman S: The role of anticoagulation in cavernous sinus thrombosis. **Neurology 38**:517-522, 1988
207. Leyvraz PF, Richard J, Bachman F, et al: Adjusted versus fixed-dose subcutaneous heparin in the prevention of deep-vein thrombosis after total hip replacement. **N Engl J Med 309**:954-958, 1983
208. Lindhagen A, Bergqvist A, Bergqvist D, et al: Late venous function in the leg after deep venous thrombosis occurring in relation to pregnancy. **Br J Obstet Gynaecol 93**:348-352, 1986
209. Lobo RA: Estrogen and the risk of coagulopathy. **Am J Med 92**:283-285, 1992 (Editorial)
210. Lockner D, Bratt G, Törnebohm E, et al: Intravenous and subcutaneous administration of Fragmin in deep venous thrombosis. **Haemostasis 16 (Suppl 2)**: 25-29, 1986
211. Lord RSA, Chen FC, Devine TJ, et al: Surgical treatment of acute deep venous thrombosis. **World J Surg 14**:694-702, 1990
212. Lowe GDO: Epidemiology of postoperative deep vein thrombosis and pulmonary embolism. **Semin Thromb Hemost 17 (Suppl)**:247-249, 1991
213. Macchi PJ, Grossman RI, Gomori JM, et al: High field MR imaging of cerebral venous thrombosis. **J Comput Assist Tomogr 10**:10-15, 1986
214. Maruishi M, Kato H, Nawashiro H, et al: Successful treatment of increased intracranial pressure by barbiturate therapy in a patient with severe sinus thrombosis after failure of osmotic therapy. A case report. **Acta Neurochir 120**:88-91, 1992
215. Maternal and Neonatal Haemostasis Working Party of the Haemostasis and Thrombosis Task: Guidelines on the prevention, investigation and management of thrombosis associated with pregnancy. **J Clin Pathol 46**:489-496, 1993
216. Mattle HP, Wentz KU, Edelman RR, et al: Cerebral venography with MR. **Radiology 178**:453-458, 1991
217. Mätzsch T, Bergqvist D, Hedner U, et al: Effects of an enzymatically depolymerized heparin as compared with conventional heparin in healthy volunteers. **Thromb Haemost 57**:97-101, 1987
218. Mätzsch T, Bergqvist D, Hedner U, et al: Effects of low molecular weight heparin and unfragmented heparin on induction of osteoporosis in rats. **Thromb Haemost 63**:505-509, 1990
219. Mayberg MR, Symon L: Meningiomas of the clivus and apical petrous bone. Report of 35 cases. **J Neurosurg 65**:160-167, 1986
220. McCarthy ST, Turner J: Low-dose subcutaneous heparin in the prevention of deep-vein thrombosis and pulmonary emboli following acute stroke. **Age Ageing 15**:84-88, 1986
221. McCarthy ST, Turner JJ, Robertson D, et al: Low-dose heparin as a prophylaxis against deep-vein thrombosis after acute stroke. **Lancet II**:800-801, 1977
222. McKenna R, Cole ER, Vasan U: Is warfarin sodium contraindicated in the lactating mother? **J Pediatr 103**:325-327, 1983
223. McLachlin J, Richards T, Paterson JC: An evaluation of clinical signs in the diagnosis of venous thrombosis. **Arch Surg 85**:738-744, 1962
224. Melissari E, Parker CJ, Wilson NV, et al: Use of low molecular weight heparin in pregnancy. **Thromb Haemost 68**:652-656, 1992
225. Menon IS, Dewar HA: Increased fibrinolytic activity in venous blood of hemiplegic limbs. **Br Med J 2**:

613-615, 1967

226. Merli GJ, Crabbe S, Doyle L, et al: Mechanical plus phamacological prophylaxis for deep vein thrombosis in acute spinal cord injury. **Paraplegia 30:**558-562, 1992
227. Merli GJ, Herbison GJ, Ditunno JF, et al: Deep vein thrombosis: prophylaxis in acute spinal cord injured patients. **Arch Phys Med Rehabil 69:**661-664, 1988
228. Messmore HL, Wehrmacher WH: Therapeutic use of low molecular weight heparins. **Semin Thromb Hemost 19 (Suppl 1):**97-100, 1993
229. Miyamoto AT, Miller LS: Pulmonary embolism in stroke: prevention by early heparinization of venous thrombosis detected by iodine-125 fibrinogen leg scans. **Arch Phys Med Rehabil 61:**584-587, 1980
230. Mohr DN, Ryu JH, Litin SC, et al: Recent advances in the management of venous thromboembolism. **Mayo Clin Proc 63:**281 290, 1988
231. Monreal M, Lafoz E, Olive A, et al: Comparison of subcutaneous unfractionated heparin with a low molecular weight heparin (Fragmin) in patients with venous thromboembolism and contraindications to coumarin. **Thromb Haemost 71:**7-11, 1994
232. Muchmore JH, Dunlap JN, Culicchia F, et al: Deep vein thrombophlebitis and pulmonary embolism in patients with malignant gliomas. **South Med J 82:** 1352-1356, 1989
233. Myllynen P, Kammonen M, Rokkanen P, et al: Deep venous thrombosis and pulmonary embolism in patients with acute spinal cord injury: a comparison with nonparalyzed patients immobilized due to spinal fractures. **J Trauma 25:**541-543, 1985
234. Myllynen P, Kivioja A, Rokkanen P, et al: Cervical spinal cord injury: the correlations of initial clinical features and blood gas analyses with early prognosis. **Paraplegia 27:**19-26, 1989
235. Narayan H, Cullimore J, Krarup K, et al: Experience with the Cardial inferior vena cava filter as prophylaxis against pulmonary embolism in pregnant women with extensive deep venous thrombosis. **Br J Obstet Gynaecol 99:**637-640, 1992
236. National Institutes of Health Consensus Conference: Prevention of venous thrombosis and pulmonary embolism. **JAMA 256:**744-749, 1986
237. Nielsen HK: Pathophysiology of venous thromboembolism. **Semin Thromb Hemost 17 (Suppl 3):** 250-253, 1991
238. Nurmohamed MT, Rosendaal FR, Büller HR, et al: Low-molecular-weight heparin versus standard heparin in general and orthopedic surgery: a meta-analysis. **Lancet 340:**152-156, 1992
239. Olin JW, Young JR, Graor RA, et al: Treatment of deep vein thrombosis and pulmonary emboli in patients with primary and metastatic brain tumors. Anticoagulants or inferior vena cava filter? **Arch Intern Med 147:**2177-2179, 1987
240. Omri A, Delaloye JF, Andersen H, et al: Low molecular weight heparin Novo (LHN-1) does not cross the placenta during the second trimester of pregnancy. **Thromb Haemost 61:**55-56, 1989
241. Padayachee TS, Bingham JB, Graves MJ, et al: Dural sinus thrombosis. Diagnosis and follow-up by magnetic resonance angiography and imaging. **Neuroradiology 33:**165-167, 1991
242. Patronas NJ, Duda EE, Mirfakhraee M, et al: Superior sagittal sinus thrombosis diagnosed by computed tomography. **Surg Neurol 15:**11-14, 1981
243. Patterson WP, Ringenberg QS: The pathophysiology of thrombosis in cancer. **Semin Oncol 17:**140-146, 1990
244. Perkash A: Experience with the management of deep vein thrombosis in patients with spinal cord injury. Part II: a critical evaluation of the anticoagulant therapy. **Paraplegia 18:**2-14, 1980
245. Perkash A, Prakash V, Perkash I: Experience with the management of thromboembolism in patients with spinal cord injury: part 1. Incidence, diagnosis and role of some risk factors. **Paraplegia 16:**322-331, 1978
246. Petäjä J, Myllynen P, Rokkanen P, et al: Fibrinolysis and spinal injury. Relationship to post-traumatic deep vein thrombosis. **Acta Chir Scand 155:**241-246, 1989
247. Petitti DB, Strom BL, Melmon KL: Duration of warfarin anticoagulant therapy and the probabilities of recurrent thromboembolism and hemorrhage. **Am J Med 81:**255-259, 1986
248. Philipps RS: The incidence of deep vein thrombosis in paraplegics. **Paraplegia 1:**116-130, 1963
249. Pineo GF, Hull RD: Prevention, diagnosis and treatment of thromboembolism in hip replacement surgery. **Curr Opin Orthopedics 3:**449-454, 1992
250. The PIOPED Investigators: Value of the ventilation/perfusion scan in acute pulmonary embolism. Results of the prospective investigation of pulmonary embolism diagnosis (PIOPED). **JAMA 263:**2753-2759, 1990
251. Powers SK, Edwards MSB. Prevention and treatment of thromboembolic complications in a neurosurgical patient, in Wilkins RH, Rengachary SS (eds): **Neurosurgery.** New York: McGraw-Hill, 1985, pp 406-410
252. Powers SK, Edwards MSB: Prophylaxis of thromboembolism in the neurosurgical patient: a review. **Neurosurgery 10:**509-513, 1982
253. Prandoni P, Lensing AW, Buller HR, et al: Comparison of subcutaneous low-molecular-weight heparin with intravenous standard heparin in proximal deep-vein thrombosis. **Lancet 339:**441-445, 1992
254. Prandoni P, Lensing AWA, Büller HR, et al: Deep-vein thrombosis and the incidence of subsequent symptomatic cancer. **N Engl J Med 327:**1128-1133, 1992
255. Prandoni P, Vigo M, Cattelan AM, et al: Treatment of deep venous thrombosis by fixed dosed of a low-molecular-weight heparin (CY216). **Haemostasis 20 (Suppl 1):**220-223, 1990
256. Puls M, Horst HM, Diaz FG: Neurosurgical patients: at high risk for pulmonary emboli. **Surg Forum 37:** 522-523, 1986
257. Ramirez LF, Thisted R: Complications and demographic characteristics of patients undergoing lumbar discectomy in community hospitals. **Neurosurgery 25:**226-231, 1989
258. Rao KCVG, Knipp HC, Wagner EJ: Computed tomographic findings in cerebral sinus and venous thrombosis. **Radiology 140:**391-398, 1981
259. Ray BS, Dunbar HS: Thrombosis of the dural venous sinuses as a cause of "pseudotumor cerebri." **Ann Surg 134:**376-386, 1951
260. Rippe DJ, Boyko OB, Spritzer CE, et al: Demonstration of dural sinus occlusion by the use of MR angiography. **AJNR 11:**199-201, 1990

261. Rosenfeld JC, Estrada FP, Orr RM: Management of deep venous thrombosis in the pregnant female. **J Cardiovasc Surg 31:**678-682, 1990
262. Rosiello RA, Chan CK, Tencza F, et al: Timing of oral anticoagulation therapy in the treatment of angiographically proven acute pulmonary embolism. **Arch Intern Med 147:**1469-1473, 1987
263. Rossi EC, Green D, Rosen JS, et al: Sequential changes in factor VIII and platelets preceding deep vein thrombosis in patients with spinal cord injury. **Br J Haematol 45:**143-151, 1980
264. Ruff RL, Posner JB: Incidence and treatment of peripheral venous thrombosis in patients with glioma. **Ann Neurol 13:**334-336, 1983
265. Ruggieri PM, Masaryk TJ, Ross JS: Magnetic resonance angiography. Cerebrovascular applications. **Stroke 23:**774-780, 1992
266. Rutherford S, Montoro M, McGhee W, et al: Thromboembolic disease associated with pregnancy: an 11-year review. **Am J Obstet Gynecol 164:**286, 1991(Abstract)
267. Rutherford SE, Phelan JP: Deep venous thrombosis and pulmonary embolism in pregnancy. **Obstet Gynecol Clin North Am 18:**345-370, 1991
268. Sackett DL: Rules of evidence and clinical recommendations on the use of antithrombotic agents. **Chest 89 (Suppl):**2S-3S, 1986
269. Sackett DL: Rules of evidence and clinical recommendations on the use of antithrombotic agents. **Chest 95 (Suppl):**2S-4S, 1989
270. Salzman EW: Low-molecular-weight heparin and other new antithrombotic drugs. **N Engl J Med 326:**1017-1019, 1992 (Editorial)
271. Salzman EW, Davies GC: Prophylaxis of venous thromboembolism. Analysis of cost effectiveness. **Ann Surg 191:**207-218, 1980
272. Salzman EW, Deykin D, Shapiro RM, et al: Management of heparin therapy. Controlled prospective trial. **N Engl J Med 292:**1046-1050, 1975
273. Sawaya R, Cummins CJ, Kornblith PL: Brain tumors and plasmin inhibitors. **Neurosurgery 15:**795-800, 1984
274. Sawaya R, Decourteen-Meyers G, Copeland B: Massive preoperative pulmonary embolism and suprasellar brain tumor: case report and review of the literature. **Neurosurgery 15:**566-571, 1984
275. Sawaya R, Zuccarello M, El-Kalliny M: Brain tumors and thromboembolism: clinical, hemostatic, and biochemical correlations. **J Neurosurg 70:**314A, 1989 (Abstract)
276. Sawaya R, Zuccarello M, El-Kalliny M, et al: Postoperative venous thromboembolism and brain tumors: Part I. Clinical profile. **J Neurooncol 14:**119-125, 1992
277. Sawaya RE, Ligon BL: Thromboembolic complications associated with brain tumors. **J Neurooncol 22:**173-181, 1994
278. Schafer AI: The hypercoagulable states. **Ann Intern Med 102:**814-828, 1985
279. Schaible TF, Alavi A: Antifibrin scintigraphy in the diagnostic evaluation of acute deep venous thrombosis. **Semin Nucl Med 21:**313-324, 1991
280. Scmidt EV, Smirnov VE, Ryabova VS: Results of the seven-year prospective study of stroke patients. **Stroke 19:**942-949, 1988
281. Scott JA, Pascuzzi RM, Hall PV, et al: Treatment of dural sinus thrombosis with local urokinase infusion. Case report. **J Neurosurg 68:**284-287, 1988
282. Scurr JH, Ibrahim SZ, Faber RG, et al: The efficacy of graduated compression stockings in the prevention of deep vein thrombosis. **Br J Surg 64:**371-373, 1977
283. Secker-Walker RH: The use of radioisotopes in the management of venous thromboembolism. **Chest 89 (Suppl):**413S-416S, 1986
284. Skillman JJ, Collins REC, Coe NP, et al: Prevention of deep vein thrombosis in neurosurgical patients: a controlled, randomized trial of external pneumatic compression boots. **Surgery 83:**354-358, 1978
285. So W, Hugenholtz H, Richard MT: Complications of anticoagulant therapy in patients with known central nervous system lesions. **Can J Surg 26:**181-183, 1983
286. Squires JW, Pinch LW: Heparin-induced spinal fractures. **JAMA 241:**2417-2418, 1979
287. Srinivasan K: Cerebral venous and arterial thrombosis in pregnancy and puerperium, a study of 135 patients. **Angiology 34:**731-746, 1983
288. Srinivasan K: Puerperal cerebral venous and arterial thrombosis. **Semin Neurol 8:**222-225, 1988
289. Stansfield FR: Puerperal cerebral thrombophlebitis treated by heparin. **Br Med J 1:**436-438, 1942
290. Strauss HS, Diamond LK: Elevation of factor VIII (antihemophilic factor) during pregnancy in normal persons and in a patient with von Willebrand's disease. **N Engl J Med 269:**1251-1252, 1963
291. Sturridge F, de Swiet M, Letsky E: The use of low molecular weight heparin for thromboprophylaxis in pregnancy. **Br J Obstet Gynaecol 101:**69-71, 1994
292. Swann KW, Black PM: Deep vein thrombosis and pulmonary emboli in neurosurgical patients: a review. **J Neurosurg 61:**1055-1062, 1984
293. Swann KW, Black PM, Baker MF: Management of symptomatic deep venous thrombosis and pulmonary embolism on a neurosurgical service. **J Neurosurg 64:**563-567, 1986
294. Symon L, Rosenstein J: Surgical management of suprasellar meningioma. Part 1: The influence of tumor size, duration of symptoms, and microsurgery on surgical outcome in 101 consecutive cases. **J Neurosurg 61:**633-641, 1984
295. Tengborn L, Bergqvist D, Mätzsch T, et al: Recurrent thromboembolism in pregnancy and puerperium. Is there a need for thromboprophylaxis? **Am J Obstet Gynecol 160:**90-94, 1989
296. Terrin M, Goldhaber SZ, Thompson B, et al: Selection of patients with acute pulmonary embolism for thrombolytic therapy. Thrombolysis in pulmonary embolism (TIPE) patient survey. **Chest 95 (Suppl):**279S-281S, 1989
297. Thoron L, Arbit E: Hemostatic changes in patients with brain tumors. **J Neurooncol 22:**87-100, 1994
298. Thron A, Wessel K, Linden D, et al: Superior sagittal sinus thrombosis: neuroradiological evaluation and clinical findings. **J Neurol 233:**283-288, 1986
299. Todd JW, Frisbie JH, Rossier AB, et al: Deep venous thrombosis in acute spinal cord injury: a comparison of ^{125}I fibrinogen leg scanning, impedance plethysmography and venography. **Paraplegia 14:**50-57, 1976
300. Tomita T, Raimondi AJ: Brain tumors in the elderly. **JAMA 246:**53-55, 1981
301. Toulemonde F: Can the bleeding potential of low molecular weight heparins be assessed and mini-

mized in postsurgery prophylaxis? **Semin Thromb Hemost 17**:351-355, 1991
302. Towbin A: The syndrome of latent cerebral venous thrombosis: its frequency and relation to age and congestive heart failure. **Stroke 4**:419-430, 1973
303. Tribe CR: Cause of death in the early and late stages of paraplegia. **Paraplegia 1**:19-47, 1963
304. Turkewitz LJ, Jacobs AK, Bidwell JK: Atypical MRI findings of venous sinus thrombosis in pregnancy: clinical significance relating to episodic vascular headache. **Headache 31**:240-243, 1991
305. Turpie AGG, Delmore T, Hirsh J, et al: Prevention of venous thrombosis by intermittent sequential calf compression in patients with intracranial disease. **Thromb Res 15**:611-616, 1979
306. Turpie AGG, Gallus AS, Beattie WS, et al: Prevention of venous thrombosis in patients with intracranial disease by intermittent pneumatic compression of the calf. **Neurology 27**:435-438, 1977
307. Turpie AGG, Hirsh J, Gent M, et al: Prevention of deep vein thrombosis in potential neurosurgical patients. A randomised trial comparing graduated compression stockings alone or graduated compression stockings plus intermittent pneumatic compression with control. **Arch Intern Med 149**:679-681, 1989
308. Turpie AGG, Levine MN, Hirsh J, et al: Double-blind randomized trial of Org 10172 low-molecular-weight heparinoid in prevention of deep-vein thrombosis in thrombotic stroke. **Lancet 1**:523-526, 1987
309. Turpie AGG, Levine MN, Hirsh J, et al: A randomized controlled trial of a low-molecular-weight heparin (Enoxaparin) to prevent deep-vein thrombosis in patients undergoing elective hip surgery. **N Engl J Med 315**:925-929, 1986
310. Valladares JB: Venous thromboembolism in neurosurgery. **Prog Neurol Surg 11**:141-164, 1984
311. Valladares JB, Hankinson J: Incidence of lower extremity deep vein thrombosis in neurosurgical patients. **Neurosurgery 6**:138-141, 1980
312. Van Dulken H, Thomeer RTWM: Mini-dose heparin. **J Neurosurg 47**:974, 1977 (Letter)
313. Villasanta U: Thromboembolic disease in pregnancy. **Am J Obstet Gynecol 93**:142-160, 1965
314. Virapongse C, Cazenave C, Quisling R, et al: The empty delta sign: frequency and significance in 76 cases of dural sinus thrombosis. **Radiology 162**: 779-785, 1987
315. Warkentin TE, Kelton JG: Heparin-induced thrombocytopenia. **Prog Hemost Thromb 10**:1-34, 1991
316. Warlow C, Ogston D, Douglas AS: Deep venous thrombosis of the legs after strokes. **Br Med J 1**: 1178-1183, 1976
317. Warlow C, Ogston D, Douglas AS: Venous thrombosis following strokes. **Lancet I**:1305-1306, 1972
318. Warlow CP, Rennie JAN, Ogston D, et al: Platelet adhesiveness and fibrinolysis after recent cerebrovascular accidents and their relationship with subsequent deep venous thrombosis of the legs. **Thromb Haemost 36**:127-132, 1976
319. Watson N: Anticoagulant therapy in the treatment of venous thrombosis and pulmonary embolism in acute spinal injury. **Paraplegia 12**:197-201, 1974
320. Weinmann EE, Salzman EW: Deep-vein thrombosis. **N Engl J Med 331**:1630-1641, 1994
321. Weitz J, Michelsen J, Gold K, et al: Effects of intermittent pneumatic calf compression on postoperative thrombin and plasmin activity. **Thromb Haemost 56**:198-201, 1986
322. Wendling LR: Intracranial venous sinus thrombosis: diagnosis suggested by computed tomography. **AJR 130**:978-980, 1978
323. Wessler S, Gitel SN: Warfarin. From bedside to bench. **N Engl J Med 311**:645-652, 1984
324. Wetzel N, Anderson MC, Shields TW: Pulmonary embolism as a cause of death in the neurosurgical patient. **J Neurosurg 17**:664-668, 1960
325. Wheeler AP, Jaquiss RDB, Newman JH: Physician practices in the treatment of pulmonary embolism and deep venous thrombosis. **Arch Intern Med 148**: 1321-1325, 1988
326. Wheeler HB: Diagnosis of deep vein thrombosis. Review of clinical evaluation and impedance plethysmography. **Am J Surg 150(4A)**:7-13, 1985
327. White RH, McGahan JP, Daschbach MM, et al: Diagnosis of deep-vein thrombosis using duplex ultrasound. **Ann Intern Med 111**:297-304, 1989
328. Wille-Jørgensen P: Prophylaxis of postoperative thromboembolism with combined methods. **Semin Thromb Hemost 17 (Suppl 3)**:272-279, 1991
329. Willis BK: Timing of anticoagulant therapy for thromboembolic complications after craniotomy for brain tumors. **Neurosurgery 28**:929-930, 1991 (Letter)
330. Wise PH, Hall AJ: Heparin-induced osteopenia in pregnancy. **Br Med J 281**:110-111, 1980
331. Woodhams BJ, Candotti G, Shaw R, et al: Changes in coagulation and fibrinolysis during pregnancy: evidence of activation of coagulation preceding spontaneous abortion. **Thromb Res 55**:99-107, 1989
332. Wright JG, Cooper P, Astedt B, et al: Fibrinolysis during normal human pregnancy: complex inter-relationships between plasma levels of tissue plasminogen activator and inhibitors and the euglobulin clot lysis time. **Br J Haematol 69**:253-258, 1988
333. Yasargil MG, Damur M: Thrombosis of the cerebral veins and dural sinuses, in Newton TH, Potts DG (eds): **Radiology of the Skull and Brain.** St Louis, MO: CV Mosby, 1974, pp 2375-2400
334. Yelnik A, Dizien O, Bussel B, et al: Systematic lower limb phlebography in acute spinal cord injury in 147 patients. **Paraplegia 29**:253-260, 1991
335. Zelikovski A, Zucker G, Eliashiv A, et al: A new sequential pneumatic device for the prevention of deep vein thrombosis. **J Neurosurg 54**:652-654, 1981

Portions of this manuscript were previously published in *Neurosurgery*[133] and have been used with the permission of the authors and the publisher.

CHAPTER 11

CEREBRAL EMBOLISM IN PREGNANT WOMEN

PATRICIA H. DAVIS, MD, MICHAEL R. JACOBY, MD, AND
HAROLD P. ADAMS, JR., MD

The diagnosis and management of cerebral embolism in a pregnant woman is a challenging endeavor because of the diverse number of potential causes (Table 1) and because of the importance of instituting therapy early to prevent recurrent embolism while avoiding potentially harmful effects to the fetus. These decisions must be accomplished in the emotionally difficult setting of a young woman facing possible major disability or death at a time when she is undertaking the responsibility of parenthood.

EPIDEMIOLOGY

The frequency of ischemic stroke as a complication of pregnancy has not been established. Studies in the United States have reported rates varying from one per 26,099 pregnancies in Rochester, Minnesota[110] to one per 10,000 in Dallas, Texas.[98] The highest rate reported in the world is one per 481 pregnancies in Madurai, India.[99] Wiebers[109] estimates that the risk of ischemic stroke increases by 13 times during pregnancy. In several case series of young adults with ischemic stroke, the event was attributed to pregnancy in 2.6% to 5% of cases overall.[16,46,50,63,69]

TABLE 1
CEREBRAL EMBOLISM ASSOCIATED WITH PREGNANCY

Cardiac Causes	Noncardiac Causes
Rheumatic heart disease	Air embolism
Prosthetic heart valves	Fat embolism
Infective endocarditis	Amniotic fluid embolism
Nonbacterial thrombotic endocarditis	Choriocarcinoma
Atrial myxoma	Arterial dissection
Paradoxical embolism	Illicit drugs
Peripartum cardiomyopathy	
Antiphospholipid antibodies	
Mitral valve prolapse	

TABLE 2

DIAGNOSTIC TESTS

All Patients	Selected Patients
Complete blood count	Antinuclear antibodies, rheumatoid factor
Erythrocyte sedimentation rate	Blood or urine toxicology
Electrolytes, blood urea nitrogen, creatinine	Fibrinogen
Prothrombin, partial thromboplastin times	Hemoglobin electrophoresis
CT scan	Anticardiolipin antibodies
Chest x-ray	Protein C
ECG	Protein S
Urinalysis	Antithrombin III
Transthoracic echocardiogram (with contrast)	VDRL
	Blood cultures
	Serum human chorionic gonadotropin level
	Carotid duplex ultrasonography
	Lower extremity Doppler studies
	MRI
	Transesophageal echocardiogram
	Cerebral arteriogram
	Holter monitoring
	Cerebrospinal fluid examination
	EEG

DIAGNOSIS

Arterial occlusions tend to occur most often during the second and third trimesters of pregnancy and during the first postpartum week.[31] The increased risk of ischemic stroke during pregnancy may be related to a presumed hypercoagulable state which is maximal in the second and third trimesters and which persists for 2 to 3 weeks after delivery.[101] It is unclear what proportion of ischemic strokes occurring during pregnancy are due to cerebral embolism, as series include small numbers of patients and the diagnosis depends on how carefully an embolic source was sought. In one series of 15 pregnant women with stroke, nine were ischemic and of these, three were felt to be due to cerebral embolism.[98]

A pregnant woman requires the same extensive diagnostic evaluation to determine the most likely etiology of ischemic stroke as would any other young adult with stroke. Table 2 lists suggested tests. Unusual causes of ischemic stroke, including unusual causes of embolism, should be considered. Most diagnostic tests pose only minimal risk to the fetus. Computed tomography (CT) of the brain can be performed with abdominal shielding, producing a fetal radiation exposure of approximately 2 mrad.[31] CT differentiates infarct from hemorrhage and may demonstrate the arterial distribution of the infarct which suggests embolism (Figure 1 *left*). A comparable amount of radiation exposure results when cerebral arteriography is performed with abdominal shielding. Arteriography may demonstrate the embolus,

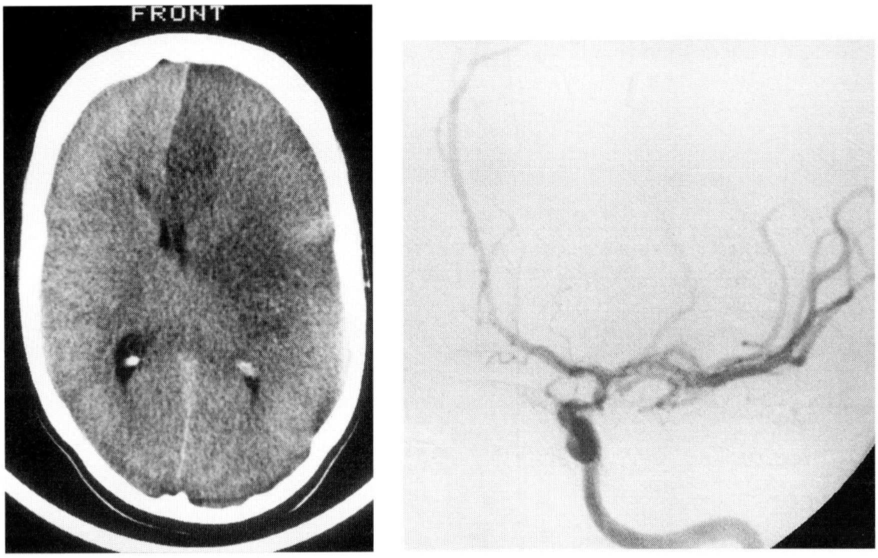

Figure 1: Left) CT scan without contrast of a 28-year-old woman at 29 weeks' gestation showing infarction in the distribution of the left middle and anterior cerebral arteries with mass effect and midline shift. **Right)** Angiogram of the same patient showing irregularity and vessel caliber variation involving the left internal, middle, and anterior cerebral arteries consistent with recanalization of an intraluminal thromboembolus.

particularly if done early; if delayed, it may show evidence of recanalization (Figure 1 *right*). In addition, arteriography may provide additional information concerning the source of embolism, such as an arterial dissection, aneurysm, or fibromuscular dysplasia. No short-term effects have been seen on the fetus with magnetic resonance imaging (MRI) but long-term risk is unknown.[31] Findings of multiple strokes in different vascular territories, a branch cortical artery occlusion, or hemorrhagic transformation may suggest the diagnosis of embolism. A thorough cardiac investigation is important and includes a careful clinical examination of the heart, chest x-ray, electrocardiogram, transthoracic echocardiography (TTE), transesophageal echocardiography (TEE), and in selected patients, cardiac rhythm monitoring and blood cultures. TTE is noninvasive and has a high yield for ventricular thrombus, mitral valve prolapse, and aortic and mitral stenosis but can miss left atrial lesions or left atrial turbulence, left atrial appendage thrombus, and thrombus or vegetations on prosthetic or native heart valves. TEE is superior for detection of these lesions and, while more invasive, can be performed safely in pregnant patients with no adverse effects on the fetus as determined by fetal monitoring.[102] While TEE has a higher yield of abnormalities than TTE, the relevance of some of these abnormalities, such as a patent foramen ovale, atrial septal aneurysm, remains unclear and spontaneous echo contrast or "smoke," as a potential cardioembolic source.

Treatment

Potential treatments for a pregnant women who has suffered an embolic stroke include antiplatelet agents, anticoagulants, antibiotics to prevent or treat endocarditis or rheumatic fever, and cardiac surgery. While aspirin has been associated with birth defects and bleeding, low-dose aspirin (60 to 150 mg) in the second and third trimesters has been shown to be safe in clinical trials of the drug in the prevention of pre-eclampsia.[23,42] The only adverse effect in a large study of 9,364 women was a slight increase in the need for blood transfusion after delivery.[23] The safety of higher doses of aspirin or its use during the first trimester is unknown.[42] Teratogenic effects have not been reported in animal studies using ticlopidine but human studies have not been performed.[88] Ticlopidine should be prescribed if there is a contraindication to aspirin therapy or a recurrence of symptoms while on aspirin. Use of dipyridamole may be indicated as an alternative to adding low-dose aspirin in patients with mechanical prosthetic heart valves who have recurrent embolism while taking warfarin.[45,106] No teratogenic effects have been observed with use of dipyridamole.[88] Warfarin crosses the placenta and its use during pregnancy is associated with an embryopathy and central nervous system anomalies. Use between 6 and 12 weeks' gestation is associated with microcephalus, mental retardation, bone stippling, and midfacial hypoplasia in 8% to 67% of exposed children.[30,42,114] The incidence is affected by how carefully these abnormalities are sought and the type of study.[41] A recent retrospective study showed no cases of embryopathy in 46 women with prosthetic heart valves who took warfarin during the first trimester, while prospective cohort studies have reported risks varying from 29% to 67%.[57,114] Central nervous system abnormalities can occur in 2% to 3% of babies exposed to warfarin at any time during the pregnancy, and include agenesis of the corpus callosum, Dandy-Walker syndrome, optic atrophy, or intracranial hemorrhage.[42] Warfarin should not be used after 36 weeks' gestation because of the risk of either maternal or fetal hemorrhage.[30] Heparin does not cross the placenta and does not appear to be associated with increased risk to the fetus.[43] Maternal complications include thrombocytopenia and osteoporosis with long-term use. In a prospective study of 14 women receiving heparin during pregnancy and 14 matched pregnant controls, bone densities were measured prior to pregnancy and postpartum; of the women receiving heparin, 36% had decreased bone density postpartum compared to none of the controls.[8] In another study, 2% of women receiving heparin during pregnancy had symptomatic vertebral fractures.[27] Preliminary data show that low-molecular weight heparin also does not cross the placental barrier and may not have the side effects of osteoporosis or thrombocytopenia seen with heparin.[75] Recommendations for anticoagulation during pregnancy include: 1) subcutaneous heparin every 12 hours to prolong activated partial thromboplastin time (aPTT) to 1.5 times control, or 2) subcutaneous heparin until the 13th week of gestation and then warfarin until the middle of the third trimester, when heparin is reinstituted until delivery.[42] If a woman becomes pregnant while taking warfarin, the drug should be stopped and treatment with heparin begun as soon as possible.

Patients with pregnancy-related ischemic stroke of undetermined cause appear to have low risk of recurrence in subsequent pregnancies and should not be treated with prophylactic anticoagulation.[31] The risk of fetal death from cardiac surgery during pregnancy is significant and is estimated to be 9% to 16%.[13]

Etiology of Embolic Stroke

Cardiogenic Causes of Cerebral Embolism

Cardiogenic causes of embolic stroke include conditions which also occur outside of the setting of pregnancy, such as rheumatic heart disease, prosthetic heart valves, atrial myxoma, paradoxical embolism, infective endocarditis, and nonbacterial thrombotic endocarditis, as well as specific conditions seen only with pregnancy, such as peripartum cardiomyopathy.

Rheumatic heart disease, while relatively uncommon, presents a risk for thromboembolism in a pregnant woman with rheumatic mitral stenosis and atrial fibrillation. If atrial fibrillation occurs for the first time during pregnancy, cardioversion should be attempted. If atrial fibrillation has been present for more than 2 days, cardioversion should be preceded by 3 weeks of anticoagulation with heparin; this should be continued until sinus rhythm has been maintained for 4 weeks.[64] A TEE study may be useful to determine if there is intracardiac thrombus; however, a negative study does not change the recommendations concerning anticoagulation. To reduce the risk of recurrent rheumatic fever during pregnancy, therapy with penicillin G benzathine (1.2 million units once a month) is recommended.[109] No fetal toxicity has been reported with this therapy. Antibiotic prophylaxis for endocarditis should be given prior to labor and delivery in these patients.

Prosthetic heart valves in pregnant patients require management which must take into account both maternal and fetal risks, which are often conflicting. The optimal antithrombotic therapy for these patients during pregnancy is controversial, as properly designed studies have not been performed.[41] Salazar et al[93] found that the risk of cerebral embolism was 2.3% in a group treated with warfarin throughout pregnancy. Patients treated with warfarin except in the first trimester and last 2 weeks of pregnancy, when heparin was substituted, had an embolic rate of 8.3%, while those on antiplatelet agents had an embolic rate of 25%. Spontaneous abortion occurred in 10.3% of women taking antiplatelet agents, 28.1% of those taking warfarin, and none of those taking heparin and warfarin. Warfarin embryopathy was seen in 7.9% of babies whose mothers took warfarin throughout the pregnancy.[93] Sbarouni et al[95] did not report any cases of warfarin embryopathy and found a much higher rate of complication, including valve thrombosis, embolic events, and bleeding in women on heparin. Women receiving heparin throughout pregnancy had a major complication rate of 48% and Sbarouni et al recommend the use of warfarin throughout pregnancy. Ginsberg and Barron[41] point out the bias associated with this retrospective study and suggest that this result may be explained by inadequate heparin dosing. They recommend that the 6-hour postinjection aPTT be monitored closely and maintained at least twice the control value. They recommend either the use of subcutaneous heparin throughout pregnancy or warfarin therapy except during 6 to 12 weeks' gestation and close to delivery.[41] In women with prosthetic valves, discussion of these management options with their attendant risks and benefits should preferably take place prior to conception. Fetal complication rates are low among women with bioprosthetic valves because anticoagulants are usually not required.[82,93,95] This has led some authors to advocate the use of bioprosthetic valves for women planning pregnancy.[17,82,93] Conversely, others suggest that the increased hemodynamic load imposed by pregnancy on bioprosthetic valves raises maternal risk to unacceptable levels because these valves are less durable.[7,94] In one study, 17 of 49 patients with bioprosthetic valves required replacement during or soon after pregnancy.[95] Patients with prosthetic aortic valves appear to have fewer complications than those with mitral valve replacements.[17] Failure of high-dose heparin therapy in the prevention of recurrent embolic strokes during pregnancy in patients with mechanical prosthetic valves has been reported.[45] The use of low-dose aspirin in addition to heparin during pregnancy has not been investigated. Another option is to add dipyridamole to heparin.[45] TEE may be helpful in identifying thrombus on a prosthetic valve. The use of transcranial Doppler ultrasound to detect clinically silent emboli may be helpful in assessing the adequacy of treatment to prevent embolism during pregnancy.[11] Antibiotic prophylaxis for endocarditis should be used prior to delivery.

Infective endocarditis is a rare complication of pregnancy.[25,85] It may complicate pre-existing cardiac diseases such as rheumatic heart disease, a prosthetic heart valve, or mitral valve prolapse,[103] and can also be related to illicit intravenous drug use.[25] The most common organisms are *Streptococcus viridans* and *Staphylococcus aureus*. Enterococcal endocarditis is seen in 8% of pregnancy-related cases, particularly in association with cesarean section and uterine curettage.[31] Diagnosis may require multiple blood cultures, and TTE or TEE may be useful in identifying vegetations. Treatment should include the appropriate antibiotic, and anticoagulants are not indicated, as recurrent stroke is unlikely with native valves after antibiotic therapy has commenced.

Nonbacterial thrombotic endocarditis with cerebral embolism during pregnancy has been reported in a previously healthy woman.[40] The presumed mechanism was a hypercoagulable state due to pregnancy. This case was diagnosed only on autopsy, and antemortem diagnosis may be difficult. TTE may not detect vegetations <4 mm[70] but TEE may be more sensitive.

A clinical picture of multisystem embolism or laboratory findings consistent with low-grade disseminated intravascular coagulation may be present. Blood cultures must be performed to exclude infection. Treatment with heparin may be instituted but is of unproven value.

Atrial myxoma is a rare cause of embolism; it can present as a stroke which occurs with or without constitutional or cardiac obstructive symptoms.[62] The diagnosis is most commonly made using TTE, which usually shows a left atrial mass. TEE may be more sensitive in detecting this lesion. The treatment is surgical removal of the tumor and should be done urgently because of the risk of recurrent embolism of either thrombus or tumor and the lack of efficacy of medical therapy.[62] The problem in pregnancy is that there is significant risk of fetal death from cardiac surgery.[13]

Paradoxical embolism can occur in the setting of a venous thromboembolism in the presence of an intracardiac or pulmonary right-to-left shunt; clots that would normally reach the lungs bypass the pulmonary circulation and reach the brain. A patent foramen ovale or atrial septal defect is common in young adults. Pregnant women are at increased risk of thrombophlebitis of the veins in the legs and the pelvis, particularly during the puerperium.[31] Puerperal ovarian vein thrombosis may be another source of embolism.[101] Increased right-to-left shunting due to elevated right atrial pressure can occur with Valsalva maneuver during delivery or pulmonary hypertension caused by pulmonary embolism. Contrast studies with injection of agitated saline during TTE or TEE may demonstrate the shunting and TEE may show a patent foramen ovale or atrial septal aneurysm. Ultrasound studies of the legs may detect asymptomatic deep vein thrombosis and ultrasound or imaging with CT or MR may detect ovarian vein thrombosis. Anticoagulant therapy should be initiated for treatment of the venous thromboembolism.

Peripartum cardiomyopathy occurs in one per 1,300 to 30,000 pregnancies in Western populations, depending on how carefully other causes of congestive heart failure are sought.[53,65] This disorder occurs more frequently in African-American women, those >30 years of age, and in association with twin births, toxemia, and postpartum hypertension.[53] It is seen during the last month of pregnancy and the first 6 months postpartum. Other causes of left ventricular dysfunction that need to be eliminated include chronic hypertension, anemia, infection, thyrotoxicosis, prior subclinical heart disease, and toxins. Postpartum cardiomyopathy has been associated with maternal cocaine abuse during pregnancy.[76] Presenting features usually are fatigue, dyspnea, and edema due to congestive heart failure, but cerebral embolism may be the initial clinical event.[52] In a literature review, neurological complications occurred in only 4.7% of patients but when stroke occurred it was associated with a mortality rate of 40%.[33] While chest x-ray, electrocardiography (ECG), and echocardiography are the primary diagnostic tools, other ancillary tests including radionucleotide ventriculography, cine-CT of the heart, and cardiac MRI may be helpful.[33] While postulated causes include hormonal changes, nutritional deficiencies, immunological factors, viral infection, and genetic predisposition, the etiology remains unknown. Anticoagulation is indicated in those with systemic embolism or atrial fibrillation, those who have ventricular thrombi detected on echocardiography, and those with the greatest hemodynamic compromise.[53] The prognosis is poor if the cardiomyopathy persists for >6 months, with a mortality rate of 85%.[53] Therapy includes bed rest, diuretics, digitalis, and angiotensin-converting enzyme inhibitors; in refractory patients, endomyocardial biopsy and treatment with immunosuppressives can be considered if myocarditis is present.[53] Cardiac transplantation has been used successfully in patients unresponsive to these therapies.[77]

Antiphospholipid antibodies (aPL) include the lupus anticoagulant and anticardiolipin antibodies and have been associated with systemic lupus erythematosis, infections, and some drugs.[5] Patients with aPL may have a history of recurrent fetal loss, venous thrombosis, arterial thrombosis, and recurrent cerebral ischemic events. Embolic strokes may occur as a result of paradoxical embolism or in association with cardiac lesions which include mitral valve degeneration and Libman-Sacks endocarditis.[5] Abnormal laboratory findings include a prolonged aPTT, false positive Veneral Disease Research Laboratory test (VDRL) and elevated anticardiolipin antibody titers of >20 IU.[18] Two cases of embolic stroke during pregnancy have been reported in patients with aPL.[18,112] Optimal therapy has not been established and therapeutic options include antiplatelet therapy, anticoagulant therapy, and corticosteroids.[5] Pregnancy may be a high-risk situation for patients known to have aPL, and prophylactic therapy with low-dose aspirin or subcutaneous heparin throughout pregnancy and for several weeks postpartum has been recommended.[18]

Mitral valve prolapse associated with stroke remains controversial. This abnormality occurs in 5% of the general population.[113] There are reports of transient ischemic attack in a pregnant woman with mitral valve prolapse[6] and a branch retinal artery occlusion.[12] It is unclear whether pregnancy increases the risk of embolic events in women with mitral valve prolapse but the absolute risk appears to be low. Antiplatelet therapy is indicated for cerebral embolic events, while anticoagulant therapy can be considered for patients with recurrent events despite antiplatelet therapy.[29]

Noncardiac Causes of Cerebral Embolism

Uncommon, noncardiac causes of cerebral embolism associated with pregnancy include air, fat, and amniotic fluid embolism, metastatic choriocarcinoma, arterial dissection, and illicit drug use. The number of cases of embolic stroke due to these entities are few.

Air embolism has been described following cesarean section,[9,14,15,28,36,37,92,108] intercourse,[84] orogenital sex,[14,34,51,84] vaginal douching,[24,84] powder insufflators,[73] knee-chest exercises,[97,108] labor,[108] and abortion.[84] During pregnancy, the vagina becomes highly distensible, allowing air to enter, pass through the cervical canal, dissect the amniotic membrane from the uterine wall, and enter the venous system. From the venous system it is believed to pass to the arterial circulation through a right-to-left shunt.[14] Neurological symptoms from air embolism are nonspecific and commonly reflect multifocal cerebral lesions with a variety of findings[60] and may also partially be due to the effects of hypotension. The most common non-neurological symptoms include sudden dyspnea and chest pain. Wheezing, rales, a harsh systolic murmur, or specific "mill-wheel" murmur may be heard.[9] Air bubbles in the retina and areas of pallor on the tongue (Liebermeister's sign) are rarely found.[15]

Air embolism may be detected by transcranial Doppler ultrasound.[36,37] Using this technique, emboli can be detected during surgery but these are infrequently clinically significant.[37] Hemodynamic changes or blood gas alterations and aspiration of air from the right atrium or pulmonary artery support the diagnosis.[10,83] A chest x-ray can show pulmonary edema or air in the heart.[84] CT of the brain may show air bubbles in a watershed distribution.[55] These findings are not always present and the diagnosis should be suspected in the appropriate clinical setting even in their absence. Early diagnosis is important since treatment can be very successful. If the event occurs during surgery, nitrous oxide should be discontinued, 100% oxygen administered, and the surgical field flooded with saline. Additionally, the patient should be placed in a left lateral Trendelenburg position.[14,30,37] If cardiopulmonary arrest occurs, closed chest compression with aspiration of air from the right heart may be attempted.[3] Transfer to a hyperbaric oxygen chamber should follow immediately if arterial embolism occurs. Hyperbaric treatment has been shown to be effective, often with complete resolution of neurological symptoms even when delayed by several days.[14,15,28]

Fat embolism to the brain is usually associated with orthopedic injuries,[32] but it has also been reported in three pregnant women. The first was an obese woman who died shortly after delivering a premature infant; fat debris was found in the brain on pathological examination. The mechanism of this complication is not known.[59] In a second case, fat embolism resulted after rupture of an ovarian dermoid cyst during labor.[89] In the final case, a pregnant woman with sickle-cell hemoglobin C (HbSC) had a sickle-cell crisis which resulted in release of fat cells into the circulation, possibly due to infarction of bone.[22] Fat embolism may be more common with HbSC than with homozygosity for hemoglobin S (HbSS) because of a higher blood viscosity associated with HbSC.[22,44] The use of pitressin, a common intravenous medication administered following delivery, has been implicated as a possible causative agent by decreasing bone blood flow.[22] Fat embolism has also been described in association with amniotic fluid embolism.[54] Patients have pulmonary, neurological, or cutaneous involvement, usually with a latent period from time of the inciting event. Pulmonary symptoms are the most common and are usually the cause of death.[32] Neurological features include focal ischemic deficits, confusion, agitation, decreased levels of consciousness, and seizures.[59] A cutaneous petechial rash involving the neck, axilla, and conjunctiva may be present.[32] Other findings include anemia, coagulopathy, and fever, but in the absence of accepted diagnostic criteria, antemortem diagnosis is often difficult.[32,59] Treatment is mostly supportive with early immobilization of fractures. Other reported therapeutic measures include anticoagulation, corticosteroids, and exchange transfusions.[22,32,39,58,91]

Amniotic fluid embolism is a well-recognized complication of pregnancy which is associated with a mortality rate as high as 86%.[80] This complication is reported to occur in between one in 8,000 births[100] to one in 80,000 births.[68] Several hundred cases have been reported in the literature.[32] Amniotic fluid embolism is often such a catastrophic event from the standpoint of cardiopulmonary collapse and disseminated intravascular coagulation that cerebral sequelae are unrecognized or of secondary importance.[87] Embolism occurs when the chorioamniotic membrane ruptures in women with uterine, cervical, or vaginal tears, releasing amniotic fluid constituents directly into venous channels.[80,105] Reported risk factors include increased patient age, multiparity, premature placental separation, intrauterine fetal death, meconium staining, and hypertonic labor.[80,87] The clinical picture is dramatic, with sudden onset of dyspnea, hypotension, and shock often followed rapidly by cardiopulmonary arrest. Survivors of the initial episode frequently develop disseminated intravascular coagulation. Central nervous system hypoxia may present with alterations in consciousness and seizures.[71,80,87] The diagnosis is supported by finding fetal debris in the buffy coat layer of blood in the appropriate clinical setting.[32] Treatment is mainly supportive as no studies have shown improved outcome with any particular therapy.[21,32,71,87,90,105] The use of anticoagulants remains controversial if disseminated intravascular coagulation is present. A few case reports suggest that aggressive supportive care may improve survival.[90]

Choriocarcinoma is a malignant tumor that arises from fetal trophoblastic tissue. It invades maternal uterine blood vessels and metastasizes to the central nervous system. Metastatic choriocarcinoma is now a well-recognized cause of single or multiple strokes.[1,2,47] Infarction[81] or hemorrhage[1,47,72] (Figure 2 *left*) due to choriocarcinoma can occur during or after normal pregnancy. Patients with a hydatidiform mole can have a year or more delay between the carcinoma and the occurrence of stroke.[2] Once metastatic cells reach the brain, they invade blood vessels[1,81] (Figure 2 *right*), leading to occlusion or rupture of cerebral blood vessels. Presentations may include stuttering stroke symptoms, focal or generalized seizures, headaches, mental status changes, neck stiffness, and sphincter disturbances.[1] The diagnosis should be considered in the appropriate clinical setting and with elevated serum chorionic gonadotrophin. Early treatment with multiagent chemotherapy, brain radiation, and surgical intervention is associated with cure rates as high as 95%.[38] Choriocarcinoma is further discussed in Chapter 12.

Arterial dissection of the internal carotid[66,111] or the vertebrobasilar[74,86,107] arteries can complicate pregnancy. Too few cases are reported to determine whether pregnancy increases the risk of dissection. As in a nonpregnant patient, dissection of the arterial wall may act as a nidus for thrombus formation which can distally embolize.[4,48,49] Strokes due to dissection appear to occur near the end of pregnancy, during labor, delivery, or in the postpartum period. The stress of labor and straining during delivery may be partly responsible for formation of an intimal tear.[107,111] An underlying arterial pathology such as fibromuscular dysplasia[35] or heritable connective-tissue disorder[96] may predispose the patient to increased risk for dissection. There may be a propensity for clot formation at the site of dissection due to the hypercoagulable state that exists during pregnancy and the puerperium.[30] The clinical syndrome usually in-

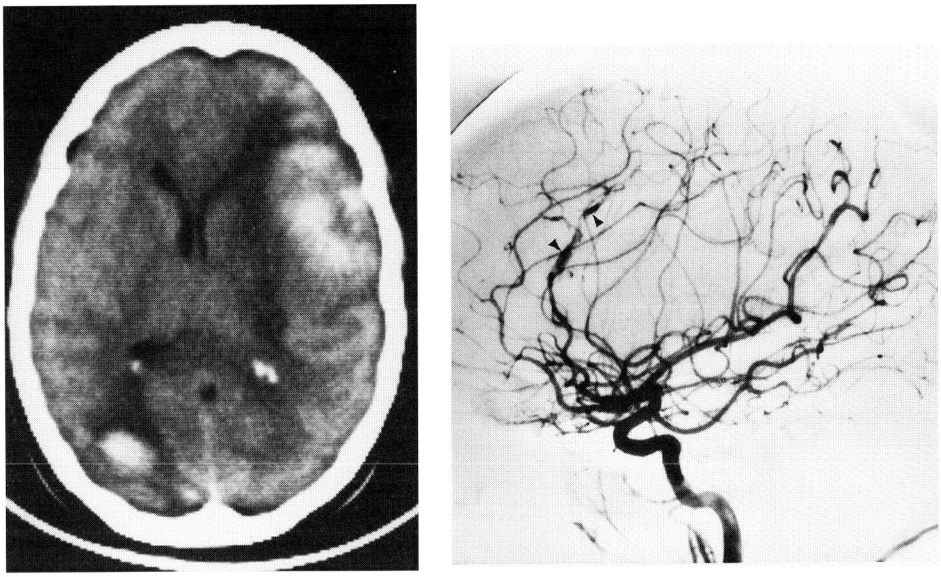

Figure 2: Left) CT scan without contrast of a 23-year-old woman 4 months postpartum with metastatic choriocarcinoma showing intracerebral hemorrhages in the left frontoparietal and right occipital regions. **Right)** Angiogram of the same patient demonstrating multiple areas of segmental dilatation and narrowing in the left carotid distribution. Additionally, there is intraluminal thrombosis and contrast extravasation (*arrows*).

volves ipsilateral head, face, or neck pain followed by neurological deficits referable to the involved artery.[48,49] A partial Horner's syndrome or cervical bruit may be detected on examination.[79] Diagnosis is confirmed with MRI or conventional angiography.[4] There is controversy regarding the most appropriate therapy; options include antiplatelet agents, anticoagulants, or surgery.[4,49] Most patients with dissection,[4,49] including those occurring during pregnancy, have a good prognosis.

Illicit drugs, including cocaine, are an increasingly recognized cause of stroke in young women. [20,56,61,67,78] Stroke associated with cocaine use can be due to thromboembolism, vasospasm, intracerebral hemorrhage, subarachnoid hemorrhage, and vasculitis.[19,61,67,78] Cocaine affects hemostasis by depleting antithrombin III and protein C and affects platelet aggregation by its action on arachidonic acid and thromboxane.[56,104] Cocaine use is associated with hypertension, myocardial ischemia, peripartum cardiomyopathy, and arrythmias which increase the risk of stroke.[26,76] These procoagulant and cardiac effects coupled with the prothrombotic state that exists during pregnancy[30] may place the pregnant patient at an increased risk of cerebral embolism. A detailed history of drug usage and a urine drug screen should be obtained in a pregnant woman presenting with stroke as this diagnosis can be overlooked.

Conclusions

Embolic stroke during pregnancy and the puerperium presents an important diagnostic challenge to the clinician because of the large number of potential causes, many of which are unusual. The most common source of embolism is the heart, and a careful cardiac evaluation is mandatory so that appropriate therapy with antiplatelet agents, anticoagulants, antibiotics, or surgery can be selected. Cardiogenic sources include bacterial endocarditis, rheumatic heart disease, prosthetic heart valve, atrial myxoma, anticardiolipin antibodies, paradoxical embolism, nonbacterial thrombotic endocarditis, and peripartum cardiomyopathy. While noncardiac causes of embolic stroke in the pregnant patient are rare, it is important to consider these entities in the setting of stroke during pregnancy. Only amniotic fluid embolism and choriocarcinoma are specifically related to pregnancy. Among the other causes of embolism, only air embolism has definitely been shown to occur more frequently during pregnancy. Awareness of these conditions may allow prompt diagnosis so that potentially lifesaving therapeutic measures may be instituted early.

REFERENCES

1. Adeloye A, Osuntokun BO, Hendrickse JP, et al: The neurology of metastatic chorion carcinoma of the uterus. **J Neurol Sci 16**:315-329, 1972
2. Aguilar MJ, Rabinovitch R: Metastatic chorionepithelioma simulating multiple strokes. **Neurology 14**: 933-937, 1964
3. Alvaran SB, Toung JK, Graff TE, et al: Venous air embolism: comparative merits of external cardiac massage, intracardiac aspiration, and left lateral decubitus position. **Anesth Analg 57**:166-170, 1978
4. Anson J, Crowell RM: Cervicocranial arterial dissection. **Neurosurgery 29**:89-96, 1991
5. The Antiphospholipid Antibodies in Stroke Study Group: Clinical and laboratory findings in patients with antiphospholipid antibodies and cerebral ischemia. **Stroke 21**:1268-1273, 1990
6. Artal R, Greenspoon JS, Rutherford S: Transient ischemic attack: a complication of mitral valve prolapse in pregnancy. **Obstet Gynecol 71**:1028-1030, 1988
7. Badduke BR, Jamieson WRE, Miyagishima RT, et al: Pregnancy and childbearing in a population with biologic valvular prostheses. **J Thorac Cardiovasc Surg 102**:179-186, 1991
8. Barbour LA, Kick SD, Steiner JF, et al: A prospective study of heparin-induced osteoporosis in pregnancy using bone densitometry. **Am J Obstet Gynecol 170**: 862-869, 1994
9. Beck DH, McQuillan PJ: Fatal carbon dioxide embolism and severe haemorrhage during laparoscopic salpingectomy. **Br J Anaesth 72**:243-245, 1994
10. Bedford RF, Marshall WK, Butler A, et al: Cardiac catheters for diagnosis and treatment of venous air embolism. A prospective study in man. **J Neurosurg 55**:610-614, 1981
11. Berger MP, Rams JJ, Davis DA, et al: Asymptomatic microemboli. **Neurology 43**:1865, 1993 (Letter)
12. Bergh PA, Hollander D, Gregori CA, et al: Mitral valve prolapse and thromboembolic disease in pregnancy: a case report. **Int J Gynaecol Obstet 27**: 133-137, 1988
13. Bernal JM, Miralles PJ: Cardiac surgery with cardiopulmonay bypass during pregnancy. **Obstet Gynecol Surv 41**:1-6, 1986
14. Bernhardt TL, Goldmann RW, Thombs PA, et al: Hyperbaric oxygen treatment of cerebral air embolism from orogenital sex during pregnancy. **Crit Care Med 16**:729-730, 1988
15. Bitterman H, Melamed Y: Delayed hyperbaric treatment of cerebral air embolism. **Isr J Med Sci 29**: 22-26, 1993
16. Bogousslavsky J, Pierre P: Ischemic stroke in patients under age 45. **Neurol Clin 10**:113-124, 1992
17. Born D, Martinez EE, Almeida PAM, et al: Pregnancy in patients with prosthetic heart valves: the effects of anticoagulation on mother, fetus, and neonate. **Am Heart J 124**:413-417, 1992
18. Branch DW: Antiphospholipid antibodies and pregnancy: maternal implications. **Semin Perinatol 14**: 139-146, 1990
19. Brown E, Prager J, Lee HY, et al: CNS complications of cocaine abuse: prevalence, pathophysiology and neuroradiology. **AJR 159**:137-147, 1992
20. Chasnoff IJ: Drug use and women: establishing a standard of care. **Ann NY Acad Sci 562**:208-210, 1989
21. Chatelain SM, Quirk JG Jr: Amniotic and thromboembolism. **Clin Obstet Gynecol 33**:473-481, 1990
22. Chmel H, Bertles JF: Hemoglobin S/C disease in a pregnant woman with crisis and fat embolization syndrome. **Am J Med 58**:563-566, 1975
23. CLASP (Collaborative Low-Dose Aspirin Study in Pregnancy) Collaborative Group: CLASP: a randomized trial of low-dose aspirin for the prevention and treatment of pre-eclampsia among 9364 pregnant women. **Lancet 343**:619-629, 1994
24. Cooke RT: Fatal air embolism due to vaginal douching in pregnancy. **Medical Memoranda 1**:1241, 1950
25. Cox SM, Hankins GDV, Leveno KJ, et al: Bacterial endocarditis. A serious pregnancy complication. **J Reprod Med 33**:671-674, 1988
26. Cregler LL, Mark H: Medical complications of cocaine abuse. **N Engl J Med 315**:1495-1500, 1986
27. Dahlman TC: Osteoporotic fractures and the recurrence of thromboembolism during pregnancy and the puerperium in 184 women undergoing thromboprophylaxis with heparin. **Am J Obstet Gynecol 168**: 1265-1270, 1993
28. Davis FM, Glover PW, Maycock E: Hyperbaric oxygen for cerebral arterial air embolism occurring during caesarian section. **Anaesth Intensive Care 18**: 403-405, 1990
29. Degani S, Abinader EG, Scharf M: Mitral valve prolapse and pregnancy: a review. **Obstet Gynecol Surv 44**:642-649, 1989
30. Digre KB, Varner MW: Diagnosis and treatment of cerebrovascular disorders in pregnancy, in Adams HP Jr (ed): **Handbook of Cerebrovascular Diseases.** New York, NY: Marcel Dekker, 1993, pp 255-286
31. Donaldson JO, Lee NS: Arterial and venous stroke associated with pregnancy. **Neurol Clin 12**:583-599, 1994
32. Dudney TM, Elliott CG: Pulmonary embolism from amniotic fluid, fat, and air. **Prog Cardiovasc Dis 36**: 447-474, 1994
33. Dyken ME, Biller J: Peripartum cardiomyopathy and stroke. **Cerebrovasc Dis 4**:325-328, 1994
34. Eckert WG, Katchis S, Dotson P: The unusual accidental death of a pregnant woman by sexual foreplay. **Am J Forensic Med Pathol 12**:247-249, 1991
35. Ezra Y, Kidron D, Beyth Y: Fibromuscular dysplasia

of the carotid arteries complicating pregnancy. **Obstet Gynecol 73**:840-843, 1989

36. Fong J, Gadella F, Druzin M: Venous emboli occurring during caesarean section: the effect of patient position. **Can J Anaesth 38**:191-195, 1991
37. Fong J, Gadalla F, Gimbel AA: Precordial Doppler diagnosis of haemodynamically compromising air embolism during caesarean section. **Can J Anaesth 37**:262-264, 1990
38. Fox MW, Harms RW, Davis DH: Selected neurologic complications of pregnancy. **Mayo Clin Proc 65**: 1595-1618, 1990
39. Fulde GWO, Harrison P: Fat embolism–a review. **Arch Emerg Med 8**:223-239, 1991
40. George J, Lamb JT, Harriman DGF: Cerebral embolism due to non-bacterial thrombotic endocarditis following pregancy. **J Neurol Neurosurg Psychiatry 47**:79-80, 1984
41. Ginsberg JS, Barron WM: Pregnancy and prosthetic heart valves. **Lancet 344**:1170-1171, 1994
42. Ginsberg JS, Hirsh J: Use of antithrombotic agents during pregnancy. **Chest 102 (Suppl 4)**:385S-390S, 1992
43. Ginsberg JS, Kowalchuk G, Hirsch J, et al: Heparin therapy during pregnancy. Risks to fetus and mother. **Arch Intern Med 149**:2233-2236, 1989
44. Godeau B, Dhainaut JF, Bachir D, et al: Pulmonary fat embolism after prostaglandin infusion in sickle cell disease with fatal outcome exchange blood transfusion. **Am J Hematol 43**:330-331, 1993 (Letter)
45. Golby AJ, Bush EC, DeRook FA, et al: Failure of high-dose heparin to prevent recurrent cardioembolic strokes in a pregnant patient with a mechanial heart valve. **Neurology 42**:2204-2206, 1992
46. Grindal AB, Cohen RJ, Saul RF, et al: Cerebral infarction in young adults. **Stroke 9**:39-42, 1978
47. Gurwitt LJ, Long JM, Clark RE: Cerebral metastatic choriocarcinoma. A postpartum cause of "stroke." **Obstet Gynecol 45**:583-588, 1975
48. Hart RG, Easton JD: Dissections. **Stroke 16**:925-927, 1985
49. Hart RG, Easton JD: Dissections of cervical and cerebral arteries. **Neurol Clin 1**:155-182, 1983
50. Hart RG, Miller VT: Cerebral infarction in young adults: a practical approach. **Stroke 14**:110-114, 1983
51. Hill BF, Jones JS: Venous air embolism following orogenital sex during pregnancy. **Am J Emerg Med 11**: 155-157, 1993
52. Hodgman MT, Pessin MS, Homans DC, et al: Cerebral embolism as the initial manifestation of peripartum cardiomyopathy. **Neurology 32**:668-671, 1982
53. Homans DC: Peripartum cardiomyopathy. **N Engl J Med 312**:1432-1437, 1985
54. Huaman A, Nice W, Merkel RL, et al: Amniotic fat embolism. New laboratory diagnosis and a case presentation. **J Kans Med Soc 73**:441-443, 1972
55. Hwang TL, Fremaux R, Sears ES, et al: Confirmation of cerebral air embolism with computerized tomography. **Ann Neurol 13**:214-225, 1983
56. Isner JM, Chokshi SK: Cocaine and vasospasm. **N Engl J Med 321**:1604-1606, 1989 (Editorial)
57. Iturbe-Alessio I, del Carmen Fonseca M, Mutchinik O, et al: Risks of anticoagulant therapy in pregnant women with artificial heart valves. **N Engl J Med 315**: 1390-1393, 1986
58. Jacobson DM, Terrence CF, Reinmuth OM: The neurologic manifestations of fat embolism. **Neurology 36**:847-851, 1986
59. Jonas EG: Maternal death due to fat-embolism. A case report. **J Obstet Gynecol 68**:479-480, 1961
60. Kashuk JL, Penn I: Air embolism after central venous catheterization. **Surg Gynecol Obstet 159**:249-252, 1984
61. Klonoff DC, Andrews BT, Obana WG: Stroke associated with cocaine use. **Arch Neurol 46**:989-993, 1989
62. Knepper LE, Biller J, Adams HP Jr, et al: Neurologic manifestations of atrial myxoma. A 12-year experience and review. **Stroke 19**:1435-1440, 1988
63. Lanzino G, Andreoli A, Di Pasquale G, et al: Etiopathogenesis and prognosis of cerebral ischemia in young adults. A survey of 155 treated patients. **Acta Neurol Scand 84**:321-325, 1991
64. Laupacis A, Albers G, Dunn M, et al: Antithrombotic therapy in atrial fibrillation. **Chest 102 (Suppl 4)**: 426S-433S, 1992
65. Lee W: Clinical management of gravid women with peripartum cardiomyopathy. **Obstet Gynecol Clin North Am 18**:257-271, 1991
66. Lepojärvi M, Tarkka M, Leinonen A, et al: Spontaneous dissection of the internal carotid artery. **Acta Chir Scand 154**:559-566, 1988
67. Levine SR, Brust JCM, Futrell N, et al: Cerebrovascular complications of the use of the "crack" form of alkaloidal cocaine. **N Engl J Med 323**:699-704, 1990
68. Lewis TLT: The changing practice of obstetrics, in Lewis TLT (ed): **Progress in Clinical Obstetrics and Gynecology.** London: Churchill Livingstone, 1964, p 48
69. Lisovoski F, Rousseaux P: Cerebral infarction in young people. A study of 148 patients with early cerebral angiography. **J Neurol Neurosurg Psychiatry 54**:576-579, 1991
70. Lopez JA, Fishbein MC, Siegel RJ: Echocardiographic features of nonbacterial thrombotic endocarditis. **Am J Cardiol 59**:478-480, 1987
71. Mainprize TC, Maltby JR: Amniotic fluid embolism: a report of four probable cases. **Can Anaesth Soc J 33**:382-387, 1986
72. Mandybur TI: Intracranial hemorrhage caused by metastatic tumors. **Neurology 27**:650-655, 1977
73. Martland HS: Air embolism. Fatal air embolism due to powder insufflators used in gynecological treatments. **Am J Surg 68**:164-169, 1945
74. Mas JL, Bousser MG, Corone P, et al: Anévrysme disséquant des artères vertébrales extracraniennes et grossesse. **Rev Neurol 143**:761-764, 1987
75. Melissari E, Parker CJ, Wilson NV, et al: Use of low molecular weight heparin in pregnancy. **Thromb Haemost 68**:652-656, 1992
76. Mendelson MA, Chandler J: Postpartum cardiomyopathy associated with maternal cocaine abuse. **Am J Cardiol 70**:1092-1094, 1992
77. Midei MG, DeMent SH, Feldman AM, et al: Peripartum myocarditis and cardiomyopathy. **Circulation 81**:922-928, 1990
78. Mody CK, Miller BL, McIntyre HB, et al: Neurologic complications of cocaine abuse. **Neurology 38**: 1189-1193, 1988
79. Mokri B, Schievink WI, Olsen KD, et al: Spontaneous dissection of the cervical internal carotid artery. Presentation with lower cranial nerve palsies. **Arch Otolaryngol Head Neck Surg 118**:431-435, 1992

80. Morgan M: Amniotic fluid embolism. **Anaesthesia 34:**20-32, 1979
81. Nakagawa Y, Tashiro K, Isu T, et al: Occlusion of cerebral artery due to metastasis of chorioepithelioma. Case report. **J Neurosurg 51:**247-250, 1979
82. Oakley C, Doherty P: Pregnancy in patients after valve replacement. **Br Heart J 38:**1140-1148, 1976
83. Orebaugh SL: Venous air embolism: clinical and experimental considerations. **Crit Care Med 20:** 1169-1177, 1992
84. OSMA Committee on Material Health: Maternal deaths due to air embolism. **Ohio State Med J:** 1105-1107, 1972
85. Payne DG, Fishburne JI Jr, Rufty AJ, et al: Bacterial endocarditis in pregnancy. **Obstet Gynecol 60:** 247-250, 1982
86. Peerier O, Cauche C, Demanet JC: Hematointramural par dissection parietale (anevrysme dissequant) du tronc basilare. **Acta Neurol Psychiatr Belg 64:**1064-1074, 1964
87. Peterson EP, Taylor HB: Amniotic fluid embolism. An analysis of 40 cases. **Obstet Gynecol 35:**787-793, 1970
88. **Physicians' Desk Reference, 48th ed.** Montvale, NJ: Medical Economics, 1994
89. Prichard RW: Generalized fat embolism: a complication of rupture of a dermoid cyst during labor: a case report. **Med Times 93:**1359-1362, 1965
90. Resnik R, Swartz WH, Plumer MH, et al: Amniotic fluid embolism with survival. **Obstet Gynecol 47:** 295-298, 1976
91. Robert JH, Hoffmeyer P, Broquet PE, et al: Fat embolism syndrome. **Orthop Rev 22:**567-571, 1993
92. Sadan O, Adler M, Ezra S, et al: Air embolism due to pulmonary barotrauma in a patient undergoing cesarean section. **Acta Obstet Gynecol Scand 70:** 511-513, 1991
93. Salazar E, Zajarias A, Gutierrez N, et al: The problem of cardiac valve prostheses, anticoagulants, and pregnancy. **Circulation 70 (Suppl I):**I169-I177, 1984
94. Sareli P, England MJ, Berk MR, et al: Maternal and fetal sequelae of anticoagulation during pregnancy in patients with mechanical heart valve prostheses. **Am J Cardiol 63:**1462-1465, 1989
95. Sbarouni E, Oakley CM: Outcome of pregnancy in women with valve prostheses. **Br Heart J 71:**196-201, 1994
96. Schievink WI, Michels VV, Piepgras DG: Neurovascular manifestations of heritable connective tissue disorders. A review. **Stroke 25:**889-903, 1994
97. Schwarz GA: Pathogenesis of certain neurologic complications following from knee-chest position in the puerperium. **Obstet Gynecol 27:**536-540, 1966
98. Simolke GA, Cox SM, Cunningham FG: Cerebrovascular accidents complicating pregnancy and the puerperium. **Obstet Gynecol 78:**37-42, 1991
99. Srinivasan K: Cerebral venous and arterial thrombosis in pregnancy and puerperium: A study of 135 patients. **Angiology 34:**731-746, 1983
100. Steiner PE, Lushbaugh CC: Maternal pulmonary embolism by amniotic fluid. As a cause of obstetric shock and unexpected deaths in obstetrics. **JAMA 117:**1340-1344, 1941
101. Stern BJ: Cerebrovascular disease and pregnancy, in Goldsten PJ, Stern BJ (eds): **Neurological Disorders of Pregnancy, 2nd ed.** Mount Kisco, NY: Futura Publishing, 1992, pp 51-84
102. Stoddard MF, Longaker RA, Vuocolo LM, et al: Transesophageal echocardiography in the pregnant patient. **Am Heart J 124:**785-787, 1992
103. Strasberg GD: Postpartum Group B Streptococcal endocarditis associated with mitral valve prolapse. **Obstet Gynecol 70:**485-487, 1987
104. Togna G, Tempesta E, Togna AR, et al: Platelet responsiveness and biosynthesis of thromboxane and prostacyclin in response to *in vitro* cocaine treatment. **Haemostasis 15:**100-107, 1985
105. Turner R, Gusack M: Massive amniotic fluid embolism. **Ann Emerg Med 13:**359-361, 1984
106. Turpie AGG, Gent M, Laupacis A, et al: A comparison of aspirin with placebo in patients treated with warfarin after heart-valve replacement. **N Engl J Med 329:**524-529, 1993
107. Van de Kelft E, Kunnen J, Truyen L, et al: Postpartum dissecting aneurysm of the basilar artery. **Stroke 23:** 114-116, 1992
108. Waldrop GS: Fatal air embolism during term labor and the puerperium. Report of a case. **Obstet Gynecol 1:**454-459, 1953
109. Wiebers DO: Ischemic cerebrovascular complications of pregnancy. **Arch Neurol 42:**1106-1113, 1985
110. Wiebers DO, Whisnant JP: The incidence of stroke among pregnant women in Rochester, Minn, 1955 through 1979. **JAMA 254:**3055-3057, 1985
111. Wiebers MD, Mokri B: Internal carotid artery dissection after childbirth. **Stroke 16:**956-959, 1985
112. Wilson JJ, Zahn CA, Ross SD, et al: Association of embolic stroke in pregnancy with the lupus anticoagulant. A case report. **J Reprod Med 31:**725-728, 1986
113. Wilterdink JL, Easton JD: Cerebral ischemia. **Adv Neurol 64:**1-11, 1994
114. Wong V, Cheng CH, Chan KC: Fetal and neonatal outcome of exposure to anticoagulants during pregnancy. **Am J Med Genet 45:**17-21, 1993

CHAPTER 12

CHORIOCARCINOMA IN PREGNANCY

MICHAEL SALCMAN, MD, FACS

Choriocarcinoma, a form of gestational trophoblastic neoplasia, is the most malignant tumor associated with pregnancy. It is preceded by a hydatidiform mole in 50% of patients, by a spontaneous abortion or an ectopic pregnancy in 30%, and by a normal term pregnancy in <20% of cases. The importance of choriocarcinoma to the neurologist and neurosurgeon derives from several unique features. First, the tumor has a very high incidence of metastatic spread to the central nervous system (CNS) and may initially present as an intracranial mass lesion. Between 10% and 15% of choriocarcinomas involve the CNS in comparison to <1% of other gynecological malignancies.[36] In many patients with metastatic choriocarcinoma, involvement of the brain is the most frequent cause of death.[10] Second, the tumor has a very high incidence of spontaneous hemorrhage and may present as postpartum stroke of unknown etiology.[26,31] Choriocarcinoma is also among the most frequent tumors associated with the formation of oncotic aneurysms and may be a cause of subarachnoid hemorrhage. Third, successful treatment of gestational choriocarcinoma metastatic to the brain with the aid of chemotherapy has important lessons to teach us in regard to the management of similar or even identical germ cell tumors arising in the testis, pituitary gland, and pineal region.[9,30,37]

INCIDENCE

The incidence of choriocarcinoma is highly variable in different populations. In the United States, from one in 20,000 to one in 40,000 pregnancies is associated with the development of a gestational trophoblastic tumor; in Southeast Asia, choriocarcinoma is observed after 1:250 to 1:3,708 pregnancy events, and the tumor represents 3% of all malignancies in Thai women.[7] Pre-existing molar pregnancy is a known risk factor for the development of choriocarcinoma and the incidence of this condition also demonstrates a striking geographic and racial variation. The incidence of molar pregnancy ranges from 1:1,200 to 1:2,500 in the United States, but may occur as frequently as 1:200 to 1:250 in Thailand. Similar figures have been suggested for Nigeria. Under the appropriate circumstances, therefore, one should be especially suspicious of the diagnosis of CNS choriocarcinoma in women of Chinese or Japanese extraction.

The incidence of CNS involvement in choriocarcinoma is not precisely known. On the basis of clinical manifestations alone, 10% to 15% of choriocarcinomas involve the CNS, compared with <1% of other gynecological malignancies.[36] The overall clinical incidence is about 20%, but cerebral metastases have been found in 40% to 66.7% of cases at autopsy.[17,31,36] In most geographic areas, choriocarcinoma is a relatively rare cause of metastatic brain tumor. In Southeast Asia, however, this lesion represented 12% (20/171) of all metastatic brain tumors encountered in a clinical series.[28] In a computed tomography (CT) study conducted in Bangkok, choriocarcinoma represented 9.3% of all tumors (four of 43) found to seed the cerebrospinal fluid (CSF) pathways.[16] In a United States registry of 1,800 cases of chorionepithelioma, 70 were found to involve the CNS.[36] Overall, the brain is the fourth most frequent site of metastatic choriocarcinoma, exceeded only by the lung, vagina, and liver.[13]

Although choriocarcinoma may follow any gestational event (i.e., hydatidiform mole, spontaneous abortion, or term pregnancy), the disease is most aggressive after a term gestation and CNS metastases are also more common with such tumors. In a series of 366 patients with choriocarcinoma, 15 (4%) developed the tumor after a term pregnancy. Systemic metastases were detected in 87% (13 patients) at the time of diagnosis,[4] seven (54%) of whom demonstrated involvement of the liver and/or brain. Conversely, the incidence of systemic metastases was only 36% (125/351) in choriocarcinoma patients with other gestational events ($p < 0.01$), and the incidence of hepatic or cerebral lesions was only 10%.[4] Similarly, there were only 14 cases of metastatic brain lesions identified in a series of more than 500 gestational (i.e., non-hydatidiform mole) cases of choriocarcinoma without preceding delivery.[33]

PATHOLOGY

Choriocarcinoma is a germ cell tumor composed of syncytotrophoblastic and cytotrophoblastic elements. It may develop from the hydatidiform mole, a pre-existing benign lesion that contains all the elements of the original conceptus including the cytotrophoblast, syncytotrophoblast, and chorionic villi. Hydatidiform moles may demonstrate an abnormal karyotype, metastasis, and malignant transformation. Of course, choriocarcinomas are much more poorly differentiated. The tumor consists of an abnormal proliferation of cuboidal and syncytial cells of the placental epithelium. In addition, the cytotrophoblasts are clearly anaplastic and the syncytotrophoblasts lack villi. The tumor demonstrates striking pleomorphism, areas of hemorrhage, and immunoreactivity for both human chorionic gonadotropin (hCG) and human placental lactogen. It usually develops as a malignant lesion in which the uterine wall is invaded by trophoblastic cells.[23] The primary lesion can be restricted or rejected, and the patient may die later from the effects of metastatic disease without sign of the primary tumor at autopsy. On occasion, even pulmonary metastases have been observed to spontaneously regress. Of course, spontaneous rejection is more common in cases of hydatidiform mole than it is in patients with malignant choriocarcinoma.

The mechanism of metastatic spread in choriocarcinoma is clearly hematogenous and is based on the propensity for normal chorionic tissue to root within the uterine wall for blood vessels to nourish the fetus. In the brain, trophoblasts invade the vasculature just as they would in the uterus or in the pulmonary capillaries. The damaged vessel may thrombose, produce an embolus, or its wall may weaken and form an aneurysmal pouch or varicosity.[31] At autopsy, some patients who present with embolic infarctions secondary to tumor cells in the vessel walls do not have evidence of parenchymal tumor.[35] Frank invasion of the walls of cerebral vessels has been demonstrated histologically in a number of case reports of oncotic aneurysms secondary to choriocarcinoma.[8,10,22,24] The abnormal vessels associated with tumor growth also have weak walls and may bleed into the tumor or into the surrounding brain. When associated aneurysms are present, subarachnoid hemorrhage is also possible. At autopsy, the majority (62.5%) of metastatic cerebral lesions are found to be hemorrhagic.[17] Next to metastatic melanoma, choriocarcinoma has the highest rate of spontaneous hemorrhage of any brain tumor and, in comparison to other types of metastatic tumor, choriocarcinoma appears to bleed at an earlier stage of implantation.[21]

The cerebral metastases of choriocarcinoma can be solitary or multiple and are usually located within the distribution of the middle cerebral artery. In a series of 24 cases, 66.7%

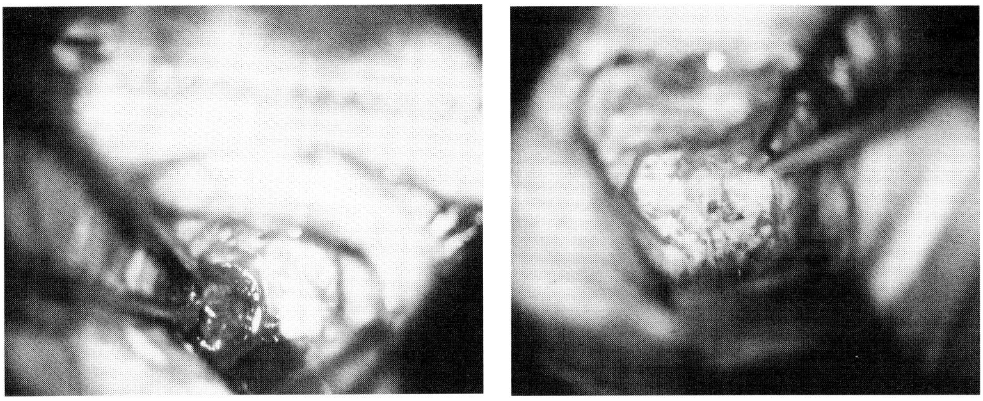

Figure 1: Appearance of metastatic choriocarcinoma at surgery. The patient was a 22-year-old white male with a known testicular tumor who presented with intracranial mass effect. At surgery, the metastasis was discovered to be grossly hemorrhagic (**left**) and the surrounding white matter was yellow and discolored from unsuspected subclinical bleeding. This finding is more obvious after removal of the hemorrhagic nidus (**right**).

were single lesions and the most frequent locations, in descending order, were the parietal, temporal, occipital, cerebellar, and frontal portions of the brain.[17] In a combined clinical and pathological study of 47 cases, the most frequent locations were parietal (45%), frontal (43%), occipital (23%), temporal (15%), and cerebellar (9%), with 4% of lesions in the brain stem.[36] Additionally, 9% of the patients had spinal metastases. In this study, only 21% of the tumors were multifocal. When choriocarcinoma gains access to the CSF pathways, it usually spreads to the lateral ventricles and the supratentorial leptomeninges.[16]

Presentation

For obvious reasons, patients with metastatic choriocarcinoma are overwhelmingly young and female. In one series of 34 patients with cerebral metastases, the average age was 33.7 years;[18] in another report of 14 cases, the average age was 21.6 years.[33] In the largest reported series, the average age was 26.9 years with a range of 13 to 49 years.[36] In a few women, CNS involvement first becomes evident in the fifth or sixth decade, well past the childbearing years, when a previously undiagnosed benign mole has undergone malignant transformation.[17,28] In a series containing such patients, the age at presentation ranged from 23 to 60 years with an average of 35.5 years.[17] In a series of 78 cases in a worldwide United States-based registry, 56% of the patients were white, 18% black, 2.7% Oriental, 2.7% Mexican, 1.4% Native American, and 19.2% were of unknown racial origin.[36] Cerebral choriocarcinoma in males usually occurs within the context of metastatic spread from a testicular tumor (Figure 1).

From the time of diagnosis of the primary tumor, metastatic involvement of the CNS occurs with a highly variable latency. In a series of 14 cases, the range reported was 1 to 30 months, with a mean of 7 months.[33] In some patients, the diagnosis is made more difficult by the fact that latencies as short as 2 days and as long as 17 years can occur between pregnancy and presentation of the primary tumor.[10] In the majority of cases, however, neurological symptoms develop within the context of known metastatic involvement of other organs. In particular, almost all cases of cerebral choriocarcinoma demonstrate prior or simultaneous pulmonary disease. In one series of cerebral metastases, 30 of 34 patients also had pulmonary involvement;[18] in another series of 14 cases, all patients with CNS lesions also had lung tumors.[33] In 74 registry cases, concomitant metastases were recorded in the lungs (97%), uterus (74%), liver (36%), kidney (26%), vagina (19%), intestine (15%), pelvis (7%), scalp (3%), and 1% in the vulva.[36] In this series, the brain was the sole apparent metastatic site in only one case. In the People's Republic of China, vaginal metastases have been seen in a little more than one third of cases of cerebral choriocarcinoma.[18]

Despite the propensity of cerebral choriocarcinoma to present in the context of systemic disease, 10% of cerebral metastases become symptomatic prior to knowledge of either the primary tumor or other metastatic sites.[5] This rate is similar to that reported for other types of primary cancers metastatic to the brain. For example, purely neurological presentations have been described in two Chinese women, a 30-year-old who became ill 1-1/2 years after a molar pregnancy and a 26-year-old who developed symptoms 5 months after a first trimester abortion.[13]

The metastatic lesions of choriocarcinoma are frequently hemorrhagic, and much of the neurological literature has emphasized this feature.[21,31] Seven of 12 patients with cerebral metastases in one series and 14 of 23 in another had a history of stroke.[1,31] Usually, an apoplectic event occurs in the context of a known hydatidiform mole or postpartum choriocarcinoma, but may also occur during the course of an otherwise normal pregnancy.[11] Intracranial hemorrhage is the most frequent mode of presentation in two-thirds of cerebral metastases.[14] On occasion, neurological symptoms precede diagnosis of the primary tumor;[13,28] this may occur in up to 10% of cases.[5] Transient focal, hemispheric, or global signs, possibly representing transient ischemic episodes secondary to embolic tumor in cerebral vessels, form a unique prodromal syndrome. This is usually followed in a month by the classic symptoms of a mass lesion.[7,27] In women of childbearing age, the triad of menstrual abnormalities, recent or remote pregnancy or abortion, and an acute cerebrovascular event with evidence of a mass lesion should suggest the diagnosis of metastatic choriocarcinoma.[7] Stroke is a leading cause of maternal death and choriocarcinoma is an important element in the differential diagnosis.[5]

Approximately 3% to 4% of all brain tumors develop intratumoral or peritumoral bleeding and an equal number of apparently spontaneous intracerebral hematomas actually are due to primary or metastatic neoplasms.[26] Among metastatic brain tumors, the incidence of spontaneous intratumoral bleeding is highest for malignant melanoma and metastatic choriocarcinoma.[32] At autopsy, the majority of choriocarcinomas in the brain are hemorrhagic.[17] When the tumor bleeds into itself, the hemorrhage may be clinically silent; bleeding into the surrounding parenchyma is almost always symptomatic. In a series of 66 registry cases, CNS involvement was asymptomatic in 8%.[36] Temporary or permanent occlusion of cerebral vessels by tumor emboli may result in cerebral infarction.

As already mentioned, choriocarcinoma in the brain has frequently been observed to invade the walls of blood vessels and, as a result, patients may present with either subarachnoid hemorrhage or intraparenchymal bleeding secondary to rupture of an oncotic aneurysm.[7,8,10,12,22,24,27] At least 18 cases of oncotic cerebral aneurysm have been tabulated;[10] some cases in earlier reports have been missed or were secondary to nongestational ovarian choriocarcinoma.[12,25] The clinical picture can be indistinguishable from that of ordinary aneurysmal subarachnoid hemorrhage. The aneurysms can be multiple and may originate from neoplastic implants in the heart.[8,27] A similar sequence of events has been reported in association with emboli from cardiac myxoma and bronchogenic carcinoma.[12] Neoplastic aneurysms usually develop at distal sites in the distribution of the middle cerebral artery.[10,24] Hemorrhage from such aneurysms may occur in the first few days of the postpartum period.[22]

The signs and symptoms of metastatic choriocarcinoma are otherwise similar to those of any secondary cerebral neoplasm and depend highly on the location of the tumor in the brain. The most frequent symptom is headache and it is present in more than one-half of patients.[18] In a series of 66 registry cases, the most frequent signs and symptoms were headache (55%), paresis (49%), cranial nerve symptoms (36%), decreased sensorium (29%), seizures (24%), nausea and vomiting (23%), aphasia (17%), meningismus (8%), and papilledema in 8%.[36]

Prognosis

In a series of 399 patients with choriocarcinoma, 50% of the 48 cases that died had metastases to the brain, liver, or peritoneal cavity when they first presented for treatment.[20] Death in patients with metastatic choriocarcinoma is associated with a pregnancy event (term pregnancy, abortion, or ectopic pregnancy) rather than a hydatidiform mole in 71% of cases, with delay in diagnosis from the pregnancy event of >4 months or a pretreatment serum beta-hCG titer of >100,000 IU/L in 64%. The most common immediate causes of death are hemorrhage from a metastatic site (42%) and pulmonary insufficiency (31%).

In a series of 78 patients with choriocarcinoma and CNS involvement, those who failed to receive chemotherapy and radiation died in 74% of cases from CNS causes.[36] In patients who received only chemotherapy, 24% survived and 58% died of CNS complications; in those who received both chemotherapy and irradiation, there was a 50% survival rate and none of the deaths were due to CNS causes.[36] Patients with post-term metastatic choriocarcinoma in the liver and brain invariably die if the diagnosis is delayed more than 4 months from the antecedent term delivery.[4]

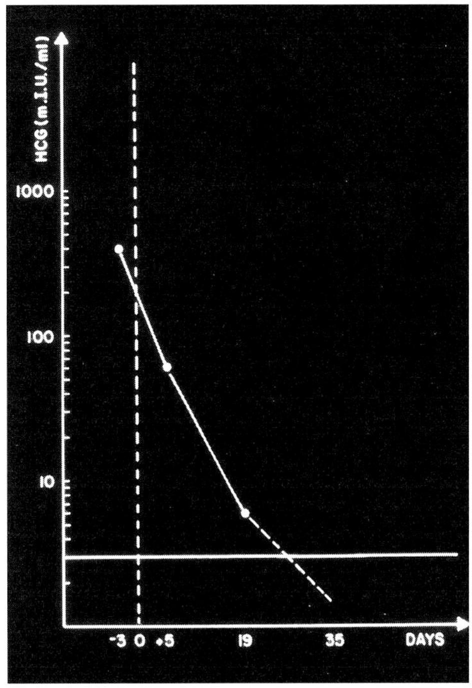

Figure 2: Use of plasma hCG levels to monitor therapy. The levels were measured 3 days prior to surgery, and at 5, 19, and 35 days postoperatively. The *vertical dotted line* indicates the time of craniotomy and the *horizontal solid line* the upper limit of normal for plasma hCG. Exponential clearing of hCG from the plasma on this semilogarithmic plot not only demonstrates the effectiveness of craniotomy but also confirms that the cerebral tumor was the only metastatic lesion in this patient (same case as Figure 1).

Diagnostic Workup

The presence of an invasive hydatidiform mole or choriocarcinoma is usually documented by pelvic examination, curettage, pelvic ultrasound, and angiography. The extent of metastatic disease is determined by chest x-ray, liver function tests, a brain CT or magnetic resonance imaging (MRI) scan, a liver isotope scan, CSF hCG level, laparoscopy, intravenous pyelography, and selective angiography of pelvic and abdominal organs. Levels of plasma hCG are monitored weekly until they are normal for 3 consecutive weeks and then monthly until normal for 12 consecutive months.[4] Plasma levels are measured by radioimmunoassay for the beta-subunit of hCG (Figure 2). Serum values of beta-hCG >40,000 mIU/ml or urine beta-hCG >100,000 IU/24 hours carry a bad prognosis.[10] Nongestational choriocarcinomas or mixed germ cell tumors of the testis and pineal gland may cause elevations in alpha-fetoprotein.[7]

In general, cerebral choriocarcinoma enhances brightly with contrast on both CT and MRI scans (Figure 3). A variable amount of peritumoral edema is observed and an angiographic blush is seen on vascular studies. The findings are nonspecific since they are typical of any highly vascular and/or hemorrhagic lesion. In particular, metastatic gestational choriocarcinoma, metastatic testicular choriocarcinoma, and primary choriocarcinoma of the pineal gland share similar radiographic features. Bleeding can be observed either in the center or at the periphery of the tumor. As previously discussed, secondary oncotic aneurysms are usually located on the distal segments of the middle

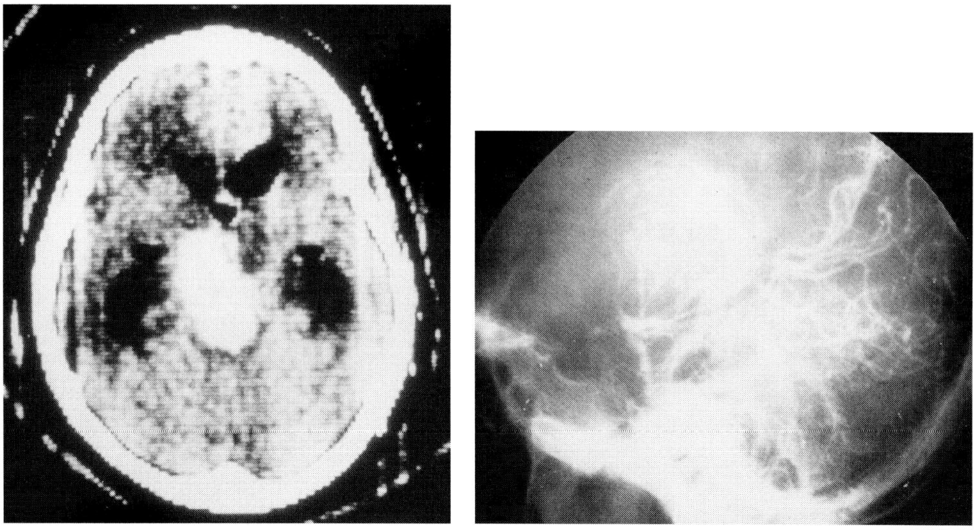

Figure 3: Radiological appearance of a primary choriocarcinoma of the pineal region. The patient was a 13-year-old white male with elevated plasma levels of hCG and signs of raised intracranial pressure. The axial CT scan (**left**) demonstrates unusually bright enhancement and hydrocephalus. This study was one of the first enhanced CT scans performed at the Neurological Institute of New York. The lateral angiogram (**right**) demonstrates the tremendous hypersaccularity of the lesion fed by the posterior choroidal arteries.

cerebral artery; the sacs can be smooth or irregular, large or small, single or multiple.

TREATMENT

Chemotherapy has a prominent role in the management of patients with choriocarcinoma. It is the primary treatment in all cases with disseminated disease, with or without CNS metastases. In the presence of multiple intracranial lesions, chemotherapy is used in combination with cranial radiation because nearly all such patients have pulmonary metastases as well. In the treatment of solitary hemorrhagic lesions, chemotherapy can be employed to consolidate the beneficial effects of craniotomy and radiation on the presumption of systemic disease and nonvisualized seedlings in the brain. Since multiagent chemotherapy is used in the initial treatment of all high-risk patients with choriocarcinoma, systemic exposure may serve a prophylactic function in the nervous system.

High-risk patients with metastatic choriocarcinoma require up-front treatment with multiagent rather than single-agent chemotherapy.[4,19] Adverse prognostic factors include high levels of serum hCG, prolonged time to diagnosis, term pregnancy as a prelesion event, previous failed therapy, and metastatic disease in the brain, liver, or small intestine.[4,20] Once instituted, the response rate to multiagent chemotherapy is only 44% for patients with metastases outside the lungs or vagina compared to 74% for more restricted disease ($p<0.05$); the response rate is 50% for patients with term pregnancies as opposed to 75% for those with abortions, and only 27% for patients with three or more risk factors in comparison to 74% ($p<0.005$) for those with better prognostic profiles.[20] It is important to recognize high-risk patients because multiagent chemotherapy as an up-front treatment has a 63% response rate but when used in a secondary manner is effective in only 30% of patients ($p<0.01$).[20] Low-risk patients usually receive single-agent chemotherapy with either 15 to 25 mg daily of intramuscular methotrexate or 12 μg/kg of intravenous actinomycin-D.[34,36]

In the 1980s, the overall response rate to standard multiagent chemotherapy stabilized at about 51%.[19,34] The regimen consists of 0.3

mg/kg of intramuscular methotrexate, 3 mg/kg of cytoxan or cyclophosphamide, and 8-10 µg/kg of intravenous actinomycin-D given over 5 days at 12- to 14-day cycles.[19] Patients with an invasive mole rather than choriocarcinoma are usually cured ($p<0.005$). In order to further improve the results, a number of other agents have been used in addition to these, especially cis-platinum, bleomycin, and etopside; these drugs are also used to treat patients in relapse after primary chemotherapy.[19] Some investigators use the Bagshawe (cyclophosphamide, hydroxyurea, actinomycin-D, methotrexate, Oncovin (vincristine), citrovorum factor, and adriamycin), or CHAM-OCA, regimen upfront in the treatment of high-risk patients.[19,20] Endpoints for multiagent chemotherapy include clearing of lesions on radiographic studies and the disappearance of measureable hCG by radioimmunoassay. Since the latter is negative in the presence of <10,000 cells, it is important to continue chemotherapy for 2 to 3 cycles beyond normalization of the hCG level.[19] Long-term surveillance is essential because some tumors can recur after more than a year of normalized hCG levels.[15]

The treatment of solitary choriocarcinoma in the brain is similar to that of other metastatic tumors. Long-term survival after surgical excision and postoperative radiation or chemotherapy has been reported on a number of occasions.[13,17,18] Multiple metastatic lesions have been removed with good results at both a single and more than one craniotomy.[13,17] When adequate treatment is delivered to the brain, patients who die from metastatic choriocarcinoma usually do not have evidence of intracranial disease.[20,36] Subarachnoid hemorrhage and intraparenchymal bleeding are treated by clot evacuation and clipping or excision of the responsible aneurysm.[8,22,24] Except in patients with cerebral aneurysm, some authors reserve the use of surgery for cases of progressive neurological deterioration and patients who need control of hemorrhage.[29,34] In other clinics, the use of surgery is considerably more aggressive; in one series of 24 cases, more than one-third underwent craniotomy.[17] Nevertheless, the 20% 1-month mortality rate in patients who present with intracranial hemorrhage has not changed for more than 20 years.[2]

Results

Complete remission has been produced in 100% of patients with nonmetastatic choriocarcinoma, in 87% of those with metastatic disease, and in 72% of those with high-risk metastatic disease.[4] Patients with metastatic choriocarcinoma to the brain have an overall survival rate of 18%.[3] If no treatment is employed, none of the patients survive and 74% die of CNS complications.[36] If only chemotherapy is employed, 24% survive and 58% die of CNS complications. For example, the use of single-agent or bivalent chemotherapy without radiation in 34 patients in China resulted in a 20.5% survival rate;[18] craniotomy was employed in four patients. In another report, the use of multiagent chemotherapy alone, consisting of cis-platinum, etoposide, actinomycin-D, and intrathecal methotrexate, produced a durable remission and allowed a 25-year-old patient to deliver a normal child almost 3 years after onset of her metastatic disease.[3]

Most effective, however, is the routine use of both cranial radiation and multiagent chemotherapy, since these can produce a 50% survival rate and a 0% incidence of CNS death.[20,36] For example, in a series of 13 cases of cerebral metastases, 3,000 to 3,600 cGy was delivered in 10 to 12 fractions of 300 cGy during induction with the combination of actinomycin-D, methotrexate, and cytoxan, and 54% of the patients were cured.[19] In an earlier series, the regimen of actinomycin-D, methotrexate, and 8 mg of oral chlorambucil, in combination with radiation therapy, produced a 50% survival rate in a series of 14 patients who were alive and well at 12 to 200 months after diagnosis.[34] The combination of chemotherapy and radiation is also the most effective treatment strategy in patients with metastatic testicular tumors.[30] Remission rates as high as 70% have been reported for patients with metastatic gestational choriocarcinoma to other sites and response rates in the brain are similar.[6,33] However, in post-term choriocarcinoma metastatic to the brain, the survival rate can be as low as 28.6%.[4]

Ingenious combinations of surgery and chemotherapy have been used to solve particularly difficult problems. For example, a 26-year-old pregnant woman developed a hemiparesis, was discovered to have three middle cerebral artery aneurysms, and survived at least 6 years after craniotomy and EMA-CO (etoposide, methotrexate, actinomycin-D, cyclophosphamide, and vincristine) chemotherapy.[8] In such a case, chemotherapy presumably was used to sterilize the cerebral vasculature after evacuation of the hematoma and excision of the oncotic aneurysms. In the presence of a solitary metastasis or sudden hemorrhage, craniotomy can be life-saving and sometimes curative. The combination of chemotherapy and craniotomy without radiation has been reported to produce 5- and 9-year survivals in two Chinese women, one of whom was subjected to two craniotomies.[13] Chemotherapy itself can produce hemorrhage and necrosis and may necessitate subsequent craniotomy for the treatment of raised intracranial pressure.

Conclusion

In summary, choriocarcinoma is the most malignant tumor associated with pregnancy and 10% to 15% of cases demonstrate metastatic spread to the brain. The diagnosis should be suspected in women of childbearing age who have a history of menstrual irregularity, recent or remote pregnancy or abortion, and evidence of a mass lesion or cerebrovascular event. Bleeding occurs in >50% of cerebral tumors and patients may present with postpartum stroke of unknown etiology. Choriocarcinoma is one of the most frequent causes of oncotic aneurysms and may cause subarachnoid hemorrhage. Almost all patients with cerebral metastases have pulmonary lesions and require multiagent chemotherapy in addition to craniotomy and postoperative radiation. The prognosis is poor in patients with disseminated choriocarcinoma, in patients with tumors associated with a term pregnancy, in cases of delayed diagnosis, and in those who do not receive a combination of multiagent chemotherapy and cranial radiation. The principles of treatment learned in the therapy of metastatic gestational choriocarcinoma also apply to testicular choriocarcinoma and primary intracranial lesions of similar histology. In addition to radiographic studies, the progress of therapy and the clinical course are easily monitored with serial determination of plasma hCG.

References

1. Adeloye A, Osuntokun BO, De V. Hendrickse JP, et al: The neurology of metastatic chorion carcinoma of the uterus. **J Neurol Sci 16:**315-329, 1972
2. Athanassiou A, Begent RHJ, Newlands ES, et al: Central nervous system metastases of choriocarcinoma. 23 years' experience at Charing Cross Hospital. **Cancer 52:**1728-1735, 1983
3. Bakri YN, Pedersen P, Nassar M: Normal pregnancy after curative multiagent chemotherapy for choriocarcinoma with brain metastases. **Acat Obstet Gynecol Scand 70:**611-613, 1991
4. Berkowitz RS, Goldstein DP, Bernstein MR: Choriocarcinoma following term gestation. **Gynecol Oncol 17:**52-57, 1984
5. Biller J, Adams HP Jr: Cerebrovascular disorders associated with pregnancy. **Am Fam Physician 33(6):** 125-132, 1986
6. Buckner JC: The role of chemotherapy in the treatment of patients with brain metastases from solid tumors. **Cancer Metastasis Rev 10:**335-341, 1991
7. Dagi TF, Maccabe JJ: Metastatic trophoblastic disease presenting as a subarachnoid hemorrhage: report of two cases and review of the literature. **Surg Neurol 14:**175-184, 1980
8. Fujiwara T, Mino S, Nagao S, et al: Metastatic choriocarcinoma with neoplastic aneurysms cured by aneurysm resection and chemotherapy. Case report. **J Neurosurg 76:**148-151, 1992
9. Furukawa F, Haebara H, Hamashima Y: Primary intracranial choriocarcinoma arising from the pituitary fossa. Report of an autopsy case with literature review. **Acta Pathol Jpn 36:**773-781, 1986
10. Giannakopoulos G, Nair S, Snider C, et al: Implications for the pathogenesis of aneurysm formation: metastatic choriocarcinoma with spontaneous splenic rupture. Case report and a review. **Surg Neurol 38:**236-240, 1992
11. Gurwitt LJ, Long JM, Clark RE: Cerebral metastatic choriocarcinoma. A postpartum cause of "stroke." **Obstet Gynecol 45:**583-588, 1975
12. Ho KL: Neoplastic aneurysm and intracranial hemorrhage. **Cancer 50:**2935-2940, 1982
13. Ilancheran A, Ratnam SS, Baratham G: Metastatic cerebral choriocarcinoma with primary neurological presentation. **Gynecol Oncol 29:**361-364, 1988
14. Ishizuka T, Tomoda Y, Kaseki S, et al: Intracranial metastasis of choriocarcinoma. A clinicopathologic study. **Cancer 52:**1896-1903, 1983
15. Jones WB, Lewis JL Jr: Late recurrence of gestational trophoblastic disease. **Gynecol Oncol 20:**83-91, 1985
16. Khanjanasthiti P, Issaragrisil R: CT findings of seeding tumors. **J Med Assoc Thai 74:**299-305, 1991
17. Kobayashi T, Kida Y, Yoshida J, et al: Brain metastasis of choriocarcinoma. **Surg Neurol 17:**395-403, 1982
18. Liu TL, Deppe G, Chang QT, et al: Cerebral metastatic choriocarcinoma in the People's Republic of China. **Gynecol Oncol 15:**166-170, 1983

19. Lurain JR, Brewer JI: Treatment of high-risk gestational trophoblastic disease with methotrexate, actinomycin D, and cyclophosphamide chemotherapy. **Obstet Gynecol 65:**830-836, 1985
20. Lurain JR, Brewer JI, Mazur MT, et al: Fatal gestational trophoblastic disease: an analysis of treatment failures. **Am J Obstet Gynecol 144:**391-395, 1982
21. Mandybur TI: Intracranial hemorrhage caused by metastatic tumors. **Neurology 27:**650-655, 1977
22. Momma F, Beck H, Miyamoto T, et al: Intracranial aneurysm due to metastatic choriocarcinoma. **Surg Neurol 25:**74-76, 1986
23. Novak E, Woodruff JD: **Novak's Gynecological and Obstetric Pathology: With Clinical and Endocrine Relations, 7th ed.** Philadelphia, PA: WB Saunders, 1974
24. Pullar M, Blumbergs PC, Phillips GE, et al: Neoplastic cerebral aneurysm from metastatic gestational choriocarcinoma. Case report. **J Neurosurg 63:**644-647, 1985
25. Punnonen R, Hori A, Okawada M, et al: Treatment and prognosis of metastatic gestational trophoblastic disease. **Acta Obstet Gynecol Scand 63:**299-302, 1984
26. Salcman M: Intracranial hemorrhage caused by brain tumor, in Kaufman HH (ed): **Intracerebral Hematomas.** New York, NY: Raven Press, 1992, pp 95-106
27. Seigle JM, Caputy AJ, Manz HJ, et al: Multiple oncotic intracranial aneurysms and cardiac metastasis from choriocarcinoma: case report and review of the literature. **Neurosurgery 20:**39-42, 1987
28. Shuangshoti S, Panyathanya R, Wichienkur P: Intracranial metastases from unsuspected choriocarcinoma. Onset suggestive of cerebrovascular disease. **Neurology 24:**649-654, 1974
29. Soper JT, Hammond CB: Role of surgical therapy and radiotherapy in gestational trophoblastic disease. **J Reprod Med 32:**663-668, 1987
30. Spears WT, Morphis JG II, Lester SG, et al: Brain metastases and testicular tumors: long-term survival. **Int J Radiat Oncol Biol Phys 22:**17-22, 1992
31. Vaughan HG Jr, Howard RG: Intracranial hemorrhage due to metastatic chorionepithelioma. **Neurology 12:**771-777, 1962
32. Wakai S, Yamakawa K, Manaka S, et al: Spontaneous intracranial hemorrhage caused by brain tumor: its incidence and clinical significance. **Neurosurgery 10:** 437-444, 1982
33. Weed JC Jr, Hammond CB: Cerebral metastatic choriocarcinoma: intensive therapy and prognosis. **Obstet Gynecol 55:**89-94, 1980
34. Weed JC Jr, Woodward KT, Hammond CB: Choriocarcinoma metastatic to the brain: therapy and prognosis. **Semin Oncol 9:**208-212, 1982
35. Xu Z: Cerebral metastatic choriocarcinoma. Analysis of 35 autopsies. **Chin Med J (Engl) 95:**273-277, 1982
36. Yordan EL Jr, Schlaerth J, Gaddis O, et al: Radiation therapy in the management of gestational choriocarcinoma metastatic to the central nervous system. **Obstet Gynecol 69:**627-630, 1987
37. Yoshida K, Toya S, Ohtani M, et al: Extraneural metastasis of choriocarcinomatous element in pineal germ-cell tumor. Case report. **J Neurosurg 63:** 463-466, 1985

CHAPTER 13

NERVE INJURIES RELATED TO CHILDBIRTH

JOHN P. LAURENT, MD

Birth-related brachial plexus injury occurs in one or two of every 1,000 live births, the result of stretch damage to the infant's neck in a descending fashion from the suprascapular nerve through C5, C6, and C7, during delivery (Figure 1).[32] Many plexus-injured infants have neurapraxic lesions which resolve spontaneously before specialist consultation can be obtained; surgical intervention is required in one or two of every 10,000 live births.

The literature of the early 20th century acknowledged the obstetrical role of brachial plexus injury[3,5,6,10,40] as physicians began to notice that the skill of the midwife influenced the condition of the neonate in long, difficult deliveries.[33,35] Until this time, brachial plexus palsy had been attributed to internal and external uterine compression of the brachial plexus.[41] Obstetrical factors known to contribute to brachial plexus injury include a multiparous mother, prolonged labor, increased birth weight, and shoulder dystocia.[15,34,44] Injury has been reported in both premature births and cesarean deliveries.[8,16,37] Breech deliveries with arm hyperextension invariably involve the upper plexus, usually bilaterally, and may affect the lower brachial plexus as well.[1,14,31] The incidence of brachial plexus injury is greater in breech deliveries than in normal vertex presentations.[25,30,37]

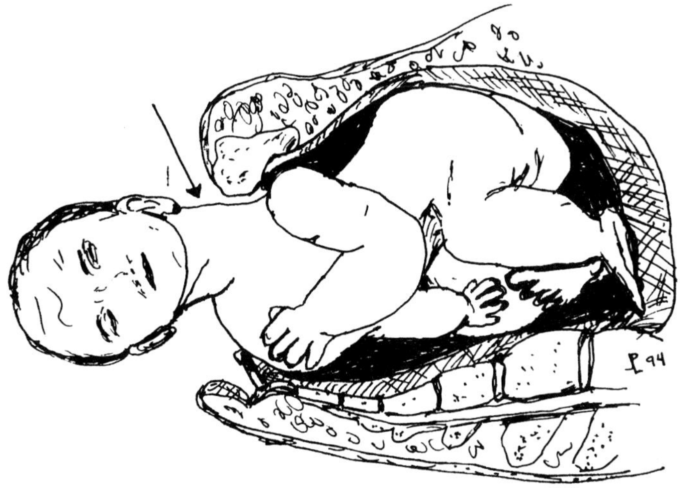

Figure 1: Stretch damage to the brachial plexus usually lateralizes to the side of the anterior shoulder pubic bone.

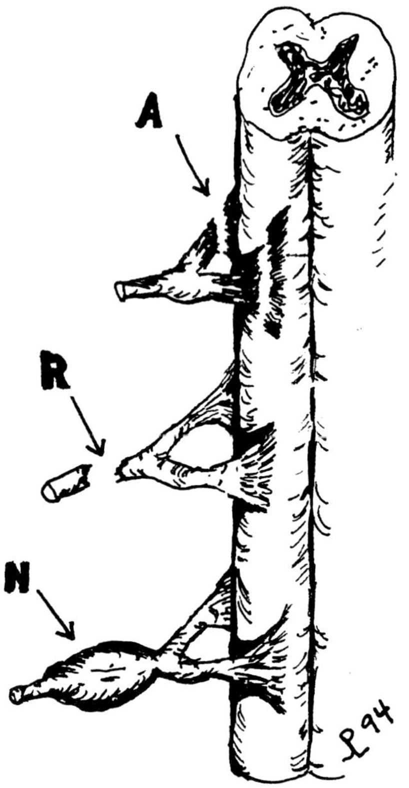

Figure 2: Schematic illustration of different types of stretch injury to the brachial plexus. A = avulsion; R = rupture; N = neuroma.

Pathophysiology

The severity of injury varies, depending on the site of the trauma, and ranges from the neurapraxia mentioned above to avulsion of nerve rootlets within the spinal cord. Once the rootlets coalesce to form the mixed nerve root that traverses and exits the root canal, injury may occur in differing degrees to the trunks, divisions, cords, and peripheral nerves of the brachial plexus (Figure 2).

Neurapraxic lesions are temporary blocks in nerve conduction without permanent structural damage; recovery is usually quick and complete. In axonotmesis, the internal neural elements are disrupted while the sheath elements remain intact. The proximal nerve growth bulb often reconnects to the distal disconnected neural elements within the neural sheath; recovery of function generally takes place 4 to 6 months after injury.

Neurotmesis, or complete rupture, disrupts both the neuronal and the sheath elements and is similar to laceration of a nerve. Partial or complete rupture may evolve into a neuroma in continuity as the sprouting neurons of the growth bulb of the proximal damaged end form a mass of fibrous tissue and disorganized neurons in an attempt to reach the distal end. Nerve conduction through a neuroma depends on the number of neurons successfully making the connection distally. Recovery of function is usually incomplete.

Avulsions are proximal lesions within the spinal cord involving nerve rootlets (anterior and/or posterior) which are torn from the spinal cord proximal to the formation of a mixed nerve root. The avulsive process may occasionally damage the spinal cord itself. Avulsed nerve rootlets do not recover their function, and surgical reconnection to the spinal cord is impossible.

Clinical Presentation

After parturition, most children with brachial plexus palsy (C5-T1) demonstrate flaccid arms. By 2 to 8 weeks of age, a dominant lesion is established (Figure 3).

In 1872, Duchenne[7] reported the physical findings in infants with birth-related brachial plexus injuries; Erb's[9] description 2 years later of an electrical stimulation point on the upper brachial plexus (C5-6) made his name synonymous with upper brachial plexus palsy. In classic Erb's palsy, which involves C5, C6, and C7, the affected arm is limp, the shoulder is adducted and internally rotated, the elbow is extended, and the forearm pronated; paralysis of the deltoid, supraspinatus, infraspinatus, teres minor, biceps, brachialis, brachioradialis, supinator, and wrist and finger extensor muscles places the wrist and fingers in the "waiter's tip" position (Figure 4).

Klumpke,[22] in 1885, described a pure lower plexus lesion (C7-T1) in which the shoulder was in relatively normal position with the arm flexed, the forearm supinated, and the wrists and fingers flaccid. A lower plexus injury at root

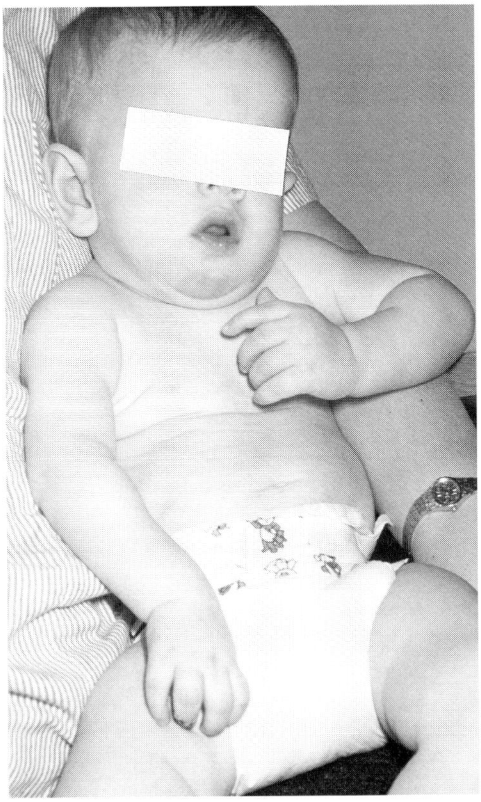

Figure 3: The initial presentation of birth-related brachial plexus palsy in this child was a flaccid right arm.

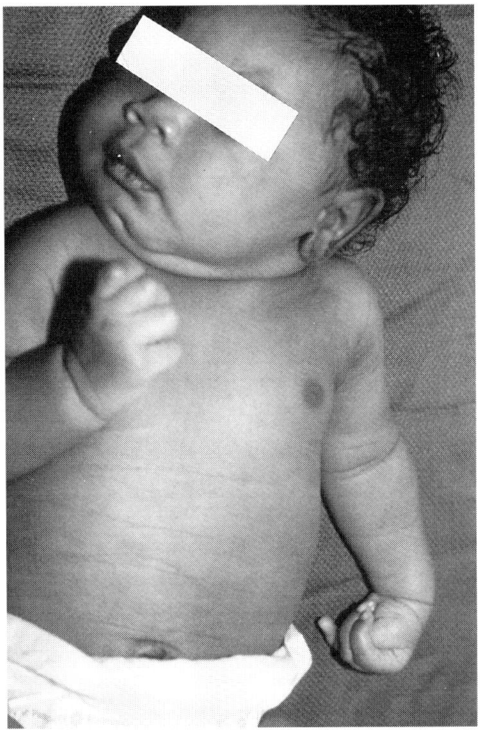

Figure 4: Classic Erb's palsy (C5-7 nerve roots) involved the left arm of this child.

level is characterized by Horner's syndrome. Pure lower plexus injuries are rare.

In our series of 400 new birth-related brachial plexus injuries consecutively evaluated in the Brachial Plexus Clinic at Texas Children's Hospital from 1987 through 1993, 74% of the lesions involved upper brachial plexus injury (C5-7) while only 2% of the injuries were lower plexus injuries (C7-T1). Combined upper and lower plexus lesions (C5-T1) comprised 20% of the injuries evaluated, and 4% of the lesions were bilateral. This distribution is similar to that reported in other series.[12]

Natural History

While reports of spontaneous recovery and good functional outcome vary widely throughout the history of literature on birth-related brachial plexus injuries,[13,15,42,43] one observation has held true: the rate of spontaneous recovery from a birth-related brachial plexus injury dictates the final functional outcome (that is, the faster the recovery, the more complete the functional return). For the infant to attain maximum functional status, spontaneous recovery should be in evidence between the ages of 2 and 6 months.[4,11,13,15,18,27,28,43] The Collaborative Perinatal Study reported complete functional return in 95% of infants with birth-related brachial plexus palsy; 93% of those exhibited some muscle improvement by 4 months of age.[15]

Reports of "good outcome" may be interpreted differently in the absence of the universal application of muscle movement standards. Gjorup[13] followed 103 nonoperated brachial plexus-injured patients over a period of 35 years; while 30% of these patients were assessed as having gained "good" recovery in the affected limb, all considered themselves handicapped. Only 56% of the patients in Wickstrom's[42] series of nonoperated brachial plexus-injured children demonstrated "satisfactory" functional return.

Clinical Assessment

Evaluation of an infant in the Brachial Plexus Clinic of Texas Children's Hospital begins with observation and reward-induced movements as muscle strength and range of motion are assessed. Functionality (the ability to flex the elbow and raise the arm to feed oneself) is regarded as more important than electrical activity recorded in the muscle. The infant is periodically graded on the British Muscle Movement Scale range (0 to 5) by at least two examiners. An antigravity score of 3 in 50% of the muscle groups for upper plexus injury (biceps, deltoid, triceps) correlated with "good" functional outcome; the same antigravity score (3) in 50% of the muscle groups for lower plexus injury (biceps, deltoid, triceps, wrist extensors, finger extensors) correlated with "good" functional outcome.

Surgery is recommended for infants who have not demonstrated improvement of at least one grade in the majority of the corresponding lesion-muscle groups by 4 to 6 months of age or in whom such improvement occurs but plateaus at less than antigravity function for a period of at least 4 months. While other authors have recommended surgical exploration of the brachial plexus at 3 months of age,[4,11,28] we have observed "good" functional recovery in some infants with onset of muscle movement during the 4th month of life and do not consider surgery before 4 months of age.

The Brachial Plexus Clinic staff is multidisciplinary and includes a pediatric neurologist, a pediatric neurosurgeon, a pediatric physiatrist, a plastic surgeon, a pediatric orthopedic surgeon, and a nurse coordinator. The clinic provides patients and their parents, many of whom live in small, isolated communities, extensive support and education in the form of written materials, video teaching aids, social work intervention, and a constantly accessible clinic coordinator who is of great importance because of the dearth of information in lay publications about birth-related brachial plexus injuries. Referring physicians may be unaware of the possibility of recovery and of treatment options.

Conservative Treatment

The majority of infants (90%-95%) with birth-related brachial plexus injuries require only physical and occupational therapy. Tendon and muscle transfers and contracture releases may be indicated in children 3 years or older; these surgeries have been extensively reported in the orthopedic and plastic surgery literature.[2,26,28,36,39]

In our series of 400 infants evaluated, 325 were not selected for surgical intervention. Of this group, 60% were seen by 3 months of age and 92% of these infants demonstrated spontaneous muscle grade improvement in the majority of the corresponding lesion-muscle group by 4 months of age; 8% exhibited initial muscle grade improvement slightly later, at 4 or 5 months of age. Of the group of infants who did not undergo surgery, 40% were seen at more than 3 months of age; a majority of these babies had already recovered satisfactory muscle function at the time of their first clinic consultation.

Preoperative Evaluation

The Texas Children's Hospital series is skewed to the more severely affected children who fail to demonstrate any neurological improvement after a period of time and who are referred to the Brachial Plexus Clinic by their private physicians. Of the 400 infants evaluated, surgical exploration was recommended for 75. In 63, the brachial plexus injury had been explored by 7 months of age; in two infants, the parents refused surgical intervention, and in another two, bilateral explorations were performed. In the total surgical group, improvement can be expected in 80% of infants undergoing early neural repair; in children operated later, Kline[21] noted improvement in only 50% to 70%. The increased functional improvement in infants undergoing earlier repair may be attributable to the shorter nerve repair length, the plasticity of the central nervous system, greater neuronal growth potential, and the growth potential of the infantile mesenchymal structures of the shoulder, arm, and hand.

Preoperative and postoperative electrodiagnostic testing (electromyogram and somatosensory evoked potentials) has been helpful in confirming or refining the clinical evaluation. In our experience this testing has not been of particular independent utility in predicting clinical outcome.

For infants undergoing surgical exploration of the brachial plexus, preoperative 1-mm overlapping spinal computed tomography (CT) scanning with metrizamide has *not* been helpful in predicting nerve rootlet avulsions. The presence of pseudomeningoceles on CT myelography may not necessarily correlate with nerve rootlet avulsions, determined intraoperatively by evoked responses.

Surgical Treatment

Repair of the birth-injured brachial plexus was first reported in 1903 by Kennedy,[20] who removed neuromas and directly sutured nerve roots in three 2-month-old infants; Clark et al[5] performed a similar operation on seven children <1 year of age in 1905. The mortality rate in both series was high. The interest in surgical exploration continued sporadically into the 1960s,[19,24,38,43] but high morbidity and mortality rates and the lack of significant postoperative improvement discouraged most surgeons from attempts at repair. Infants were usually referred to physical therapists and orthopedic or plastic surgeons.

In 1987, Gilbert and Tassin[11] reported successful early interventional surgery for birth-related brachial plexus injuries. Since that time, pediatric neurosurgical approaches to the problem have evolved and the operative morbidity rate has dropped significantly, refined by such technological improvements as the operating microscope, nontraumatic suture needles, ultrafine nonfibrosing sutures, and intraoperative electrodiagnostic testing.[23,29]

Neurosurgical techniques for repairing damaged neural elements include external neurolysis or neuroplasty, internal neurolysis (fascicles identified), nerve grafting, neuroma dissection and removal, and direct end-to-end nerve repair (coaptation). The infantile brachial plexus is explored under general anesthesia via a supraclavicular incision which exposes the plexus from exiting nerve roots C3 through T1.

Neuroplasty, or removal of scar tissue produced by adherence of the omohyoid and scalene muscles to the brachial plexus, with complete mobilization of the plexus is required prior to electrodiagnostic testing; the phrenic nerve is frequently involved in these adhesions. Electromyography and sensory- and motor-evoked potentials (antigrade motor-evoked potentials) to C1, C2, and the parietal region determine which of the procedures described above are required. Multiple procedures are usually performed in a single brachial plexus operation.

Excision of neuroma in continuity is determined by neural conduction. If conduction, measured by amplitude of electromyogram of the appropriate muscle, is decreased by >50% across the neuroma, the lesion is excised and an intact nerve root is grafted distally. Because direct suturing is usually not possible after neuroma removal, the gap between neural elements is bridged with interpositional cable grafts of sural nerve, which serve as conduits to guide the proximal sprouting neural growth bulb to the severed distal ends. If conduction across the neuroma is marginally decreased (25%-45%), internal neurolysis with removal of intervening scar tissue and identification of individual nerve fascicles is carried out.

Experience

In their operative series, Boome and Kaye[4] observed recovery of at least antigravity function in >95% of the deltoids and 80% of the biceps within 2 years of repair. Hunt[17] reported "good" outcome within 5 years postoperatively in 80% of pure upper plexus lesions (C5-6), 45% of Erb's palsy cases (C5-7), and 35% of complete plexus lesions (C5-T1). Gilbert and Whitaker[12] measured a single muscle action, abduction of the shoulder, and reported that >90% of the brachial plexus-injured patients demonstrated improvement following surgery at 3 months of age; >80% of infants with pure upper plexus involvement, 75% of those with

Erb's palsy, and <45% of infants with complete lesions attained the shoulder abduction movement.

In our series of 73 infants undergoing neurosurgical exploration at 2 to 6 months of age, 90% with pure upper plexus injury (C5-6) demonstrated an increase of at least one grade (range 0 to 5) in the majority of the corresponding lesion-muscle group (deltoid, biceps, triceps) by 1 year postoperatively; these children continued to improve. Eighty-two percent of infants with Erb's palsy improved by the same measurements; 92% had antigravity function of the deltoid and 87% exhibited antigravity movement of the biceps by 2 years postoperatively. Only 67% of infants in our series with combined lesions (C5-T1) had improved at least one grade in the majority of the corresponding lesion-muscle group by 1 year after surgery, and, beyond this time, only the deltoid and biceps muscles continued to improve. In the infants with combined brachial plexus lesions, antigravity function was attained by 2 years postoperatively in 80% of deltoids and in 85% of biceps.

No surgical fatalities occurred, and no permanent increase in neurological deficits was seen postoperatively. Morbidity consisted of a transient diaphragm paralysis and a wound infection in one patient each. Of the 75 plexi, eight (in six infants) were not repairable. Two of the six infants had bilateral injuries with cerebrospinal fluid filling the nerve roots (C3-T1). Intercostal nerves (C3-4) were coapted to the distal phrenic nerve in these two infants, who both are now respirator-independent.

Neuroma formation was present in 95% of the plexi explored, 90% involving the upper trunk complex (C5-6) and 40% involving the middle and lower trunk complex (C7-T1). Eight-two percent of the avulsions occurred at the C7-8 nerve rootlet level, and 88% of the ruptures occurred at the C5-6 nerve root level. The primary donor nerve roots for grafting were C5 and C6.

Summary

Technological advances in microsurgical and neuroelectrodiagnostic testing methods have re-established the role of the pediatric neurosurgeon in the treatment of infants with birth-related brachial plexus injuries. We have described our experience during a 6-year period in the Brachial Plexus Clinic of Texas Children's Hospital in the evaluation and treatment, both nonsurgical and surgical, of 400 brachial plexus-injured infants.

Of the infants operated on in our series, 80% demonstrated antigravity muscle movement in the majority of the corresponding lesion-muscle group assessed at least 1 year following surgery. Improvement in proximal muscle function (arm and forearm) exceeded distal improvement (wrist and hand). The infants in our operative series would not have attained antigravity function without early brachial plexus repair, and would have remained severely handicapped using historical data for comparative analysis.

References

1. Adler JB, Patterson RL: Erb's palsy. Long-term results of eighty-eight cases. **J Bone Joint Surg (Am) 49**:1052-1064, 1967
2. al-Rajeh S, Corea JR, al-Sibai MH, et al: Congenital brachial palsy in the eastern province of Saudi Arabia. **J Child Neurol 5**:35-38, 1990
3. Bailey P: Brachial plexus palsy. **Bull Lying In Hosp NY 4**:119, 1908
4. Boome RS, Kaye JC: Obstetric traction injuries of the brachial plexus. Natural history, indications for surgical repair and results. **J Bone Joint Surg (Br) 70**:571-576, 1988
5. Clark LP, Taylor AS, Prout TP: A study on brachial birth palsy. **Am J Med Sci 130**:670-674, 1905
6. Darling HCR: The surgery of the brachial plexus. **Med J Aust 6**:335, 1915
7. Duchenne GBA: **De l'Electrisation Localisée et de son Application à la Pathologie et à la Thérapeutique, ed 3.** Paris: Balliére,1872, pp 357-362
8. Eng GD, Kock B, Smokvina MO: Brachial plexus palsy in neonates and children. **Arch Phys Med Rehabil 59**:458-464, 1978
9. Erb W: Über eine eigenthümliche Localisation von Lähmungen im Plexus brachialis. **Verh Naturhistr Med Heidelberg 2**:130, 1874
10. Fairbanks HAT: Birth palsy: subluxation of the shoulder-joint in infants and young children. **Lancet 1**:1217, 1913
11. Gilbert A, Tassin JL: Obstetrical palsy: a clinical, pathologic, and surgical review, in Terzis JK (ed): **Microreconstruction of Nerve Injuries.** Philadelphia, PA: WB Saunders, 1987, pp 529-553
12. Gilbert A, Whitaker I: Obstetrical brachial plexus lesions. **J Hand Surg (Br) 16**:489-491, 1991
13. Gjorup L: Obstetrical lesions of the brachial plexus. **Acta Neurol Scand 18**:9-38, 1965

14. Gordon A: An unusual form of birth palsy. **JAMA 63**:2282, 1914
15. Gordon M, Rich H, Deutschberger J, et al: The immediate and long-term outcome of obstetric birth trauma. I. Brachial plexus paralysis. **Am J Obstet Gynecol 117**:51-56, 1973
16. Hardy AE: Birth injuries of the brachial plexus. Incidence and prognosis. **J Bone Joint Surg (Br) 63**: 98-102, 1981
17. Hunt D: Surgical management of brachial plexus birth injuries, **Dev Med Child Neurol 30**:824-828, 1988
18. Jackson ST, Hoffer MM, Parrish N: Brachial-plexus palsy in the newborn. **J Bone Joint Surg (Am) 70**: 1217-1220, 1988
19. Janec M, Siman J, Majesky I: Ergebnisse der chirurgischen Revision perinataler Schadigungen des Plexus brachialis. **Int Z Kinderchir** 1968
20. Kennedy R: Suture of the brachial plexus in birth paralysis of the upper extremity. **Br Med J 1**: 298-301, 1903
21. Kline DG: Perspectives concerning brachial plexus injury and repair. **Neurosurg Clin North Am 2**: 151-164, 1991
22. Klumpke A: Contribution à l'étude des paralysies radiculaires du plexus brachial. **Rev Med 5**:591, 1885
23. Laurent JP, Shenaq S, Lee R, et al: Upper brachial plexus birth injury, in Marlin AE (ed): **Concepts in Pediatric Neurosurgery, Vol 10.** Basel: S Karger, 1990, pp 156-178
24. Lauwers ME: Le traitement chirurgical de la paralysie obstétricale. **J Chir 36**:161-174, 1930
25. Merger R, Judet J: Paralysie obstétricale du plexus brachial. Prévention et traitement. **Nouv Presse Med 2**:1935-1938, 1973
26. Meyer RD: Treatment of adult and obstetrical brachial plexus injuries. **Orthopedics 9**:899-903, 1986
27. Nagano A, Tsuyama N, Hara T, et al: Brachial plexus injuries. Prognosis of postganglionic lesions. **Arch Orthop Trauma Surg 102**:172-178, 1984
28. Narakas A, Herzberg G: Neuro-neural intraplexal transfers in traumatic radicular avulsions of the brachial plexus. Report of fifteen cases. **Ann Chir Main 4**:211-218, 1985
29. Piatt JH Jr, Hudson AR, Hoffman HJ: Preliminary experiences with brachial plexus exploration in children: birth injury and vehicular trauma. **Neurosurgery 22**:715-723, 1988
30. Rubin A: Birth injuries: incidence, mechanisms, and end results. **Obstet Gynecol 23**:218-221, 1964
31. Scaglietti O: The obstetrical shoulder trauma. **Surg Gynecol Obstet 66**:868-877, 1938
32. Sever JW: Obstetric paralysis. Its etiology, pathology, clinical aspects and treatment, with a report of four hundred and seventy cases. **Am J Dis Child 12**: 541-542, 1916
33. Sever JW: Obstetric paralysis. Report of eleven hundred cases. **JAMA 85**:1862-1870, 1925
34. Sharpe W: The operative treatment of brachial plexus paralysis. **JAMA 66**:876-884, 1916
35. Smellie WJ: **Collection of Cases and Observation in Midwifery, 4th ed.** 1768, Vol 2, pp 504-505
36. Solonen KA, Vastarmäki M, Ström B: Surgery of the brachial plexus. **Acta Orthop Scand 55**:436-440, 1984
37. Tan KL: Brachial palsy. **J Obstet Gynaecol Br Commonwealth 80**:60-62, 1973
38. Taylor AS: Brachial birth palsy and injuries of similar type in adults. **Surg Gynecol Obstet 30**:495-502, 1920
39. Terzis JK, Liberson WT, Levine R: Our experience in obstetrical brachial plexus palsy, in Terzis J (ed): **Microreconstruction of Nerve Injuries.** Philadelphia, PA: WB Saunders, 1987, pp 513-528
40. Thomas JJ: Two cases of bilateral birth paralysis of the lower arm type. **Boston Med Surg 153**:43, 1905
41. Thomas TT: The relation of posterior subluxation of the shoulder-joint to obstetrical palsy of the upper extremity. **Ann Surg 59**:197-200, 1914
42. Wickstrom J: Birth injuries of the brachial plexus. Treatment of defects in the shoulder. **Clin Orthop 23**:187-196, 1962
43. Wyeth JA, Sharpe W: The field of neurological surgery in a general hospital. **Surg Gynecol Obstet 24**: 29-36, 1917
44. Zancolli EA: Classification and management of the shoulder in birth palsy. **Orthop Clin North Am 12**:433-457, 1981

CHAPTER 14

Idiopathic Intracranial Hypertension (Pseudotumor Cerebri), Hydrocephalus, and Ventriculoperitoneal Shunts in Pregnancy

Timothy C. Ryken, MD

Idiopathic Intracranial Hypertension

Idiopathic intracranial hypertension (IIH), also known as pseudotumor cerebri, benign intracranial hypertension, or meningeal hydrops, was first described in 1897 by Quincke. It is a relatively common condition of unknown etiology.[50] Foley first used the term "benign intracranial hypertension,"[15] although a high incidence of visual deterioration has more recently become associated with this condition, and the term "benign" has largely been dropped.[9] For unknown reasons these patients develop subacute increased intracranial pressure (ICP) without localizing signs over several weeks or months. The majority present with headaches, although blurred vision, dizziness, diplopia, or facial numbness have also been described as the presenting symptom. Upon examination, these patients generally demonstrate marked papilledema and visual alterations; they may also exhibit a sixth cranial nerve palsy. Lumbar puncture will show increased cerebrospinal fluid (CSF) pressures in the 200-450 mm range.[7] Fluctuations of CSF pressures in roughly 20- to 30-minute cycles occur, characterized by a gradual increase and followed by a precipitous decline to near normal levels.[24] The symptoms of headache do not appear to correspond with the transient peaks of ICP. IIH has been described primarily in obese adolescent girls and young women of childbearing age and has been associated with a variety of medical conditions. The association of pregnancy and pseudotumor cerebri has been suggested by several clinical investigators.[14,21,31,34,45,46] More recent reviews suggest that pregnancy occurs in pseudotumor cerebri in about the same rate as the general population.[11,13,18,50] Nonetheless, this is a condition that does affect women of childbearing years and is occasionally encountered in the pregnant patient. A review of the available literature highlights the signs, symptoms, pathophysiology, and treatment considerations of IIH in pregnancy.

Incidence and Associated Conditions

In a review by Durcan et al[13] of several state populations, the annual incidence of newly diagnosed IIH in the general population was approximately 0.9 per 100,000. This was increased over threefold to 3.5 per 100,000 in women ranging from 15 to 44 years of age. In women whose body weight is >20% over ideal, the incidence increased dramatically to 19 per 100,000.

Conditions that diminish the flow of CSF through the arachnoid granulations or that result in venous hypertension will result in intracranial hypertension. A number of conditions have been reported in association with IIH; however, many represent anecdotal case reports and only a few have been investigated with controlled studies.[6,12,14,15,18,20-22,31,34,44,46,49,50,55,60,63,65] The association of pregnancy and IIH is most likely a result of rapid weight gain, rather than a direct result of pregnancy.[11,13,14,18,21,31,34,45,46,50] Digre et al[11] found that the IIH patients were more likely to be obese than their age- and parity-matched controls. Giuseffi et al[18] described a high correlation between the diagnosis of IIH and a rapid weight gain in the year prior to diagnosis. These authors found no association of IIH with pregnancy, irregular menses, medication, or endocrine conditions. There does appear to be an association of IIH with rapid steroid withdrawal, Addison's disease, hypothyroidism, and certain medications (including vitamin A, anabolic steroids, certain anti-inflammatory medications, nalidixic acid, nitrofurantoin, and lithium).[20,55,62] Several case control studies failed to show an association of IIH with the use of oral contraceptives, multivitamins, antibiotics, or corticosteroids.[18,31]

From the available literature, it appears that IIH may be associated with obesity and rapid weight gain; however, the majority of other reported associated factors are common conditions found in women of childbearing age and probably are not involved in the specific etiology.

Pathophysiology

The etiology of IIH is unknown. Interstitial and intracellular cerebral edema has been described and may indicate a reduced absorption of CSF.[53] Some authors have postulated that this reduction in absorption is compensated with an increase in ICP to overcome the reduced CSF absorption, thus increasing the hydrostatic pressure of the CSF.[12,14] Interestingly, despite the increased pressure and reduction in CSF outflow, the ventricular size remains normal or is reduced.[41,48,64] Alterations in cerebrovascular hemodynamics with a rise in cerebral blood volume and reduced cerebral blood flow have been postulated to play a role in the increased ICP, but experimental studies examining this hypothesis have met with mixed results.[3,19,39,47]

Symptoms and Signs

Generalized increased ICP without focal neurological deficit should raise the suspicion of IIH. Common complaints in patients with documented IIH include headache, visual disturbance or deterioration, diplopia, and retrobulbar pain. Giuseffi et al[18] reported that 94% of patients with IIH complained of headache at the time of initial diagnosis. Diplopia was noted in 38% and visual loss was observed in 30%.

Headaches in patients with IIH are diverse in presentation and do not appear to correspond directly with alterations in ICP.[32] The headache is often severe, long lasting (several hours), and associated with nausea and vomiting.[59] Visual alterations (or transient visual obscurations) also do not appear to be directly related to ICP alterations.[27,52] These episodes may consist of blurry vision, occur in one or both eyes, and are not generally associated with a permanent loss of vision.[9,10,60,61] These transient episodes of visual disturbance may be related to transient ischemia of the optic nerve head following cyclic fluctuations in the CSF pressure.[52]

Of the patients interviewed by Giuseffi et al,[18] 60% complained of pulsatile intracranial noise, similar to pulsatile tinnitus; this was relieved with ipsilateral jugular compression and was attributed to intensified vascular pulsations transmitted to the wall of the venous sinuses.[18] Approximately 20% to 40% of patients with IIH report horizontal diplopia and exhibit sixth cranial nerve palsies secondary to diffuse ICP elevation.[60] Involvement of other cranial nerves with elevated ICP should prompt reconsideration of the diagnosis of IIH. Afferent pupillary defects are seen in only about 20% of patients with IIH, probably due to the relatively symmetrical elevation in CSF pressure seen by the optic nerve heads.[9,26]

Papilledema is the most characteristic sign of IIH and suggests chronic elevation of ICP. Transient elevations of ICP generally do not result in florid papilledema. Long-standing papilledema has been associated with visual deterioration secondary to edema of the optic nerve head. However, in IIH the severity of visual loss does not always appear to directly correlate with the severity of papilledema.[60] Early papilledema can be difficult to recognize by direct ophthalmoscopy, and accurate diagnosis may depend on indirect ophthalmoscopy with serial funduscopic photography.[16] Standard visual acuity testing is relatively insensitive to alterations in papilledema until late in the course of the disease.[60] Other neuro-ophthalmological testing methodology, particularly contrast sensitivity, may contribute more significant information on visual deterioration.[58,60] Alterations in color vision response and visual evoked responses are not felt to be reliable methods for detecting or following visual field deficits in IIH.[58,60]

Visual field testing with Goldmann perimetry is likely the most sensitive testing method for following patients with IIH.[9,56,60] In a prospective study of 50 patients, Wall et al[60] documented visual loss in one or both eyes in 96% of IIH patients, approximately 25% of whom were unaware of the deficit. Commonly seen visual field deficits include enlargement of the blind spot, inferonasal visual field deficits, scotomas, and other nerve fiber bundle defects. Visual field deterioration may be progressive and result in complete loss of vision if left untreated.[9,60,61]

Evaluation

Following a complete neurological examination, serum chemistries (erythrocyte sedimentation rate, acetylneuraminic acid, Venereal Disease Research Laboratory test, fluorescent treponemal antibody absorption test, serum cortisol, and electrolytes) should be obtained to rule out other inflammatory or autoimmune etiologies. Patients presenting with signs of increased ICP should be evaluated with neuroimaging. Evaluation for other etiologies of elevated ICP is important, as IIH remains a diagnosis of exclusion once structural lesions such as tumor or hemorrhage have been excluded from consideration. The findings with computed tomography (CT) or magnetic resonance imaging (MRI) of the brain in IIH are nonspecific.[41,48,64] The ventricular system may be normal or compressed symmetrically. The arachnoid cisterns may be obliterated, suggesting elevated ICP. Evidence of diffuse cerebral edema with increased white matter T2-weighted signal on MRI may be present and an empty sella may be seen. In selected cases, cerebral angiography may be warranted to exclude venous sinus thrombosis.

Once a structural lesion has been excluded, a lumbar puncture should be performed with measurement of opening pressure and evaluation of routine CSF chemistries.[7,19,24,32,57] The opening pressure in IIH is typically >200 mm water. The patient who has evidence of increased ICP in the absence of lateralizing neurological findings, who has an elevated opening pressure on lumbar puncture, and who has no known etiology after thorough clinical evaluation and neuroimaging satisfies the generally accepted criteria for IIH.[6,7,10,34,44,50,57,60,63]

As the primary morbidity of IIH is loss of vision, a major portion of the evaluation and follow-up of these patients should be focused on the evaluation of visual function. Although visual acuity testing and visual evoked responses have been used, some authors believe that these are insensitive tests for the long-term follow-up of IIH patients.[58,60] Visual field testing with perimetry appears to be the method of choice for long-term surveillance of these patients.[9,56,60]

Treatment

A wide variety of treatments have been proposed for IIH. Some authors believe that in cases of IIH associated with pregnancy, there appears to be little difference in outcome regardless of the type of treatment employed. Some cases improve without treatment, while others progress to visual deterioration.[21,44,46] The pregnant patient with IIH should probably be monitored closely with serial visual field examinations, and treatment instituted in the setting of visual deterioration.

Obesity has been associated with the onset of IIH and has been associated with visual deterioration secondary to IIH.[7,9,11,18,22,31,60,65] A supervised weight-loss program has been reported to improve visual symptoms in patients with IIH.[42] In the pregnant patient, caloric restriction should be recommended with caution and employed under careful observation with a weight gain goal of approximately 20 pounds, depending on the body habitus of the patient.

Drug therapy of IIH has focused on the use of diuretics and corticosteroids. Corticosteroids have been reported to improve visual function in several series.[44,63] Caution must be used in the tapering dosages, as rapid withdrawal has been associated with the onset or worsening of symptoms of IIH. In the pregnant patient, any drug must be given with caution. Corticosteroids have been associated with birth defects in laboratory animals and with low birth weight in humans.[11] Acetazolamide has been reported to lower ICP by reducing CSF production, and may be useful in the treatment of IIH.[11,24] Dosages of 2 to 4 gm per day have been used with success. Digre et al[11] suggest that acetazolamide may be used after 20 weeks' gestation as earlier use was associated with a single case of sacrococcygeal teratoma. There are no studies directly addressing the safety of acetazolamide in human pregnancy, and its use should probably be avoided, particularly in the first trimester, unless the expected results outweigh the potential risk, as may be the case with rapid visual deterioration.

A variety of surgical procedures have been attempted to alleviate the symptoms of increased ICP and visual deterioration in IIH. Historically, subtemporal and suboccipital decompression have been attempted but were abandoned with the advent of alternate techniques. Repeated lumbar punctures have also been attempted in the treatment of IIH, but are uncomfortable and often impractical.[63] In addition, the CSF is generally replenished within several hours and therefore lumbar puncture does not result in long-term improvement. Temporary reduction in ICP can be obtained by the insertion of a lumbar subarachnoid catheter to an external drain until a definitive procedure is elected. Lumboperitoneal shunting and optic nerve sheath fenestration have both been used with success in the treatment of IIH, and can be performed safely in the pregnant patient. Lumboperitoneal shunting can effectively reduce ICP but suffers from the complications inherent to a shunting procedure: occlusion, infection, and local irritation.[6,50,51] Optic nerve sheath fenestration has been described as an effective means for reversing visual deterioration and protecting the optic nerve from additional insult.[4,8,10,33,54] This technique appears to be effective by a combination of decompressing the subarachnoid space around the optic nerve, with subsequent scarring and fibrosis closing the potential subarachnoid space.[33]

Summary

IIH, or pseudotumor cerebri, is a condition of unknown etiology which results in elevation of the ICP and can result in visual deterioration secondary to optic nerve ischemia. IIH is seen most frequently in obese women of childbearing age. Although associated with pregnancy, it is likely that this association is a result of rapid weight gain rather than a direct result of pregnancy. Headache, papilledema, and diplopia are common findings and serial visual field testing appears to be the most sensitive method of following IIH patients for visual deterioration. A review of the available literature suggests that pregnant patients with IIH may improve with expectant management following delivery. In general, pregnant patients with IIH can be managed in a similar fashion to nonpregnant patients, with the exception of carefully managed caloric restriction and cautious use of drug therapy. In patients with rapid visual deterioration, most authors recommend aggressive treatment with steroids and either lumboperitoneal shunting or optic nerve fenestration.

Hydrocephalus and Ventriculoperitoneal Shunting

Advances in the treatment of hydrocephalus with shunting of the CSF to other body cavities have improved the survival of hydrocephalic infants and children.[1,25,35] As a result, these patients have an increased chance of surviving

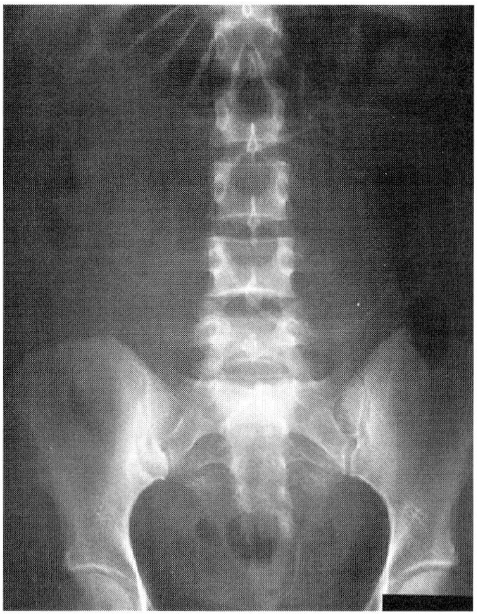

Figure 1: Abdominal radiograph of a 30-year-old female with a ventriculoperitoneal shunt, placed in childhood for aqueductal stenosis, presenting with obtundation and loss of upgaze. A shunt series was obtained and revealed a fetus in a cephalic presentation. The patient was not aware of the pregnancy at the time of presentation.

to childbearing age and may come to the attention of obstetricians (Figure 1). The majority of these shunts are placed from the ventricular system to the peritoneum (ventriculoperitoneal). In general, the complication rate of ventriculoperitoneal shunting appears to be lower than other types, such as ventriculoatrial, ventriculopleural, or lumboperitoneal shunting procedures.[1,23,25,35,37] The available literature on maternal hydrocephalus and pregnancy is limited to a series of case reports documenting a variety of presentations and complications related to hydrocephalus, shunting procedures, and pregnancy.[17,30,36,40,43,66]

Etiology

Extracranial shunting procedures are used to treat failure of the CSF to drain via normal CSF pathways. Obstruction of the CSF pathways resulting in hydrocephalus occurs for a variety of reasons, including congenital anomalies, central nervous system infection, subarachnoid hemorrhage, neoplasms, or trauma.[25] Problems with hydrocephalus during pregnancy may develop in the setting of known hydrocephalus with an existing shunt or in a previously asymptomatic patient developing symptoms of hydrocephalus during pregnancy.[66] This latter group appears to be the result of physiological changes in CSF dynamics in patients with compensated or arrested hydrocephalus. Extracranial shunts have a one-way valve system which is preset to drain CSF distally when the ICP exceeds this preset limit. Low-, medium-, and high-pressure valve systems have been used depending on the reason for shunt insertion. In patients with ventriculoperitoneal shunts it has been suggested that the rise in intra-abdominal pressure with advancing pregnancy may play a role in the development of shunt malfunction by impeding drainage into the peritoneum.[36] The possible etiology of ventriculoatrial shunt malfunction with pregnancy is less clear. In fact, due to the limited number of reported cases and the relatively high incidence of shunt malfunctions in the general population, it has been stated that the incidence of shunt-related problems may not actually be increased with pregnancy.[30] In contrast, Wisoff et al[66] reported that 58% of pregnant patients with shunts demonstrated signs of increased ICP. In their series, pregnant patients with extracranial shunts frequently developed problems related to increased intracranial pressure. They proposed that an increase in intracerebral fluid content with venous distention occurs during pregnancy, which compromises intracranial compliance and results in symptoms of increased ICP.

Symptoms and Signs

In general, the signs and symptoms of reported cases of shunt malfunction in pregnant patients with extracranial shunts are similar to those described in nonpregnant patients with shunt malfunction.[66] The symptoms of increased ICP include headache, nausea and vomiting, memory disturbance, altered sensorium, and seizures. In four patients with newly diagnosed hydrocephalus described by Wisoff et al,[66] three became symptomatic during the last two trimesters of pregnancy. In an additional 17 patients with pre-existing shunts, 76% developed neurological complications. These included severe headache with and without documented increased ICP (65%), nausea and vomiting (35%), lethargy (29%), ataxia (18%), and gaze paresis (18%). Three patients (18%) experienced the new onset of seizures and two patients had an exacerbation of a previous seizure disorder. These authors observed no relationship between the type of shunting procedure and the type or incidence of neurological symptoms.[66]

Management

Prenatal care for pregnant patients with hydrocephalus should include an assessment of fetal risk for developing hydrocephalus. A search for a hereditary component of the maternal hydrocephalus is indicated. If the mother has a neural tube defect, the risk of her baby being similarly affected has been estimated at 2% to 3%.[5,28] Amniocentesis for alpha-fetoprotein can then be performed to assist in the assessment of fetal risk. Less common inheritable causes include aqueductal stenosis and Dandy-Walker syndrome, although these conditions may be secondary to sporadic genetic events and may not place the fetus at an increased risk for the development of hydrocephalus.[17] Other causes for maternal hydrocephalus, such as post-infectious or post-hemorrhagic hydrocephalus, are unlikely to have a genetic component. Serial ultrasound monitoring can also be performed to monitor the development of the fetal ventricular system.

In the patient with known hydrocephalus and an extracranial shunt, careful observation to detect the early signs of shunt malfunction is warranted to avoid a delay in diagnosis. Signs of increased ICP, including severe headache, lethargy, gaze paresis, nausea and vomiting, ataxia, nystagmus, or seizures, should be aggressively evaluated to exclude a shunt malfunction. The differential diagnosis of these signs in various combinations should include pre-eclampsia/eclampsia, pseudotumor cerebri, hyperemesis gravidarum, intracranial hemorrhage, or neoplasm.[6,25,45,66] Cerebral CT or MRI prior to conception and the development of symptoms is useful to allow comparison of ventricular size if symptoms develop.

The presence of signs or symptoms suggestive of increased ICP warrants radiographic evaluation with CT or MRI to assess the ventricular size and exclude other intracranial pathology. The clinical status of the patient must be judged against any potential risk to the fetus with imaging studies. Direct measurement of the ICP and an assessment of proximal and distal patency can be obtained by tapping the ventricular reservoir, which also allows the collection of CSF for cell count, CSF chemistries, Gram stain, and culture to exclude an infectious etiology of the shunt malfunction. A nuclear medicine radioisotope shunt study may also be useful to document the rate of flow of the CSF from the reservoir to the peritoneum and has been used in these patients (Figure 2).[66]

If the symptoms are not associated with elevated ICP or evidence of shunt obstruction or infection, conservative measures with bed rest and mild fluid restriction (taking care to avoid dehydration and precipitation of early labor), steroids, and diuretics have resulted in improvement.[17,30,36,40,43,66] Manual pumping of the shunt valve, if possible, has also been described to improve symptoms in selected patients as a short-term measure (Figure 3).[36] A review by Wisoff et al[66] included seven symptomatic patients undergoing conservative treatment with normal ICP and evidence of a functioning shunt; all seven patients were delivered vaginally with resolution of symptoms postpartum. If the symptoms do not improve with conservative measures, these authors recommend early delivery via cesarean section once fetal lung maturity is documented, as symptoms often resolve postpartum.

In the patient with enlarging ventricular size or obstruction of the shunt system with elevated ICP, surgical revision of the shunt is warranted. Ventriculoperitoneal shunting appears to be safe in the first and second trimesters, avoiding the use of the shunt-passing trocar if possible.[17,66] Although clinical information is limited, ventriculoatrial or ventriculopleural shunting could be considered in the third trimester, if not otherwise contraindicated. In the review by Wisoff et al,[66] five patients underwent shunting proce-

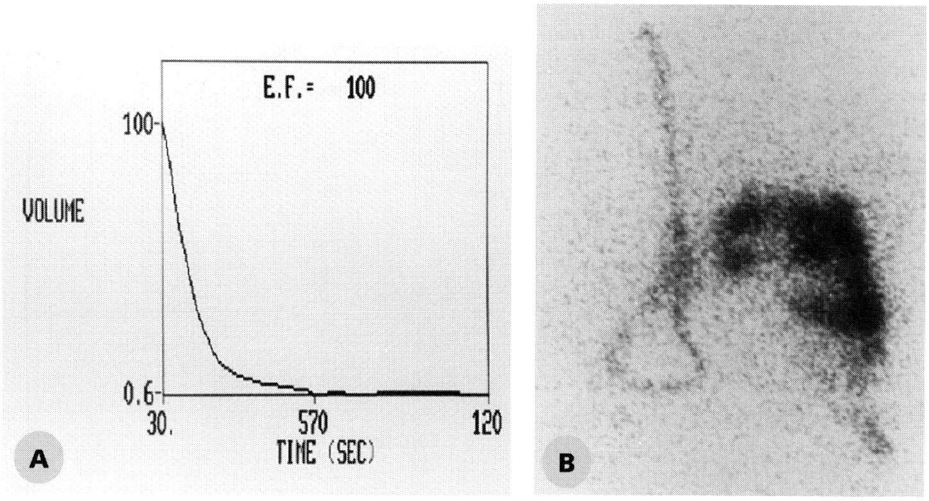

Figure 2: Radionuclide ventriculoperitoneal shunt study. Following injection of technetium-99M diethylenetriamine penta-acetic acid into the ventricular reservoir, the tracer can be followed to assess the patency and flow rate of the shunt system. **A**) Plot of volume versus time for amount of tracer present in the ventricular reservoir. The tl/2 can be calculated to assess the rate of CSF flow. In this example, the tl/2 is approximately 2.5 minutes, indicating adequate flow. **B**) Antero-posterior radioimage of the abdomen 10 minutes following injection into the ventricular reservoir. The accumulation of tracer in the peritoneum suggests patency of the distal shunt system but does not exclude the presence of a loculated intraperitoneal CSF cyst.

dures during pregnancy without neurosurgical, obstetrical, or perinatal complications.

The delivery of a neonate in patients with an extracranial shunt is dependent on the status of the patient at the time of delivery. The management of an asymptomatic patient with a functioning intracranial shunt at the time of delivery should be similar to any other obstetrical patient. Concern for transient obstruction of ventricular drainage during the elevated intra-abdominal pressures with labor has been discussed but does not appear to represent a significant risk, as the elevations are intermittent and the one-way valves of the shunting systems do not allow backflow.[29,30,36,38,40] The majority of reported cases have resulted in a vaginal delivery, about one-half by spontaneous vaginal delivery and one-half by elective low forceps to minimize second-stage labor. In Wisoff's review,[66] three of 20 patients required cesarean section for an unstable neurological condition. These were performed in patients who became symptomatic near term or during labor. The authors recommend the use of general anesthesia with careful volume monitoring in these cases. Epidural catheters are contraindicated in patients with increased ICP.

Previous authors have addressed the use of prophylactic antibiotics in pregnant patients with extracranial shunts at the time of delivery.[17,30,36,40,43,66] There is no controlled study and the evidence for or against the use of antibiotics in the delivery of a neonate in patients with an extracranial shunt is anecdotal. The incidence of asymptomatic puerperal bacteremia in a series of 1,779 cultures from 396 patients was reported as 0.5%.[2] This rate is probably increased in patients requiring invasive fetal heart rate monitoring. The shunt catheter does represent a foreign body and a site for bacterial seeding. Septicemia is a potentially life-threatening complication of extracranial shunting, particularly with venticuloatrial catheters. Although direct clinical studies are lacking, the majority of authors addressing this subject are in favor of prophylaxis. The choice of antibiotics is best tailored to the sensitivities and infection profiles of each specific institution. If this information is unavailable, coverage should be directed toward the coliform bacteria, with administration of

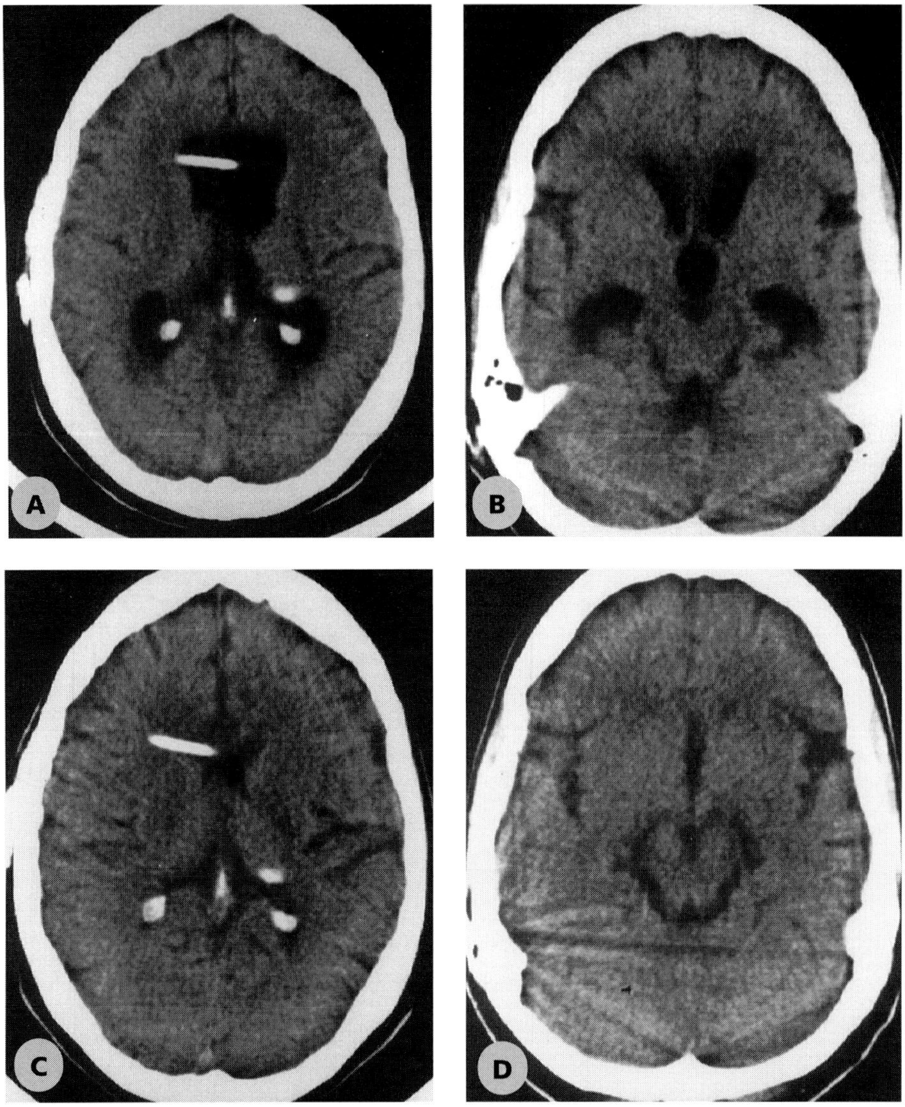

Figure 3: Axial CT scans of a pregnant female with a ventriculoperitoneal shunt presenting with headache, diplopia, and diminished sensorium. **A** and **B**) These scans were obtained at the time of presentation. Note the markedly enlarged ventricles and the presence of a right ventricular catheter. The patient was managed conservatively with observation, bed rest, and pumping of the shunt valve. **C** and **D**) Following 48 hours of conservative measures, the ventricular size is markedly improved. This patient eventually was delivered of a healthy infant without complication, but required revision of her shunt several months postpartum.

ampicillin and gentamicin during labor and for 48 hours postpartum.[40,66]

Literature Review

As the number of reported cases of hydrocephalus and ventriculoperitoneal shunting in the pregnant woman is limited, a brief review highlighting the available literature will provide insight into the specific problems encountered by physicians caring for these patients. Due to the variety of complications which are encountered with pregnancy, hydrocephalus, and extracranial shunts, care must be individualized and specific guidelines are difficult to define. Wisoff et al[66] outlined an overall approach to the pregnant patient with hydrocephalus after a careful review of the available literature. This is the most extensive review published on this subject and is summarized below with other selected case reports.

Monfared et al[40] reported two cases of pregnancy in women with extracranial shunts in 1979. The first was a 25-year-old woman who presented with headaches and nausea and vomiting at 27 weeks' gestation. Neurological investigation revealed noncommunicating hydrocephalus with obstruction of the fourth ventricle, presumably of infectious etiology. A ventriculoatrial shunt was placed with resolution of her symptoms and she was delivered vaginally with low forceps at 41 weeks without complication. The second patient was a 19-year-old woman who had had a ventriculoperitoneal shunt placed 4 years previously for progressive noncommunicating hydrocephalus of unknown etiology and who first presented for perinatal care at 33 weeks' gestation. Her course had been complicated by "blackout spells." She was treated with anticonvulsants and was delivered with low forceps vaginally at 40 weeks without complication. These authors concluded that the presence of an extracranial shunt does not preclude standard obstetrical management, but postulated that the use of low forceps delivery to shorten second stage labor and avoid prolonged intra-abdominal pressure elevation may be desirable. The use of antibiotic prophylaxis for delivery was recommended.

Howard and Herrick[30] reported two cases of pregnancy in patients with ventriculoperitoneal shunts in 1981. The first patient was a 24-year-old woman with hydrocephalus secondary to bacterial meningitis as a child, requiring placement of a ventriculoperitoneal shunt. Following premature rupture of membranes at 32 weeks' gestation, labor was induced with pitocin and she was delivered of a healthy infant by normal spontaneous vaginal delivery. Her postpartum course was complicated by *Proteus mirabilis* sepsis treated successfully with a cephalosporin and gentamicin. The second patient was a 25-year-old woman who was initially seen at 16 weeks' gestation, following placement of a ventriculoperitoneal shunt for an incomplete congenital aqueductal stenosis with symptoms of memory disturbance and facial paresthesias. Her symptoms resolved following shunting and she was delivered spontaneously at 41 weeks without complication. These authors favored vaginal delivery and point out that the Valsalva maneuver probably elevates both intra-abdominal pressure and ICP proportionally, which tends to lessen any potential harmful effects of increased intra-abdominal pressure in the presence of an extracranial shunt. The use of antibiotic prophylaxis for delivery was also recommended.

Gast et al[17] described two cases of maternal hydrocephalus in pregnancy in 1983. The first patient was a 25-year-old woman with a posterior fossa tumor treated with radiation 4 years prior to presentation. A ventriculoatrial shunt was placed 1 year later for symptoms of headache, tinnitus, and visual disturbance. She became pregnant and was delivered of a healthy infant with a low forceps delivery for poor expulsive efforts, with no evidence of shunt malfunction. The second patient was a 23-year-old woman with a ventriculoatrial shunt placed at age 7 years for aqueductal stenosis. At 6 months' gestation she developed signs of increased ICP with headache, nausea and vomiting, diminished sensorium, and ataxia. Evaluation of the shunt revealed normal ICP and a patent system. She was treated conservatively and was delivered spontaneously at term. Eight months postpartum she became pregnant again and her symptoms recurred. A CT scan revealed enlarged ventricles and her ICP was mildly elevated at 220 mm CSF. The atrial catheter was noted to be obstructed, and the catheter and valve were replaced. The second infant was delivered spontaneously at term without further complications. Antibiotic prophylaxis was used for both deliveries. These authors point out that an increasing number of women with intracranial shunts are becoming pregnant and that these women may have an uncomplicated delivery with careful monitoring for signs of shunt malfunction. They also point out the need for prenatal screening for hereditary causes of hydrocephalus and patient counseling.

Kleinman et al[36] described two cases of successful pregnancy in patients with ventriculoperitoneal shunts in 1983. Both patients experienced symptoms of shunt malfunction in the third trimester, apparently related to anatomical changes in the abdomen. The first case was a 20-

year-old woman first seen at 29 weeks' gestation. She had had a ventriculoatrial shunt placed at the age of 8 months for communicating hydrocephalus. In the early part of the third trimester she developed severe headaches, vomiting, and loss of upgaze. The shunt appeared to be functional and she was treated by serially pumping the shunt with resolution of her symptoms. She was delivered spontaneously at term without further difficulties. She was kept in a sitting position during labor to facilitate CSF drainage, was allowed to push through second stage labor, and received no antibiotic prophylaxis. The second patient was a 30-year-old woman who presented at 20 weeks' gestation. She had a ventriculoatrial shunt in place for hydrocephalus diagnosed after the onset of seizures 12 years previously. She presented at 29 weeks' gestation with severe bifrontal headaches and vomiting. Her shunt appeared to be functional after evaluation. Her symptoms also resolved with pumping of the shunt valve. She was delivered spontaneously at 36 weeks' gestation without complication. She was allowed to push through second stage labor without signs of increased ICP and received no antibiotic prophylaxis. These authors concluded that in selected cases conservative treatment with pumping of the shunt valve may be attempted to obviate the need for extensive evaluation and shunt revision late in pregnancy. Although no antibiotic prophylaxis was used, these authors state that they would not argue against the use of antibiotics in these patients.

Nugent and Hoshek[43] described a complication of peritoneal catheter placement during pregnancy which resulted in a large extra-abdominal cyst. A 30-year-old woman underwent placement of a ventriculoperitoneal shunt for hydrocephalus secondary to a cysticercosis infection at 7 weeks' gestation. She delivered without further difficulty; however, 3 weeks postpartum she returned with a slowly enlarging mass over her abdominal incision. Upon exploration, a 10-cm extraperitoneal cyst was found with the intraperitoneal portion of the catheter coiled inside. The catheter was replaced in the peritoneum without difficulty and she was discharged without further complication. The authors state that a 20-inch length of catheter was initially placed and they believe that increasing intra-abdominal pressure associated with pregnancy and labor had displaced the catheter into its extraperitoneal position. They suggest using longer segments of intra-abdominal catheter to avoid this complication in young women requiring shunting early in pregnancy.

In the most comprehensive review of CSF shunts in pregnancy published to date, Wisoff et al[66] reported the outcome of 11 new pregnancies and reviewed reports of 10 previously published pregnancies in a total of 18 patients. In this combined series, 14 patients had shunts in place prior to pregnancy and four required shunting during pregnancy for symptoms of increased ICP. Neurological complications occurred in 76% of all patients with pre-existing shunts in the combined series, and in 58% of their personal series. Four of these patients had a new shunt placed during pregnancy and one required revision of a previous shunt, all without complication. In asymptomatic patients, they recommend prenatal counseling and careful surveillance for signs of shunt malfunction. If symptoms develop, they recommend aggressive evaluation for shunt occlusion and elevated ICP. Patients with a documented shunt occlusion or malfunction should undergo shunt revision. Patients without elevated ICP are managed conservatively, with the goal of a vaginal delivery. These authors were not impressed with the effects of pumping the shunt, but recommended bed rest, fluid restriction and, in selected cases, diuretics and steroids. These authors favored a shortened second stage of labor for vaginal deliveries with the use of antibiotic prophylaxis. If the patient is at or near term and is neurologically unstable, they recommended a cesarean section under general anesthetic. By combining the previously published cases with their personal series, the numbers and statistics are difficult to follow in this paper; nonetheless, this represents the most comprehensive review of CSF shunt problems in pregnancy and serves as a guide for management in these unique patients.

Summary

Improvement in the management of hydrocephalus has allowed more patients to assume a normal lifestyle with the expectation of raising children. Consequently, pregnant women with CSF shunts will come to the attention of their obstetrician. The challenges unique to these patients combine the problems of pregnancy with the complications of hydrocephalus and extracranial shunting procedures. As no controlled studies are available, the physician encountering these patients can be guided only by review of the available literature. Each presentation and clinical situation represents a challenge to individualized care and promotes a successful outcome for the mother and child. The available literature suggests that in the majority of cases, pregnancy is not a contraindication to extracranial shunting and the presence of an extracranial shunt is not a contraindication to a labor and vaginal delivery. The role of antibiotic prophylaxis for delivery remains controversial, but the majority of authors appear to favor their use to avoid the complications of shunt infection and septicemia.

REFERENCES

1. Amacher AL, Wellington J: Infantile hydrocephalus: long-term results of surgical therapy. **Childs Brain 11:**217-229, 1984
2. Baker TH, Machikawa JH, Stapleton JJ: Asymptomatic puerperal bacteremia. **Am J Obstet Gynecol 94:**903-905, 1966
3. Brooks DJ, Beaney RP, Leenders KL, et al: Regional cerebral oxygen utilization, blood flow, and blood volume in benign intracranial hypertension studied by positron emission tomography. **Neurology 35:** 1030-1034, 1985
4. Brourman ND, Spoor TC, Ramocki JM: Optic nerve sheath decompression for pseudotumor cerebri. **Arch Ophthalmol 106:**1378-1383, 1988
5. Carter CO, Evans K: Children of adult survivors with spina bifida cystica. **Lancet 2:**924-929, 1973
6. Corbett JJ: Problems with the diagnosis and treatment of pseudotumor cerebri. **Can J Neurol Sci 10:** 221-229, 1983
7. Corbett JJ, Menta MP: Cerebrospinal fluid pressure in normal obese subjects and patients with pseudotumor cerebri. **Neurology 33:**1386-1388, 1983
8. Corbett JJ, Nerad JA, Tse DT, et al: Results of optic nerve sheath fenestration for pseudotumor cerebri. The lateral orbitotomy approach. **Arch Ophthalmol 106:**1391-1397, 1988
9. Corbett JJ, Savino PJ, Thompson HS, et al: Visual loss in pseudotumor cerebri. Follow-up of 57 patients from five to 41 years and a profile of 14 patients with permanent severe visual loss. **Arch Neurol 39:** 461-474, 1982
10. Corbett JJ, Thompson HS: The rational management of idiopathic intracranial hypertension. **Arch Neurol 46:**1049-1051, 1989
11. Digre KB, Varner MW, Corbett JJ: Pseudotumor cerebri and pregnancy. **Neurology 34:**721-729, 1984
12. Donaldson JO: Endocrinology of pseudotumor cerebri. **Neurol Clin 4:**919-927, 1986
13. Durcan FJ, Corbett JJ, Wall M: The incidence of pseudotumor cerebri. Population studies in Iowa and Louisiana. **Arch Neurol 45:**875-877, 1988
14. Fishman RA: The pathophysiology of pseudotumor cerebri. An unsolved puzzle. **Arch Neurol 41:** 257-258, 1984
15. Foley J: Benign forms of intracranial hypertension– "toxic" and "otitic" hydrocephalus. **Brain 78:**1-41, 1955
16. Frisén L: Swelling of the optic nerve head: a staging scheme. **J Neurol Neurosurg Psychiatry 45:**13-18, 1982
17. Gast MJ, Grubb RL Jr, Strickler RC: Maternal hydrocephalus and pregnancy. **Obstet Gynecol 62(Suppl):** 29S-31S, 1983
18. Giuseffi V, Wall M, Siegel PZ, et al: Symptoms and disease associations in idiopathic intracranial hypertension (pseudotumor cerebri): a case-control study. **Neurology 41:**239-244, 1991
19. Gjerris F, Soelberg-Sørenson P, Vorstrup S, et al: Intracranial pressure, conductance to cerebrospinal fluid outflow, and cerebral blood flow in patients with benign intracranial hypertension (pseudotumor cerebri). **Ann Neurol 17:**158-162, 1985
20. Greer M: Benign intracranial hypertension. II. Following corticosteroid therapy. **Neurology 13:** 439-441, 1963
21. Greer M: Benign intracranial hypertension. III. Pregnancy. **Neurology 13:**670-672, 1963
22. Greer M: Benign intracranial hypertension. VI. Obesity. **Neurology 15:**382-388, 1965
23. Grosfield JL, Cooney DR, Smith J, et al: Intra-abdominal complications following ventriculoperitoneal shunt procedures. **Pediatrics 54:**791-796, 1974
24. Gücer G, Viernstein L: Long-term intracranial pressure recording in the management of pseudotumor cerebri. **J Neurosurg 49:**256-263, 1978
25. Hammon WM: Evaluation and use of the ventriculoperitoneal shunt in hydrocephalus. **J Neurosurg 34:** 792-795, 1971
26. Hayreh SS: Optic disc edema in raised intracranial pressure. V. Pathogenesis. **Arch Ophthalmol 95:** 1553-1565, 1977
27. Hayreh SS, Hayreh MS: Optic disc edema in raised intracranial pressure. II. Early detection with fluorescein fundus angiography and stereoscopic color photography. **Arch Ophthalmol 95:**1245-1254, 1977
28. Holmes LB, Driscoll SG, Atkins L: Etiologic heterogeneity of neural-tube defects. **N Engl J Med 294:** 365-369, 1976
29. Hopkins EL, Hendricks CH, Cibils LA: Cerebrospinal fluid pressure in labor. **Am J Obstet Gynecol 93:** 907-916, 1965
30. Howard TE Jr, Herrick CN: Pregnancy in patients with ventriculoperitoneal shunts: report of two cases. **Am J Obstet Gynecol 141:**99-101, 1981
31. Ireland B, Corbett JJ, Wallace RB: The search for causes of idiopathic intracranial hypertension. A preliminary case-control study. **Arch Neurol 47:**315-320, 1990
32. Johnston I, Paterson A: Benign intracranial hypertension. II. CSF pressure and circulation. **Brain 97:**

301-312, 1974
33. Keltner JL, Albert DM, Lubow M, et al: Optic nerve decompression. A clinical pathologic study. **Arch Ophthalmol 95:**97-104, 1977
34. Keltner JL, Miller NR, Gittinger JW, et al: Pseudotumor cerebri. **Surv Ophthalmol 23:**315-322, 1979
35. Keucher TR, Mealey J Jr: Long-term results after ventriculoatrial and ventriculoperitoneal shunting for infantile hydrocephalus. **J Neurosurg 50:**179-186, 1979
36. Kleinman G, Sutherling W, Martinez M, et al: Malfunction of ventriculoperitoneal shunts during pregnancy. **Obstet Gynecol 61:**753-754, 1983
37. Leem W, Miltz H: Complications following ventricular atrial shunts in hydrocephalus. **Adv Neurosurg 6:** 1-7, 1978
38. Marx GF, Zemaitis MT, Orkin LR: Cerebrospinal fluid pressures during labor and obstetrical anesthesia. **Anesthesiology 22:**348 354, 1961
39. Mathew NT, Meyer JS, Ott EO: Increased cerebral blood volume in benign intracranial hypertension. **Neurology 25:**646-649, 1975
40. Monfared AH, Koh KS, Apuzzo MLJ, et al: Obstetric management of pregnant women with extracranial shunts. **Can Med Assoc J 120:**562-563, 1979
41. Moser FG, Hilal SK, Abrams G, et al: MR imaging in pseudotumor cerebri. **AJR 150:**903-909, 1988
42. Newborg B: Pseudotumor cerebri treated with/by rice reduction diet. **Arch Intern Med 133:**802-807, 1974
43. Nugent P, Hoshek S: Large extra-abdominal cyst as a postpartum complication of peritoneal shunt. Case report. **J Neurosurg 64:**151-152, 1986
44. Paterson R, DePasquale N, Mann S: Pseudotumor cerebri. **Medicine 40:**85-99, 1961
45. Pearlman RL, Riser JB, Riser ES: Pseudotumor cerebri mimicking hyperemesis gravidarum. **Int J Gynaecol Obstet 37:**52, 1992 (Letter)
46. Powell JL: Pseudotumor cerebri and pregnancy. **Obstet Gynecol 40:**713-718, 1972
47. Raichle ME, Grubb RL Jr, Phelps ME, et al: Cerebral hemodynamics and metabolism in pseudotumor cerebri. **Ann Neurol 4:**104-111, 1978
48. Reid AC, Matheson MS, Teasdale G: Volume of the ventricles in benign intracranial hypertension. **Lancet 2:**7-8, 1980
49. Reid AC, Thomson JA: Absence of significant endocrine deficiencies in benign intracranial hypertension. **J Neurol Neurosurg Psychiatry 44:**731-734, 1981
50. Repka MX, Miller NR, Savino PJ: Pseudotumor cerebri. **Am J Ophthalmol 98:**741-746, 1984
51. Rosenberg M, Corbett JJ, Smith C, et al: Cerebrospinal fluid diversion procedures in pseudotumor cerebri. **Neurology 43:**1071-1072, 1993
52. Sadun A, Currie J, Lessell S: Transient visual obscurations with elevated optic discs. **Ann Neurol 16:**489-494, 1984
53. Sahs AL, Joynt RJ: Brain swelling of unknown cause. **Neurology 6:**791-803, 1956
54. Sergott RC, Savino PJ, Bosley TM: Modified optic nerve sheath decompression provides long-term visual improvement for pseudotumor cerebri. **Arch Ophthalmol 106:**1384-1390, 1988
55. Sheldon RS, Becker WJ, Hanley DA, et al: Hypoparathyroidism and pseudotumor cerebri: an infrequent clinical association. **Can J Neurol Sci 14:**622-625, 1987
56. Smith TJ, Baker RS: Perimetric findings in pseudotumor cerebri using automated techniques. **Ophthalmology 93:**887-894, 1986
57. Spence JD, Amacher AL, Willis NR: Benign intracranial hypertension without papilledema: a role of 24-hour cerebrospinal fluid pressure monitoring in diagnosis and management. **Neurosurgery 7:**326-336, 1980
58. Verplanck M, Kaufman DI, Parsons T, et al: Electrophysiology versus psychophysics in the detection of visual loss in pseudotumor cerebri. **Neurology 38:** 1789-1792, 1988
59. Wall M: The headache profile of idiopathic intracranial hypertension. **Cephalalgia 10:**331-335, 1991
60. Wall M, George D: Idiopathic intracranial hypertension. A prospective study of 50 patients. **Brain 114:** 155-180, 1991
61. Wall M, George D: Visual loss in pseudotumor cerebri. Incidence and defects related to visual field strategy. **Arch Neurol 44:**170-175, 1987
62. Walsh FB: Papilledema associated with increased intracranial pressure in Addison's disease. **Arch Ophthalmol 47:**86, 1952
63. Weisberg LA: Benign intracranial hypertension. **Medicine 54:**197-207, 1975
64. Weisberg LA: Computed tomography in benign intracranial hypertension. **Neurology 35:**1075-1078, 1985
65. Wilson DH, Gardner WJ: Benign intracranial hypertension with particular reference to its occurrence in fat young women. **Can Med Assoc J 95:**102-105, 1966
66. Wisoff JH, Kratzert KJ, Handwerker SM, et al: Pregnancy in patients with cerebrospinal fluid shunts. A report of a series and review of the literature. **Neurosurgery 29:**827-831, 1991

CHAPTER 15

Operative Positioning and Fetal Monitoring Considerations

Jerry Day, MD, and H. Hunt Batjer, MD

An estimated 1.6% to 2.2% of pregnant women undergo a surgical procedure at some time during pregnancy.[31,49] Perhaps as many as 50,000 pregnant women undergo surgery of some type each year in the United States. Several factors account for a surprisingly large percentage of neurosurgical procedures in these patients.[31,46-49] Maternal mortality has progressively declined over the past four decades due to improved management of the major obstetric complications of hemorrhage, infection, and toxemia.[38,39] These developments have resulted in a relative increase in maternal deaths from nonobstetric causes. Prominent among nonobstetric causes of maternal morbidity are subarachnoid hemorrhage and intracranial tumor. Subarachnoid hemorrhage, secondary to ruptured intracranial aneurysm or arteriovenous malformation, now ranks high as a cause of maternal morbidity and mortality.[6,9,11,15-17,36-41,54] Subarachnoid hemorrhage of various etiologies is reported to cause between 4% and 24% of maternal deaths.[9,16,38-40]

Less common during childbearing years are primary and metastatic tumors; however, their clinical course may be accelerated and/or aggravated by pregnancy, probably related to extracellular fluid retention or direct hormonal influence. Thus, surgery is often required to ensure the delivery of a viable infant.[12-14,18,38,39,52,55] Other neurosurgical disorders such as cranial and/or spinal trauma, cerebral cysts or abscesses, sinus thrombosis, hydrocephalus, spinal column and spinal cord tumors, and disc disease of the spine occur frequently enough to warrant mention among the considerations for anesthetic management.[2,3,8,10,20,23,28,30,33-35,38,39,42,44,51,53] This chapter attempts to review pertinent physiology of pregnancy and to provide general guidelines for patient positioning and maternal and fetal monitoring for and during neurosurgical procedures. Specific recommendations for procedures relevant to neurosurgical disorders are detailed following a discussion of the striking physiological changes associated with pregnancy and the general principles of neuroanesthesia during pregnancy.

The objectives of neuroanesthetic management of pregnant women during the early and mid stages of pregnancy include: 1) assuring maternal safety; 2) avoiding teratogenic drugs; 3) prevention of fetal asphyxia; and 4) avoiding induction of preterm labor.[38,39] These objectives may conflict with the goals of anesthesia during labor and delivery, which are largely concerned with the provision of analgesia without endangering the fetus or aggravating the maternal neurological disorder.[38,39] Recognition of the necessity for a multidisciplinary approach toward the pregnant patient with neurological disease is the initial crucial step toward assuring the best possible outcome for the mother and fetus. Informational and technical input from the obstetrician, obstetric anesthesiologist, and often the neonatalogist is critical to assist the neurosurgeon and the neuroanesthesiologist in planning the diagnostic evaluation and neurosurgical treatment of the individual patient.

Physiological Changes of Pregnancy

Major alterations in nearly every organ system occur during pregnancy. In general, changes in the early stages of pregnancy result from hormonal secretions from the corpus luteum and placenta. The mechanical effects of the gravid uterus play a predominant role in the second and third trimesters.

Blood Volume and Components

Plasma and erythrocyte volume begin to increase between sixth and 12th weeks of pregnancy, culminating in a plasma volume increase of 40% to 50% and a total blood volume increase of 25% to 40% by the end of gestation.[31,49] Erythrocyte volume increases only by approximately 20%, which accounts for the relative reductions in erythrocyte count, hemoglobin, and hematocrit. These hemodynamic alterations provide some protection to the mother and fetus during preoperative or intraoperative hemorrhage. Minimal acceptable values for hemoglobin and hematocrit are 11-12 g/dL and 33% to 35%, respectively.[31,49] The total leukocyte count remains 8,000-10,000 throughout pregnancy and the platelet count increases from a mean nonpregnant value of 187,000/mm^3 to 210,000/mm^3 in the first trimester, 276,000/mm^3 in the second trimester, and 316,000/mm^3 in the third trimester.[31]

Plasma proteins are also affected by hemodilution; their total concentration declines to less than 6 g/dL at term, while the total amount in circulation increases.[31,49] This results in an increase of the free fraction of highly protein-bound drugs, such as diazepam and dilantin, thereby enhancing their effect and the risk of toxicity.[31,49]

Fibrinogen content increases throughout pregnancy from 250-300 mg/dL to 450 mg/dL.[31] Coincident with this change and the increased number of platelets, there is a definite marked increase in activity of several clotting factors. These factors render the blood hypercoagulable and thus predispose the pregnant woman to thromboembolic phenomena.[31]

The concentration and subsequent activity of pseudocholinesterase are also reduced by hemodilution. Activity decreases approximately 21% during the first trimester and remains fairly stable thereafter.[31,49]

Hemodynamic Changes

To meet the metabolic demands of pregnancy, the cardiovascular system becomes hyperdynamic.[49] Simultaneous reductions in systemic and uterine vascular resistance are the result of vascular relaxation induced by increased progesterone and, possibly, prostaglandin levels.[31,49,50] Uterine blood flow is approximately 3% of the total cardiac output during the first trimester and increases to approximately 10%-15% during the third trimester.[50] These factors contribute to an increased cardiac output that reaches a level approximately 30%-40% above the nonpregnant level by 30 weeks of gestation. Cardiac output is also redistributed with increased blood flow to the placenta, uterus, skin, kidneys, and mammary glands.[37] Uterine blood flow at term is about 700 ml/min, 70% to 90% of which perfuses the placenta and the remainder supplying the myometrium. The uterine vascular bed, almost maximally vasodilated under normal conditions, has very little capacity to dilate further. Uterine blood flow is not autoregulated, so it is proportional to the mean perfusion pressure. Conversely, the uterine blood vessels are capable of marked vasoconstriction.[39] Systemic arterial blood pressure normally remains unchanged or decreases slightly with advancing pregnancy because of the decrease in peripheral resistance which exceeds the increase in cardiac output.[31,50]

The enlarging uterus can mechanically produce compression of the great vessels (inferior vena cava and descending aorta) against the spine during the second and third trimesters, especially when the pregnant patient is in the supine position.[36,50] This situation results in decreased venous return and cardiac output. Arterial pressure is maintained by a compensatory increase in peripheral resistance, especially in the uteroplacental vasculature, with potential harmful effects on the fetus in this position.[36,50] Vena caval compression can begin to develop during the second trimester and becomes maximum at 36 to 38 weeks' gestation. There is a relative decrease thereafter due to the descent of the fetal head into the pelvis. These factors must be carefully considered when surgery is contemplated during the time periods. Vena caval compression is responsible for the "supine hypotensive syndrome," initially reported in 1953.[19] This phenomenon occurs in 10% to 15% of pregnant women and is manifested by arterial hypotension, tachycardia, pallor, and faintness. Radiographic studies have revealed complete inferior vena caval obstruction in approximately 90% of women at term while lying supine.[21] In this instance venous blood from the lower half of the body reaches the heart through the superior vena cava after diversion via the intervertebral venous plexus and the azygous vein. The resultant engorgement of the intervertebral venous plexus reduces the epidural and subarachnoid spaces, with a consequent decrease in the drug requirement for regional anesthesia.[31] There is approximately a 30% decrease in the amount of local anesthetic required to produce a given level of block from mid pregnancy to term.[39] Aortography has demonstrated compression of the descending aorta in the supine position.[4] This affects primarily the renal and uteroplacental blood flow.

Thus, after the first trimester the supine position must be avoided intraoperatively, even in the absence of maternal arterial hypotension.[31,50] This is accomplished by utilizing the left lateral decubitus position, placing a wedge or blanket roll beneath the right hip, and/or by rotating the operating table to the left to induce left lateral tilt of the uterus. Such measures should displace the gravid uterus off the major abdominal vessels without compromising the position of the operative field.[39,50]

Electrocardiogram

Left axis deviation results from upward displacement of the diaphragm by the enlarging uterus. As well, there is an increased tendency toward premature ventricular contractions, sinus tachycardia, and paroxysmal supraventricular tachycardia. Unless underlying cardiac disease is present, these arrhythmias do not ordinarily alter the normal course of pregnancy and pose no significant maternal hazard during anesthesia.[31]

Respiratory System

Capillary venous engorgement of the oropharynx and respiratory tract makes nasal breathing difficult for some women and increases the difficulty of nasotracheal and endotracheal intubation should general anesthesia become necessary. The trauma of repeated attempts at laryngoscopy may result in oropharyngeal and/or laryngeal edema and bleeding, thus further compromising the patient's airway.[31,49]

Lung volumes undergo progressive changes beginning in the fifth month of pregnancy. There is a reduction in expiratory reserve volume, residual volume, and functional residual capacity.[31] At term, functional residual capacity is 20% less than in the nonpregnant state owing to an increase in tidal volume and a decrease in expiratory reserve volume.[31,39] A coincident increase in inspiratory reserve capacity and inspiratory reserve volume allows total lung capacity to remain unchanged. In fact, there is a 15% increase in O_2 consumption, which places the mother at risk for developing hypoxemia during periods of apnea or hypoventilation.[31] Ventilation increases early in pregnancy and is maximum by the second or third month. At term, tidal volume is increased by 40%, respiratory rate by 15%, with a net minute ventilation approximately 50% above the nonpregnant level. Alveolar ventilation at term is approximately 70% more than in the nonpregnant state.[31] It is increased 25% at 16 weeks' gestation and more at term because of increased tidal volume in the face of unchanged total lung capacity.[38]

Basal O_2 consumption increases during pregnancy but is compensated by hyperventilation, resulting in an increase in maternal arterial O_2 tension to a mean of 106 mm Hg and a decrease of the mean maternal arterial CO_2 tension to 32 mm Hg.[31] Concomitantly, plasma bicarbonate decreases to 22 mEq/L, keeping maternal pH close to 7.4.[31,39]

These respiration changes have significant anesthetic implications. The combination of increased alveolar ventilation and decreased functional residual capacity enhances maternal uptake and elimination of inhalational anesthetics.[31] The sedative effects of progesterone and increased levels of endogenous opiates are thought to contribute further to reduction in the minimal alveolar concentration of up to 25% for halothane and 40% for isoflurane respectively.[24,25,29]

Decreased Oxygen Reserve

A decreased functional residual capacity combined with increased O_2 consumption predisposes the mother to hypoxemia even during a brief period of airway obstruction.[39] Even with rapid intubation and only 30 seconds of apnea, PaO_2 can fall to 50 mm Hg if preoxygenation is not performed.[38] This rapid development of hypoxemia is avoided by administering 100% O_2 for 3 to 5 minutes before induction and intubation or taking four vital capacity breaths of 100% O_2 in rapid sequence.[31,39,49]

Prevention of Fetal Asphyxia

A review of the anesthetic implications for uterine blood flow is relevant at this time. Reduction of uterine blood flow can cause serious fetal hypoxia with disastrous results. Mechanical ventilation can profoundly affect uterine blood flow and the fetus. Especially pertinent to neurosurgery is the use of hyperventilation. A study of nonanesthetized pregnant ewes revealed a 25% decrease in uterine blood flow during hyperventilation-induced hypocarbia and, with the addition of CO_2 to the respiratory gases, during normocarbia and hypercarbia.[22] Maternal blood pressure was unchanged during hyperventilation and the decrease in uterine blood flow was thought to result from the mechanical effects of the positive pressure ventilation, inducing a decrease in venous return and cardiac output.[22] A similar study revealed a decrease in uterine blood flow with the production of respiratory alkalosis by hyperventilation in anesthetized ewes.[27] Maternal hyperventilation and respiratory alkalosis also decrease fetal oxygen content and arterial O_2 tension despite increases in maternal oxygenation.[22,27] Maternal alkalosis similarly reduces umbilical blood flow by direct vasoconstriction. A left shift of the maternal O_2 hemoglobin dissociation curve (increased maternal affinity for hemoglobin) is the likely cause for fetal hypoxia in maternal acidosis.

As previously mentioned, uterine blood flow is directly proportional to mean perfusion pressure. Specifically, placental blood flow is directly proportional to the net perfusion pressure across the intervillous space (uterine arterial blood pressure minus intrauterine pressure minus uterine venous pressure). Placental blood flow is inversely proportional to the resistance of spiral arterioles supplying the intervillous space combined with the resistance imparted to these vessels by the myometrial tension. Any anesthetic procedure or agent that decreases the perfusion pressure and/or increases vascular resistance may result in placental hypotension and fetal asphyxia.[31,38,39]

Fetal asphyxia results in damage to the fetal central nervous system, heart, and lungs.[38] Fetal monkeys who sustained asphyxia of intermediate severity and duration with consequent acidosis incurred permanent brain injury, producing lesions similar to human cerebral palsy.[5] Severe asphyxia resulted in death from myocardial failure.[5] The goal of intraoperative fetal monitoring is to detect the earliest evidence of this potentially tragic complication.

Hypotension

Maternal systemic hypotension and, thus, uteroplacental hypotension may result from several causes. This may be induced by sympathetic blockade (epidural or spinal anesthesia), hypovolemic shock, supine hypotensive syndrome, or iatrogenically (sodium nitroprusside, deep halothane, or isoflurane anesthesia). Although hypotensive techniques have been safely used in some cases the "success" reported is often measured by a live birth with no documented assessment of fetal neurological status or pediatric follow-up.[7,26,56] Other reports have documented fetal death or distress (based on fetal heart rate monitoring) associated with these anesthetic techniques.[1,32,37] Light halothane or isoflurane anesthesia does not result in a significant reduction in uterine blood flow because of the concomitant decrease in uterine vascular resistance.[38]

In supine pregnant women, the hypotensive effect of autonomic blockade depends primarily on increased venous capacitance and pooling of blood, thereby decreasing blood return to the heart (decreased preload) and diminishing cardiac output.[38] When it becomes necessary to induce hypotension in pregnant patients, the uterus should be adequately displaced to the left and blood pressure reduction should be limited in depth and duration to the minimum required.[38] The fetal heart rate should be closely monitored because fetal tolerance depends on fetoplacental reserve, and failure of this compensatory mechanism will be quickly evident by fetal distress.[38] Frequent measurement of maternal arterial pH is necessary to avoid severe fetal or maternal compromise.

Monitoring During Craniotomy

In addition to the standard maternal monitors of an intra-arterial catheter, a Doppler air-embolism monitor, and a right atrial catheter to monitor central venous pressure, the fetus and uterus need to be continuously monitored during positioning and craniotomy. An external fetal heart rate monitor should be employed after the 16th week of pregnancy.[39] During operations performed at term, direct fetal scalp electrodes can be placed if amniotomy has occurred or simultaneous delivery is planned. Fetal heart rate monitoring provides an indication of fetal well-being and early detection of abnormalities in maternal ventilation and/or uterine perfusion. Diligent observation and control of maternal blood pressure with prompt correction of hypoxia and hypotension are mandatory for the fetus to have the greatest chance of survival with an intact nervous system.

The choice of specific anesthetic agents for pregnant women undergoing neurosurgical procedures should not be unduly influenced by concerns of teratogenicity.[43,45] Susceptibility of various fetal organ systems to these agents is clearly maximum in the first trimester. Anesthetics that readily traverse the placenta diminish the normal beat-to-beat variability of fetal heart rate and it should be kept in mind that the fetus is also being put to sleep. With induced hypothermia, the decrease in fetal heart rate parallels the reduction in maternal heart rate and does not threaten organ systems due to decreases in metabolic rate. Patterns of fetal bradycardia are direct evidence of maternal hypoxia and/or hypotension. A maternal systolic blood pressure of less than 100 mm Hg may be associated with pathological fetal bradycardia, usually beginning a few minutes after the onset of hypotension and sometimes preceded by mild fetal tachycardia. Fetal tachycardia is also recognized as an early sign of maternal hypoxia in the third trimester of pregnancy and severe fetal distress in the full-term infant.[39]

An external tocodynamometer to monitor uterine tone is indicated when the uterine fundus is above the level of the umbilicus and a surgical procedure is required.[39] The fetal heart rate and uterine tone should be monitored for at least 24 hours postoperatively or until the mother's condition is considered stable. It should be remembered that anesthesia and analgesia alter the pregnant woman's perception of uterine contractions.

Monitoring During Other Neurosurgical Procedures

The basic guidelines that are detailed for craniotomy apply to general anesthesia for any neurosurgical procedure performed during pregnancy. Diligence in displacing the gravid uterus from the retroperitoneal vessels must be maintained when using various positions for surgery. Prudent practice for all pregnant patients undergoing surgical procedures under spinal, epidural, or local anesthesia dictates the need for continuous maternal heart rate, blood pressure, and oxygen saturation monitoring. Fetal heart rate and uterine tone should be continually monitored as well.

A thoughtful and team-oriented approach to patient positioning and maternal and fetal monitoring based on the well-described physiological changes accompanying pregnancy will result in the best possible outcome for "both" patients involved.

Positioning for Neurosurgical Procedures

The preceding discussion has emphasized the dramatic physiological derangements associated with pregnancy and many of the implications of these changes for standard anesthetic management with regard to general and regional anesthetic techniques. The concluding section will deal with the specific positioning techniques that have been found to be safe once a decision is made to embark upon a surgical procedure. The neurosurgeon must always keep in mind that he or she is responsible for two patients during the entire perioperative period. As implied by the earlier discussion, patient positioning is a critical maneuver that can readily jeopardize the mother and fetus if not performed carefully and with attention to maternal and fetal mechanical and physiological problems.

Craniotomy

Concerns for patient positioning start during transport to the operating suite. Beginning with the second trimester, the pregnant woman must not be transported on a gurney supine. The vascular compression syndromes can be avoided by utilizing the sitting or left lateral decubitus position. The risk of emesis and aspiration is also high in the supine position due to elevated gastrin levels, decreased gastric pH, and incompetence of the gastroesophogeal junction.[39] The legs should also be fitted with wrapping bandages or pneumatic compression devices to minimize the risk of thromboembolism.

When a frontal or frontotemporal craniotomy is required and the supine position mandatory, displacement of the gravid uterus must be performed. For a right-sided craniotomy, this can be easily accomplished by a right shoulder and right hip roll mobilizing the uterus to the left. When a left-sided approach is required, consideration should be given to using the lateral position to allow adequate gravitational displacement of the gravid uterus. When this is not possible a large left hip roll should be employed and continuous fetal monitoring be vigilantly studied prior to surgical draping to ensure that the vascular decompression is adequate.

When posterior fossa surgery is required it is our strong preference to utilize the lateral or park-bench position and preferably the left lateral position for right-sided or midline pathology. The prone or concorde positions are obviously contraindicated due to the presence of the gravid uterus. The sitting position is also suboptimal due to the maternal venous pooling which will be exacerbated, increasing the risk of decreased cardiac output and poor fetal perfusion.

The surgeon must also be cognizant of some of the anesthetic limitations during advanced pregnancy. As previously described, severe maternal hyperventilation can gravely diminish placental perfusion. Therefore, when access to basal subarachnoid spaces will be required for vascular or neoplastic conditions, some provision for brain relaxation (other than hyperventilation) must be made. While spinal cerebrospinal fluid drainage is feasible, one must keep in mind the physiological venous engorgement which increases the risk of lumbar puncture-induced epidural hematoma. Due to this concern it is our preference to achieve brain relaxation by either early sylvian fissure dissection for anterior procedures or cisterna magna opening for suboccipital approaches. The use of direct ventricular puncture is also used routinely in this situation in our practice.

Postoperative care also requires attention to these patient-positioning principles. The left lateral decubitus position with the mother's head elevated should be used in concert with fetal heart rate monitoring to minimize the risk of fetal hypoxia and maternal emesis and aspiration.

Spinal Procedures

While many spinal conditions are clearly aggravated by the ligamentous laxity associated with pregnancy (as discussed in Chapter 6), most can be managed conservatively until the pregnancy is concluded. Occasionally, however, this is not possible, as in the case of traumatic injury, discogenic cauda equina syndrome, or progressive neurological deterioration related to intra- or extra-axial tumor progression.

When surgery is required it is our preference, when possible, to utilize regional anesthesia with spinal or epidural techniques. These procedures minimize the systemic risks of the general anesthetic agents to the pregnant woman and fetus and can usually provide adequate anesthesia for lumbar procedures.

For the above-mentioned reasons, the lateral position (particularly the left lateral position) is strongly preferred whether regional or general anesthesia is employed. The surgeon must anticipate the engorgement of epidural venous structures, which can complicate all of these procedures. The issues of preoperative, transport-related, and postoperative positioning previously described do not differ from those for the craniotomy patient except that more aggressive postoperative analgesic management may be required.

Summary

This chapter has attempted to detail the relevant physiological changes of normal pregnancy and their implications for anesthetic, maternal and fetal monitoring, and surgical positioning concerns. We have not dealt with the vitally important ethical judgments encountered with catastrophic maternal neurosurgical emergencies, but these will be discussed by Kaufman et al in Chapter 18. In addition, we did not discuss the importance of surgical judgment in attempting to defer all elective procedures until after the birth of the infant. As "captain of the ship," the neurosurgeon must keep in mind the direct responsibility for two patient lives, one of whom is completely dependent on the other. To maximize the chances for successful patient outcome, it is critical to recruit input from appropriate consultants from the time of diagnostic procedures through the perioperative period.

References

1. Aitken RR, Drake CG: A technique of anesthesia with induced hypotension for surgical correction of intracranial aneurysms. **Clin Neurosurg 21:**107-114, 1974
2. Aker JG, Parker KE: Anesthetic management for emergent caesarean section in a patient with penetrating head injury. **Nurse Anesthesia 4:**125-129, 1993
3. Alexander JT, McCormick PC: Pregnancy and discogenic disease of the spine. **Neurosurg Clin North Am 4:**153-159, 1993
4. Bieniarz J, Crottogini JJ, Curuchet E, et al: Aortocaval compression by the uterus in late human pregnancy. II. An arteriographic study. **Am J Obstet Gynecol 100:**203-217, 1968
5. Brann AW Jr., Myers RE: Central nervous system findings in the newborn monkey following severe *in utero* partial asphyxia. **Neurology 25:**327-338, 1975
6. Buckley TA, Yau GHM, Poon WS, et al: Caesarean section and ablation of a cerebral arterio-venous malformation. **Anaesth Intensive Care 18:**248-251, 1990
7. Cannell DE, Botterell EH: Subarachnoid hemorrhage and pregnancy. **Am J Obstet Gynecol 72:**844-855, 1956
8. Daley MD, Rolbin SH, Hew EM, et al: Epidural anesthesia for obstetrics after spinal surgery. **Reg Anaesth 15:**280-284, 1990
9. Dias MS, Sekhar LN: Intracranial hemorrhage from aneurysms and arteriovenous malformations during pregnancy and the puerperium. **Neurosurgery 27:** 855-865, 1990
10. Drost TF, Rosemurgy AS, Sherman HF, et al: Major trauma in pregnant women: maternal/fetal outcome. **J Trauma 30:**574-578, 1990
11. El Gawly RM: Ruptured intracranial aneurysm in pregnancy: a case report and review of the literature. **Eur J Obstet Gynecol Reprod Biol 46:**150-153, 1992
12. Fraser GC, Blair GK, Hemming A, et al: The treatment of simultaneous choriocarcinoma in mother and baby. **J Pediatr Surg 27:**1318-1319, 1992
13. Fujiwara T, Mino S, Nagao S, et al: Metastatic choriocarcinoma with neoplastic aneurysms cured by aneurysm resection and chemotherapy. Case report. **J Neurosurg 76:**148-151, 1992
14. Giannakopoulos G, Nair S, Snider C, et al: Implications for the pathogenisis of aneurysm formation: Metastatic choriocarcinoma with spontaneous splenic rupture. Case report and a review. **Surg Neurol 38:**236-240, 1992
15. Gill TE, Manis S, Dessables DR: Anesthetic management of cerebral aneurysm clipping during pregnancy: A case report. **J Am Assoc Nurse Anesthetists**

61:282-286, 1993
16. Holcomb WL Jr, Petrie RH: Cerebrovascular emergencies in pregnancy. **Clin Obstet Gynecol 33:**467-472, 1990
17. Horton JC, Chambers WA, Lyons SL, et al: Pregnancy and the risk of hemorrhage from cerebral arteriovenous malformations. **Neurosurgery 27:** 867-872, 1990
18. Hove B, Andersen BB, Christiansen TM: Intracranial oncotic aneurysms from choriocarcinoma. Case report and review of the literature. **Neuroradiology 32:**526-528, 1990
19. Howard BK, Goodson JH, Mengert WF: Supine hypotensive syndrome of late pregnancy. **Obstet Gynecol 1:**371-377, 1953
20. Joubert J, Durrheim DN, Copley IB: Cervical intraspinal lipoma in a pregnant patient. **Br J Neurosurg 7:**437-441, 1993
21. Kerr MG, Scott DB, Samuel E: Studies of the inferior vena cava in late pregnancy. **Br Med J 1:**532-533, 1964
22. Levinson G, Shnider SM, de Lorimier AA, et al: Effects of maternal hyperventilation on uterine blood flow and fetal oxygenation and acid-base status. **Anesthesiology 40:**340-347, 1974
23. Lopate G, Black JT, Grubb RL Jr: Cavernous hemangioma of the spinal cord: report of 2 unusual cases. **Neurology 40:**1791-1793, 1990
24. Lyrenäs S, Nyberg F, Lindberg B, et al: Cerebrospinal fluid activity of dynorphin-converting enzyme at term pregnancy. **Obstet Gynecol 72:**54-58, 1988
25. Merryman W, Boiman R, Barnes L, et al: Progesterone "anesthesia" in human subjects. **J Clin Endocrinol Metab 14:**1567-1569, 1954 (Letter)
26. Minielly R, Yuzpe AA, Drake CG: Subarachnoid hemorrhage secondary to ruptured cerebral aneurysm in pregnancy. **Obstet Gynecol 53:**64-70, 1978
27. Motoyama EK, Rivard G, Acheson F, et al: The effect of changes in maternal pH and PcO_2 on the PO_2 of fetal lambs. **Anesthesiology 28:**891-903, 1967
28. Okagaki A, Kanzaki H, Moritake K, et al: Case report: pregnant woman with a ventriculoperitoneal shunt to treat hydrocephalus. **Asia Oceania J Obstet Gynaecol 16:**111-113, 1990
29. Palahniuk RJ, Shnider SM, Eger EI II: Pregnancy decreases the requirements for inhaled anesthetic agents. **Anesthesiology 41:**82-83, 1974
30. Paonessa K, Fernand R: Spinal cord injury and pregnancy. **Spine 16:**596-598, 1991
31. Pedersen H, Finster M: Anesthetic risk in the pregnant surgical patient. **Anesthesiology 51:**439-451, 1979
32. Pevehouse BC, Boldrey E: Hypothermia and hypotension for intracranial surgery during pregnancy. **Am J Surg 100:**633-634, 1960
33. Poungvarin N, Bhoopat W: Symptomatic vertebral haemangiomas: report of two cases. **J Med Assoc Thai 74:**363-368, 1991
34. Preul MC, LeBlanc R, Tampieri D, et al: Spinal angiolipomas. Report of three cases. **J Neurosurg 78:** 280-286, 1993
35. Redekop GJ, DelMaestro RF: Vertebral hemangioma causing spinal cord compression during pregnancy. **Surg Neurol 38:**210-215, 1992
36. Robinson JL, Hall CJ, Sedzimir CB: Arteriovenous malformations, aneurysms, and pregnancy. **J Neurosurg 41:**63-70, 1974
37. Robinson JL, Hall CJ, Sedzimir CB: Subarachnoid hemorrhage in pregnancy. **J Neurosurg 36:**27-33, 1972
38. Rosen MA: Anesthesia for neurosurgery during pregnancy, in Shnider SM, Levinson G (eds): **Anesthesia for Obstetrics, 3rd ed.** Baltimore, MD: Williams & Wilkins, 1993, pp 551-561
39. Rosen MA: Cerebrovascular lesions and tumors in the pregnant patient, in Newfield P, Cottrell JE (eds): **Neuroanesthesia: Handbook of Clinical and Physiologic Essentials, ed 2.** Boston, MA: Little, Brown, 1991, pp 230-248
40. Sadasivan B, Malik GM, Lee C, et al: Vascular malformations and pregnancy. **Surg Neurol 33:**305-313, 1990
41. Samson DS, Clark K, Hodosh RM: Treatment of subarachnoid hemorrhage, in Rosenberg RN (ed): **The Treatment of Neurological Diseases.** New York, NY: SP Medical and Scientific Books, 1979, pp 117-142
42. Shephard RH: Spinal arteriovenous malformations and subarachnoid haemorrhage. **Br J Neurosurg 6:** 5-12, 1992
43. Shnider SM, Webster GM: Maternal and fetal hazards of surgery during pregnancy. **Am J Obstet Gynecol 92:**891-900, 1965
44. Singounas EG, Sakas DE, Hadley DM, et al: Paraplegia in a pregnant thalassemic woman due to extramedullary hematopoiesis: successful management with transfusions. **Surg Neurol 36:**210-215, 1991
45. Smith BE: Fetal prognosis after anesthesia during gestation. **Anesth Analg 42:**521-528, 1963
46. Smith LG Jr, Moise KJ Jr, Dildy GA III, et al: Spontaneous rupture of liver during pregnancy: current therapy. **Obstet Gynecol 77:**171-175, 1991
47. Smoleniec J, James D: General surgical problems in pregnancy. **Br J Surg 77:**1203-1204, 1990
48. Sorensen VJ, Bivins BA, Obeid FN, et al: Management of general surgical emergencies in pregnancy. **Am Surg 56:**245-250, 1990
49. Steinberg ES, Santos AC: Surgical anesthesia during pregnancy. **Int Anesthesiol Clin 28:**58-66, 1990
50. Strickland RA, Oliver WC Jr, Chantigian RC, et al: Anesthesia, cardiopulmonary bypass and the pregnant patient. **Mayo Clin Proc 66:**411-429, 1991
51. Tekkök IH, Açìkgoz B, Saglam S, et al: Vertebral hemangioma symptomatic during pregnancy – report of a case and review of the literature. **Neurosurgery 32:**302-306, 1993
52. Tokuda Y, Hatayama T, Sakoda K: Metastasis of malignant struma ovarii to the cranial vault during pregnancy. **Neurosurgery 33:**515-518, 1993
53. Trost HA, Seifert V, Stolke D: Advances in diagnosis and treatment of spinal hemangioblastomas. **Neurosurg Rev 16:**205-209, 1993
54. Whitburn RH, Laishley RS, Jewkes DA: Anaesthesia for simultaneous caesarean section and clipping of intracerebral aneurysm. **Br J Anaesth 64:**642-645, 1990
55. Wilkinson AG, Sellar RJ: Case report: Cerebral metastases from choriocarcinoma in the absence of detectable extracranial disease. **Clin Radiol 43:** 278-279, 1991
56. Wilson F, Sedzimir CB: Hypothermia and hypotension during craniotomy in a pregnant woman. **Lancet 2:**947-949, 1959

CHAPTER 16

Intrauterine Diagnosis of Developmental Neurosurgical Disorders

Michael G. Muhonen, MD, and Hans E. Bakken, MD

Current techniques in antenatal diagnosis allow detection of many congenital anomalies. The frequency of central nervous system (CNS) anomalies is approximately two in 1,000 newborns, with a recurrence risk in subsequent pregnancies of approximately 2%. With the advent of more sophisticated diagnostic techniques, disorders requiring neurosurgical intervention can be diagnosed more readily, thus facilitating possible intervention. The detection of fetal neurological defects is accomplished using maternal blood sampling, amniocentesis, chorionic villus sampling, fetal blood sampling, ultrasonography, and occasionally magnetic resonance imaging (MRI). Potential neurosurgical disorders generally do not require fetal blood or chorionic villus sampling, but these tests may be useful for diagnosing other congenital anomalies. In this chapter, we discuss how to establish antenatally the diagnosis of a multitude of neurosurgical problems using maternal blood sampling, ultrasonography, MRI, and amniocentesis. Specific neurosurgical developmental disorders are discussed, including spina bifida, myelodysplasia, hydrocephalus, encephalocele, CNS tumors, and cerebral anomalies.

Methods of Antenatal Diagnosis

Maternal Blood Sampling/ Alpha-Fetoprotein

Analysis of maternal serum allows broad screening for potential congenital anomalies and infections. In addition to antibodies and infection titers, the substance most commonly measured is alpha-fetoprotein. This allows a relatively simple but nonspecific antenatal screen for open neural tube defects. Alpha-fetoprotein is a glycoprotein which can be detected in the human fetus by 29 days after conception. During pregnancy, it is transferred to the mother across the placenta and across fetal membranes. Alpha-fetoprotein production is not increased in fetal abnormalities, but increased transfer into amniotic fluid is responsible for elevated maternal serum alpha-fetoprotein. Normal levels in maternal serum are about 25 mg/ml at 16 weeks' gestation. Levels then increase approximately 15% per week until about 30 weeks' gestation, remain steady for 5 additional weeks, and then fall rapidly (Figure 1). Small women,

TABLE 1

REASONS FOR ELEVATED MATERNAL SERUM ALPHA-FETOPROTEIN*

Normal pregnancy
Multiple gestation
More advanced gestational dates
Fetal abnormalities
- Open neural tube defect
- Threatened abortion/demise
- Hydrops/ascites
- Cystic hygroma
- Ventral wall defects
- Esophageal or duodenal atresia
- Urinary tract disease, congenital nephrosis, polycystic disease, obstructive lesion
- Integumental defects, epidermolysis bullosa
- Miscellaneous abnormalities, amniotic band syndrome, teratomas, ectopia cordis

Placental abnormalities
- Placental lakes, hemangiomas of the placenta and cord
- Retroplacental hemorrhage

Maternal disease
- Primary liver cancer, yolk sac tumors, and occasionally other tumors
- Acute viral hepatitis (usually peaks within 6 weeks of onset)
- Rhesus or other sensitization (e.g., Kell)
- Lupus autoantibody present

*From Simpson and Elias.[36]

TABLE 2

INDICATIONS FOR ANTENATAL ULTRASOUND OF INFANT CENTRAL NERVOUS SYSTEM*

- Elevated maternal serum or amniotic fluid alpha-fetoprotein
- Low serum or amniotic fluid alpha-fetoprotein
- History of neurological deficit in siblings of infant
- Maternal diabetes mellitus
- Exposure to teratogenic agent
- Amniotic fluid volume abnormalities: polyhydramnios or oligohydramnios
- Intrauterine growth retardation/fetal death
- Suspicion of anomaly on routine obstetric examination

*From Sabbagha.[33]

African-American women, and twin pregnancies tend to have higher levels of alpha-fetoprotein.[9,39,41] Mothers who are insulin-dependent diabetics have alpha-fetoprotein levels about 40% lower than average.[25] The most common cause of elevated alpha-fetoprotein is normal pregnancy. However, abnormally high levels can indicate serious abnormalities, including fetal death (Table 1). Even in the presence of normal ultrasound imaging and amniocentesis studies, abnormally elevated maternal serum alpha-fetoprotein screening can be associated with adverse pregnancy outcomes.[11]

Ultrasound of Fetal Nervous System

Diagnostic ultrasound poses no known biological risk to humans. It has become the standard diagnostic tool used to detect structural fetal congenital anomalies. Not all pregnancies require ultrasound of the infant, and only a minority require viewing of the CNS. The most frequent indications that warrant antenatal ultrasound of infantile CNS structures are listed in Table 2. Ultrasound is most commonly used to diagnose abnormalities in the presence of elevated maternal serum alpha-fetoprotein. When alpha-fetoprotein is elevated, the purpose of ultrasound is to perform a targeted study of the CNS in an attempt at locating congenital anomalies. Images targeted include the cranium, lateral ventricles, third ventricle, thalami, posterior fossa, and the entire spine. If any of these structures are abnormal or not well visualized on the initial ultrasound study, that area should be imaged again. The major CNS anomalies that can be detected by ultrasound include anencephaly, microcephaly, spina bifida, myelomeningocele, encephalocele, hydrocephalus, posterior fossa abnormalities, and intracerebral cysts.[34]

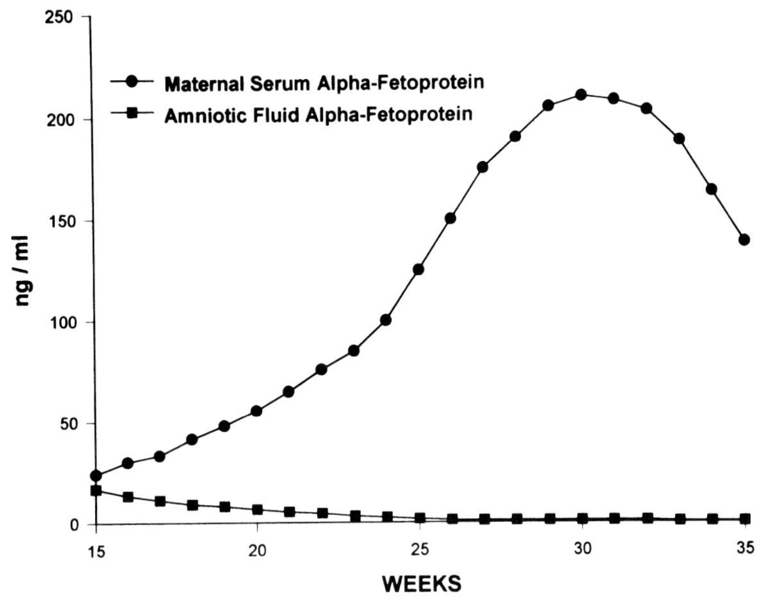

Figure 1: Levels of alpha-fetoprotein in maternal serum and amniotic fluid at corresponding weeks of pregnancy. These levels refer to routine assays from 40,000 pregnancies.[10]

Amniocentesis

A large prospective study performed by the National Institute of Child Health and Human Development concluded that midtrimester amniocentesis is an accurate and highly safe procedure that does not add significant risk to the pregnancy.[27] However, there can be complications for the mother and the infant. Maternal risks include spotting, vaginal leakage of amniotic fluid, amnionitis, and injury to an intra-abdominal viscus. Fetal risks include spontaneous abortion, needle puncture injuries, placental abruption, chorioamnionitis, and preterm labor.[13,21] In qualified hands, these risks are minimal and do not significantly change the morbidity and mortality rates of pregnancy.

Amniocentesis is not required for the evaluation of most developmental neurosurgical disorders. It is used primarily as an adjunct in the work-up of anomalies found on ultrasound. Hydrocephalus, for example, is associated with abnormal fetal karyotype in approximately 25% of cases. It may be a part of trisomies,[13,18,21] triploidy, Apert's syndrome, Roberts syndrome, or thanatophoric (deadly) dwarfism. Prenatal genetic work-up by amniocentesis has traditionally been performed at around 15 weeks' gestation. At this time a sufficient volume of amniotic fluid (approximately 200 ml) exists to permit 20 to 30 ml to be withdrawn safely. Also, the ratio of viable to nonviable cells in the amniotic fluid is relatively high and the time before fetal viability is adequate to complete diagnostic studies.[12]

Alpha-fetoprotein analysis should be performed on all amniotic samples. While maternal serum alpha-fetoprotein levels rise throughout most of pregnancy, mean amniotic fluid alpha-fetoprotein levels show a steep rise during the 12th week and peak at the 13th week.[7] Amniotic fluid alpha-fetoprotein then decreases by about 12% per week (Figure 1). Amniotic fluid alpha-fetoprotein levels are predictive of the same types of problems as maternal serum alpha-fetoprotein screening, and the ability to monitor amniotic fluid alpha-fetoprotein is one of the advantages of early amniocentesis. The most common reason for an elevated amniotic fluid alpha-fetoprotein level is fetal blood con-

TABLE 3

REASONS FOR ELEVATED AMNIOTIC FLUID ALPHA-FETOPROTEIN*

- Fetal blood contamination
- Normal pregnancy
- Early gestational dates
- Fetal demise
- Open neural tube defect
- Ventral wall defect
- Cystic hygroma
- Hydrops/ascites
- Upper gastrointestinal obstruction
- Urinary tract obstruction
- Congenital nephrosis, amniotic band syndrome, chromosome abnormality, teratoma

* Amniotic fluid alpha-fetoprotein levels elevated <2.0 multitudes of the median (MoM). From Simpson and Elias.[36]

tamination. Fetal blood contamination can be associated with fetal anomalies, particularly anencephaly. Other causes of elevation of amniotic fluid alpha-fetoprotein are listed in Table 3. It should be emphasized that maternal disease tends to result in a very high maternal serum alpha-fetoprotein and normal amniotic fluid alpha-fetoprotein. Amniotic fluid analysis for acetylcholinesterase is an additional measure taken in the case of elevated amniotic fluid alpha-fetoprotein. A positive result significantly increases the risk for abnormalities, including neural tube defects, ventral wall defects (gastroschisis), cystic hygroma, hydrops, and other rare anomalies.[8,37]

Magnetic Resonance Imaging

In utero MRI of the fetal nervous system may be useful when limitations of ultrasonography are reached. The accuracy of ultrasonography is limited in the late stages of pregnancy, particularly in the presence of maternal obesity or oligohydramnios. In addition, ultrasonography is limited in its ability to characterize different types of soft tissue.[2] In these situations, MRI of the fetus may provide superior imaging. However, MRI is constrained by the time required to obtain an image and by degradation of the image during fetal movements. MRI is exquisitely sensitive to fetal motion and lacks the spatial resolution inherent in real-time sonography. Pancuronium bromide injections are typically used to obtain fetal paralysis. However, fetal curarization requires the use of cordocentesis or direct fetal injection and may be associated with hematoma and infection. Because of these and other potential adverse events, some authors advocate MRI without curarization.[30] Based upon our review, we feel that the value of antenatal MRI of the fetus is to allow better evaluation of functional outcome and to assist in making therapeutic decisions.[13]

DEVELOPMENTAL NEUROSURGICAL DISORDERS

Hydrocephalus

Antenatal diagnosis of hydrocephalus relies on ultrasound findings (Figure 2). The ratio of ventricular width to hemispheric width is used to gauge hydrocephalus. The threshold for imaging the lateral ventricles is approximately 12 weeks' gestation. At 15 weeks' gestation, the lateral ventricles are easily visualized and, except for the anterior horns, are filled with choroid plexi. The occipital horns cannot be visualized at this time. Normal ventricular to hemispheric ratios range from an average of 50% ± 10% early in the second trimester to 33% ± 4% later in the second trimester.[29] The ratio of lateral ventricular to hemispheric width is not as sensitive to early ventriculomegaly during the first half of pregnancy due to large deviations for the normal values. This criterion is more reliable if repeat ultrasound examinations show a continued rise in the ratio instead of the normal decline. Second-trimester diagnosis of hydrocephalus is usually made by noting that the choroid plexi appear small compared with the ventricular cavities. Because the relatively hyperechoic choroid plexi occupy the entire ventricle posterior to the foramen of Monro, the lateral

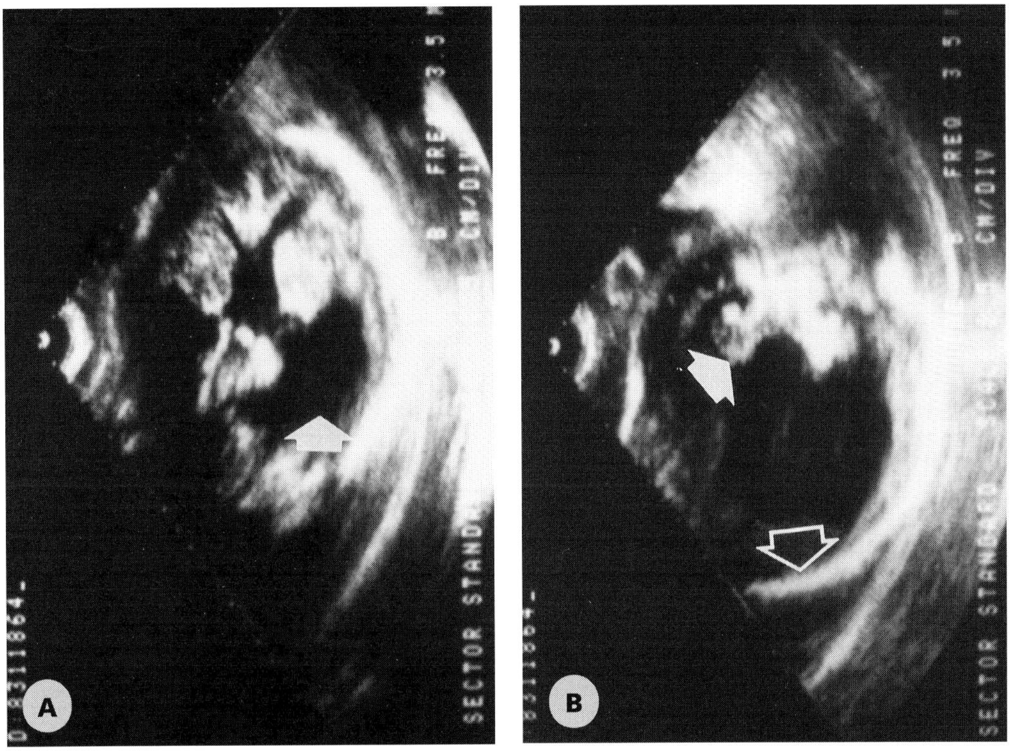

Figure 2: A) Axial ultrasound of fetus showing massive dilatation of the lateral ventricles, especially the atrium (*arrow*). **B**) Coronal ultrasound of same patient showing thin cortical rim (*open arrow*) and thalami (*closed arrow*) compressed by large ventricles. Images courtesy of Dr. Mohammed Abu-Yousef.

ventricular wall can be obscured, causing the cerebral mantle to appear as a dilated ventricle, especially when the hyperintense subarachnoid space is mistaken for compressed brain tissue.

In general, the diagnosis of hydrocephalus is more easily made as gestational age increases. The biparietal diameter remains within normal range until involvement is quite severe. Associated intracranial anomalies are present in approximately one-third of infants with fetal hydrocephalus, while extracranial malformations and chromosomal aberrations are associated with approximately two-thirds of these infants.[14] The presence of additional pathology is associated with high infant mortality rates and mental retardation. Thickness of the cortical mantle is not a valid prognosticator of future mental retardation. Compressed cortical mantle has tremendous potential for expansion following ventricular decompression (Figure 3).

If the diagnosis of hydrocephalus is established, a work-up for associated malformations should be performed. A thorough ultrasound examination of the fetus should be performed to rule out the presence of other anomalies including spina bifida, encephalocele, Dandy-Walker malformation, and other cerebral anomalies. Amniocentesis should be performed to measure alpha-fetoprotein and karyotype, and to determine the sex (relevant information for possibility of x-linked hydrocephalus). The amniotic fluid and maternal serum should be analyzed for congenital infections such as toxoplasmosis, rubella, cytomegalovirus, and syphilis.

Serial ultrasonography can indicate progressive hydrocephalus, dictating induction of labor. However, the fetus with hydrocephalus should not be delivered until fetal lung maturity is acceptable. Biparietal diameter is near normal in the majority of cases, so vaginal delivery may be performed if indicated. Conversely, with a fetus in which a fatal outlook is anticipated, intrapartum fetal distress should not be considered an indication for cesarean section. Cephalocentesis has an extremely high perinatal mortality

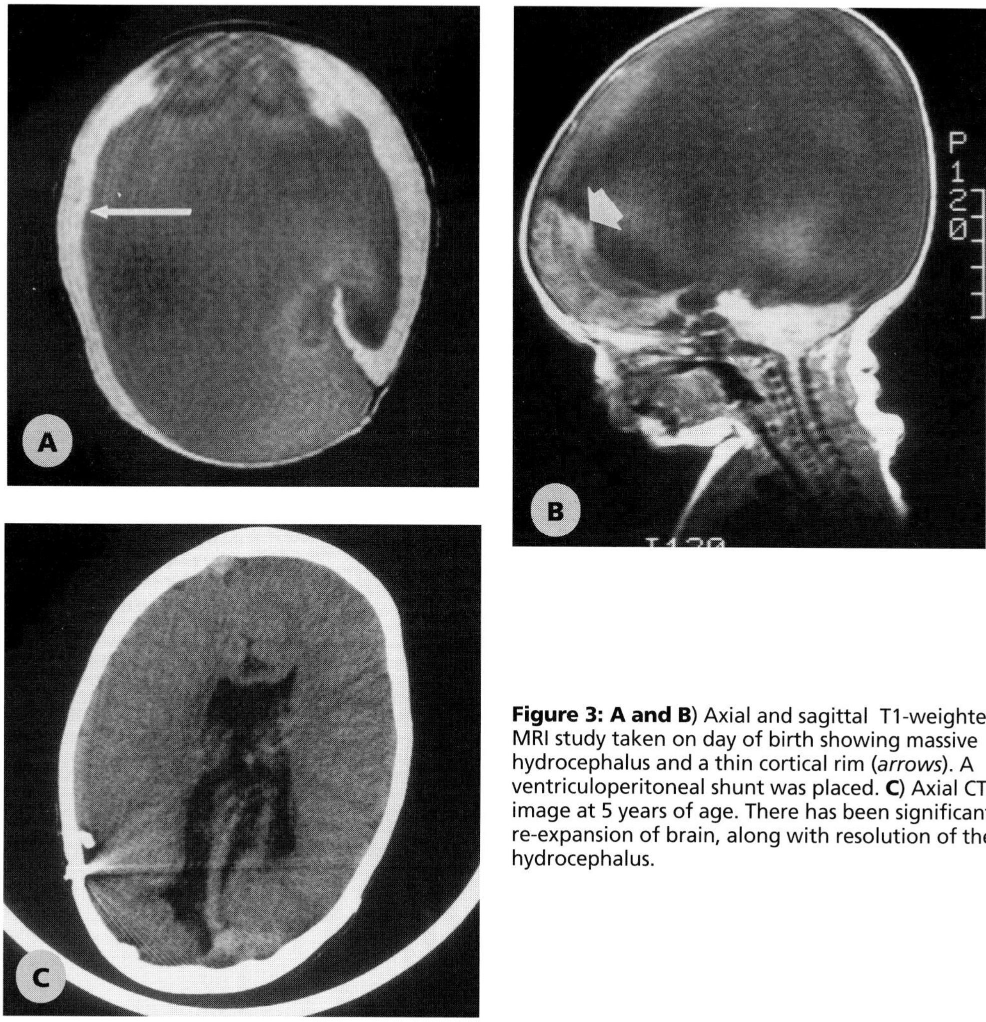

Figure 3: A and B) Axial and sagittal T1-weighted MRI study taken on day of birth showing massive hydrocephalus and a thin cortical rim (*arrows*). A ventriculoperitoneal shunt was placed. **C**) Axial CT image at 5 years of age. There has been significant re-expansion of brain, along with resolution of the hydrocephalus.

rate (see below) and should not be used as an attempt to avoid cesarean section unless the fetus has associated conditions incompatible with life.[5]

Because long-term outcome of neonatal hydrocephalus is improved by shunting the ventricles, it would seem logical to treat the hydrocephalus antenatally.[24] This has been performed by several different methods including serial percutaneous cephalocentesis and ventriculo-amniotic shunts, but with only limited success. In a series of 41 cases of hydrocephalus diagnosed in utero, 39 were treated by ventriculo-amniotic shunting and two by serial ventricular punctures.[23] Seven (18%) of the fetuses died, one before birth, secondary to needle trauma to the brain stem. Six died after birth, three resulting from premature labor presumed to be secondary to chorioamnionitis from shunt placement. The procedure-related mortality rate was 10%. Twelve of the infants were normal.

There are also theoretical concerns regarding the issue of antenatal treatment of hydrocephalus. First, infantile ventriculomegaly does not necessarily correlate with eventual psychomotor development. Second, cerebrospinal fluid flow may be necessary for the development of cerebrospinal fluid pathways. Early shunting of cerebrospinal fluid could then conceivably create irreversible hydrocephalus. At present, we do not feel that there are adequate data to support in utero shunting of the ventricles.

Neural Tube Defects

Spina bifida and anencephaly are two of the most common types of neural tube defects. These malformations occur within the first month of gestation, and their prevalence varies both geographically and by race. In the United States, the incidence is approximately 3.2 per 10,000 births, a decrease from 5.9 per 10,000 births in 1984.[3] There is a familial predisposition to the occurrence of spina bifida. In North America, the risk of having a child with spina bifida is less than 0.05%. If one sibling has spina bifida, the risk of a subsequent child having spina bifida is about 5%. If there are two siblings with spina bifida, the risk increases to about 15%.[15] Because neural tube defects recur in families, a genetic mechanism may be responsible for its occurrence. On the basis of pedigree analysis, Jorde et al[20] proposed that spina bifida occulta may be related to an autosomal dominant trait with a 75% penetrance. Neural tube defects also occur in genetic syndromes, increasing the possibility of a genetic component to the development of spina bifida.[31]

Neural tube defects can be classified as either open or closed, depending on the presence of skin covering the defect. The neural tube defect is open in 85% to 90% of myelodysplastics and in >99% of anencephalics.[36] Differentiating between open and closed neural tube defects in utero can require multiple diagnostic modalities, but can be a critical step in management. Open spina bifida requires surgical repair within 24 to 72 hours postpartum to prevent drying and infection of exposed neural tissues. Antenatal confirmation of the diagnosis allows a proper work-up to determine if other detectable anomalies exist that may affect the treatment plan, and facilitates a timely operative procedure. Early in pregnancy, evaluation of maternal serum alpha-fetoprotein levels is combined with ultrasound examinations. Ultrasound is capable of detecting mass lesions and bony defects but is unable to assess the integrity of the skin. Alpha-fetoprotein level is generally abnormally elevated in open spina bifida but not in closed spina bifida. Later in pregnancy, modalities such as MRI may be utilized to supplement the shortcomings of ultrasound, as maternal serum alpha-fetoprotein becomes increasingly elevated due to the pregnancy itself.[26]

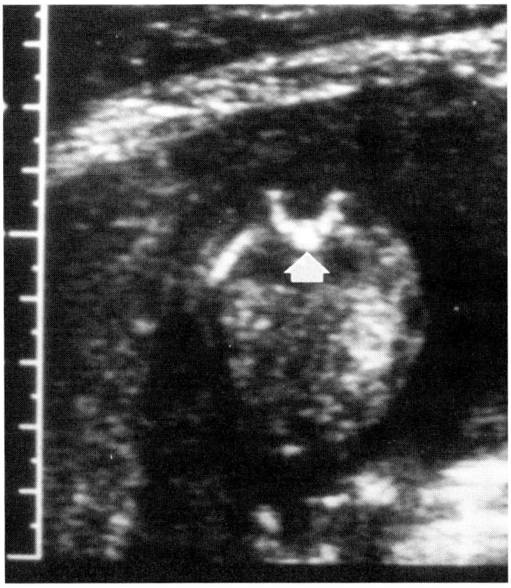

Figure 4: Antenatal ultrasound showing a lower lumbar vertebra (*arrow*) with findings classical for spina bifida. There is no spinous process, and there is widening of the lamina of the vertebra. Image courtesy of Dr. Mohammed Abu-Yousef.

The number of cases of spina bifida detected antenatally has increased dramatically since the advent of high-resolution ultrasonography (Figure 4) and routine screening of maternal serum alpha-fetoprotein. Using this information to coordinate multidisciplinary pre- and postnatal care programs has been shown to improve outcomes in some cases. Prenatal screening leading to early intrauterine diagnosis allows the parents to prepare for the birth of a child with spina bifida. For parents electing to complete pregnancy, the route of delivery of a fetus with spina bifida becomes an important issue. Some studies suggest that prelabor elective cesarean section has no significant advantage over vaginal delivery.[6,35] In the absence of an extremely large head or a large, protruding spinal lesion vaginal delivery can be employed.

The decision to perform cesarean section should then be based on obstetric indications such as a breech presentation.

Encephaloceles are neural tube defects that occur less commonly than those in the spinal axis. It is useful to diagnose this condition antenatally, as it is very anxiety-provoking in the parents, has an unpredictable course, and difficulty exists in making any predictions about outcome. Encephaloceles are related to a disorder in the closure of the primitive neural tube. The encephalocele sac may contain cerebellum, brain stem, lobes of the cerebral hemispheres, vascular structures, or only cerebrospinal fluid and glial remnants.[4] The solid structures which may herniate into the sac tend to show various degrees of disorganization. The prenatal diagnosis of encephalocele is made by ultrasound scanning. The ultrasound examination can outline the sac, its location, herniation of cerebral contents, and other structural abnormalities.[42] Based upon the size and contents of the sac, the skull size and shape, and the presence of hydrocephalus, certain prognostic implications can be made. If the sac is filled with cerebrum, for example, a more dismal prognosis is implied. If the sac is filled with spinal fluid, the problem may be more cosmetic. If the head is very small, the prognosis is relatively more poor. In addition, ultrasound can define other defects such as corpus callosum agenesis, Dandy-Walker malformation, and porencephaly.

Virtually all children born with an occipital encephalocele require operative obliteration of the lesion. The sac is grossly disfiguring, tends to expand in size, and, because of progressive hydrocephalus, there is a threat to intracranial nervous tissue. The larger encephaloceles (Figure 5) should be managed on an elective basis and only if a reasonable prognosis is anticipated. Most encephaloceles are subjected to early operative repair and early or interval treatment of the hydrocephalus.

Anencephaly/Exencephaly

Anencephaly is the absence of the cerebral hemispheres and the overlying meninges, skull, and scalp. Exencephaly is a rare, related condition in which the calvarium and other tissues are absent, but a large volume of disorganized brain tissue exists. Exencephaly has been shown to degenerate to anencephaly in some cases, but this progression does not always occur, and the reasons for this are unknown. Both conditions are now diagnosable in the first trimester with the use of high-frequency vaginal transducers in transvaginal ultrasound. The fetal cranium is not fully calcified before 10 to 11 weeks' gestational age, so the diagnosis of exencephaly lies with the recognition of the absence of normal anatomical structures such as the developing rhombencephalon, lateral ventricles, midline falx, and choroid plexus. Also, the ultrasound study may be notable for the disorganized appearance of the gyri and prominence of the midline.[22]

Cranial and Craniocervical Masses

Ultrasound can diagnose a variety of cranial and craniocervical cystic masses when the defect in the neural tube is not apparent. At times, the neural tube defect is too small to be resolved by the transducer or it may simply not be well visualized. In these cases, the echogenic characteristics of the mass can be used to assist in antenatal diagnosis. Masses visualized under these circumstances include meningocele, fetal edema, intrauterine fetal death, cystic hygroma, and stunted twin gestational sac.[34]

Meningoceles can be present even without a demonstrable neural tube defect, and the characteristic finding is a very thin echo pattern (1-2 mm) at the outer margin of the structure, even if the tissue is covered by fetal integument. The diagnosis of meningocele should not be ruled out simply due to inability to locate a neural tube defect with ultrasound. The appearance of fetal edema is that of a cystic structure with a thick outer margin and uniform semicircular shape, simulating the contour of the fetal head and neck. In these cases, ascites is usually also present on the ultrasound examination. This appearance is nearly identical with that of intrauterine fetal death, but the two can be differentiated by dynamic imaging of the fetal heart. Cystic hygroma is also seen as a thick-walled cystic structure on ultrasound, but due to the fact that it arises from the deep lymphatic

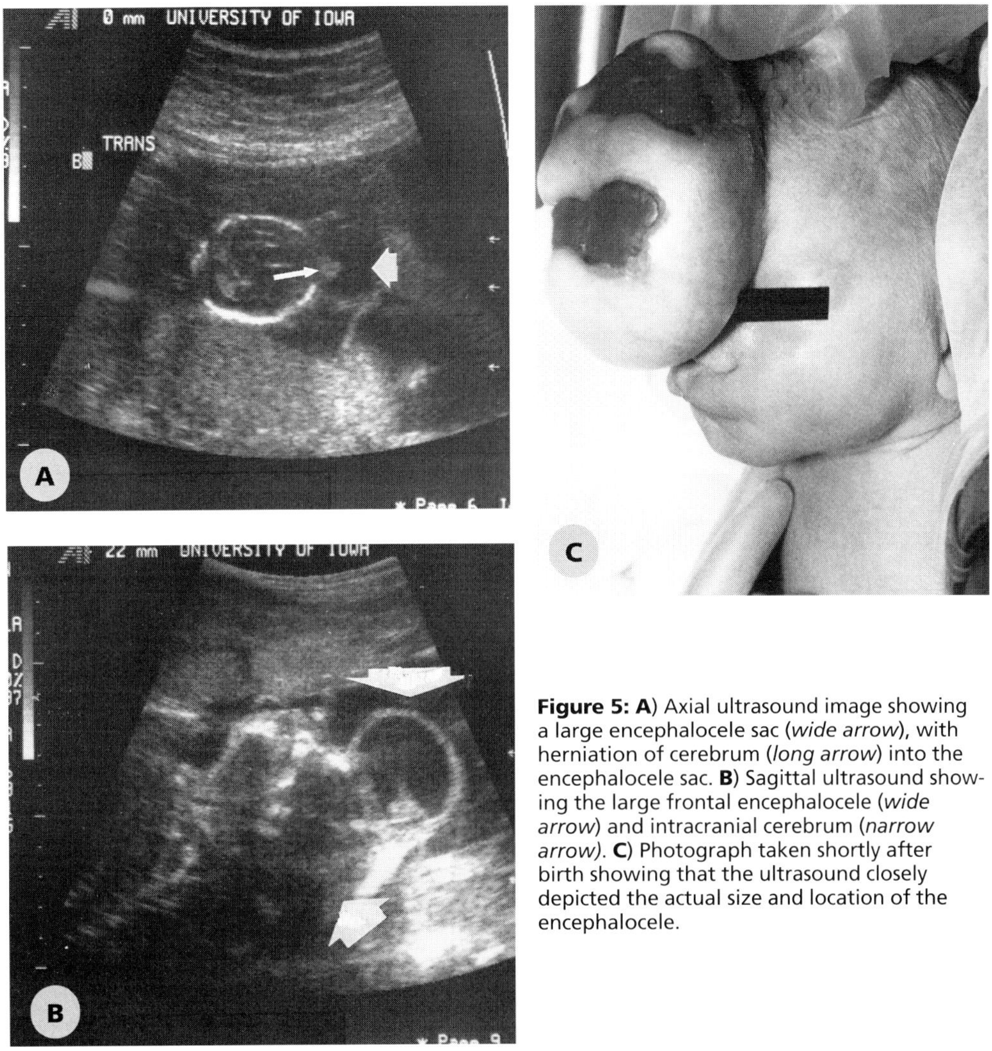

Figure 5: A) Axial ultrasound image showing a large encephalocele sac (*wide arrow*), with herniation of cerebrum (*long arrow*) into the encephalocele sac. **B**) Sagittal ultrasound showing the large frontal encephalocele (*wide arrow*) and intracranial cerebrum (*narrow arrow*). **C**) Photograph taken shortly after birth showing that the ultrasound closely depicted the actual size and location of the encephalocele.

vessels adjacent to the vertebral column, it is usually circular in structure and contained within the craniocervical area. In addition, multiple striations representing lymphatic channels can at times be observed.[16] A difficult lesion to differentiate from meningocele is that of a stunted twin gestational sac. This condition is recognized by its lack of motion in conjunction with that of the fetus. Another more uncommon misdiagnosis is that of conjoined twins for a cephalic mass.[43]

Great Vein of Galen Aneurysm

"Great vein of Galen aneurysm" is the generic term for midline arteriovenous fistula malformations associated with aneurysmal dilatation of the vein of Galen.[32] The clinical features associated with this abnormality include cardiomegaly with congestive heart failure, increased intracranial pressure, and hydrocephaly. The classic appearance of this anomaly is a midline hypoechoic structure, but variations range from single large dilatations to multiple communications between the vein and the carotid and vertebrobasilar systems. Hydrocephalus occurs through multiple mechanisms, including compression of the aqueduct, "steal" phenomena with resulting parenchymal atrophy, and absence of heart rate variability secondary to cerebral hypoxia.[19] Other less likely diagnoses with similar appearances on ultrasound examination include colloid cysts, choroid plexus cysts, porencephalic cysts, pineal tumors, intracerebral hematoma, and choroid plexus papillomas.[32] The unique finding in the case of a vein of Galen aneurysm is the presence of high-velocity flow within the structure on Doppler ultrasound examination. Right-sided cardiomegaly and distended jugular veins reinforce the diagnosis.

Intracerebral and Posterior Fossa Cysts

Choroid plexus cysts are another of the CNS malformations that can be detected in utero. While they may present as asymptomatic findings in children, antenatal diagnosis appears to be associated with chromosomal anomalies, particularly trisomy 18 and 21.[17] These cysts are usually round, <1 cm in largest diameter, and can be distinguished from papillomata of the choroid plexus (which can occur in the same location) by the hyperechogenicity of the latter.[28] When cysts of the choroid plexus are detected in utero, karyotypic and detailed sonographic examination can be performed to provide crucial information useful in the planning for future treatment.[18]

Posterior fossa cyst, enlarged cisterna magna, and Dandy-Walker malformation can be diagnosed by ultrasound. In Dandy-Walker malformation, there is typically absence of the roof of the fourth ventricle. The fourth ventricle communicates with a posterior fossa cyst, appearing as herniation of the fourth ventricle toward the cisterna magna. The Dandy-Walker syndrome should be differentiated from a mega cisterna magna. Abnormal enlargement of the cisterna magna is seen in fetuses with trisomy 18 and in fetuses of gravidas infected with human immunodeficiency virus.[1,38]

TABLE 4
Indications for Amniocentesis (and Not Maternal Serum Screening)*

- Maternal age >34 years
- Previous child with chromosome abnormality
- Parent has chromosome rearrangement or mosaic pattern
- Previous child or parent with genetic disease that can be diagnosed by DNA or biochemical tests
- Previous child or parent with neural tube defect
- Mother on anticonvulsant medications
- Multiple spontaneous abortions, drugs, radiation

*From Simpson and Elias.[36]

Conclusions

Maternal serum alpha-fetoprotein screening should be performed on all pregnant women. A small percentage of women who fit the established criteria (Table 4) ought to undergo amniocentesis, obviating the need for maternal serum alpha-fetoprotein screening. A normal maternal serum alpha-fetoprotein level does not guarantee the absence of an open neural tube defect. It will identify approximately 80% of fetuses with open spina bifida and 90% of anencephalics. The maternal blood sample should not be taken before 15 weeks' gestation. It should also be taken before 20 weeks' gestation to allow sufficient time to complete additional testing if necessary. Open spina bifida is most likely to be detected between 16 and 18 weeks.[41] If the maternal serum alpha-fetoprotein is elevated on two separate occasions, an ultrasound should be used to confirm a live pregnancy, determine gestational dates, rule out congenital anomalies, and to identify the possibility of multiple fetuses. Nearly 90% of fetal anomalies can be detected with a detailed ultrasound examination. If sonographic results are normal and corrections for weight, race, gestational age, multiple gestations, placental bleeding, and other anomalies (omphalocele, gastroschisis) are not explanatory, amniocentesis is recommended. Normal levels of alpha-fetoprotein and acetylcholinesterase in amniotic fluid have a positive predictive value of 97% or greater and a false-positive rate of 0.4% for women with elevated maternal serum alpha-fetoprotein levels.[40,41] If the antenatal work-up is equivocal or the ultrasound findings unclear, MRI may assist in making therapeutic decisions.

REFERENCES

1. Byrd SE, Naidich TP: Common congenital brain anomalies. **Radiol Clin North Am 26**:755-772, 1988
2. Catizone FA, Gesmundo G, Montemagno R, et al: The non-invasive methods of prenatal diagnosis: the role of ultrasonography and MRI. **J Perinat Med 19 (Suppl 1)**:42-49, 1991
3. Centers for Disease Control: Spina bifida incidence at birth—United States. **MMWR 41**:497, 1992
4. Chapman PH, Swearingen B, Caviness VS: Subtorcular occipital encephaloceles. Anatomical considerations relevant to operative management. **J Neurosurg 71**:375-381, 1989
5. Chervenak FA, Berkowitz RL, Tortora M, et al: The management of fetal hydrocephalus. **Am J Obstet Gynecol 151**:933-942, 1985
6. Cochrane D, Aronyk K, Sawatzky B, et al: The effects of labor and delivery on spinal cord function and ambulation in patients with meningomyelocele. **Childs Nerv Syst 7**:312-315, 1991
7. Crandall BF, Hanson FW, Tennant F, et al: Alpha-fetoprotein levels in amniotic fluid between 11 and 15 weeks. **Am J Obstet Gynecol 160**:1204-1206, 1989
8. Crandall BF, Kasha W, Matsumoto M: Prenatal diagnosis of neural tube defects: experiences with acetylcholinesterase gel electrophoresis. **Am J Med Genet 12**:361-366, 1982
9. Crandall BF, Lebherz TB, Schroth PC, et al: Alpha-fetoprotein concentrations in maternal serum: relation to race and body weight. **Clin Chem 20**:531-533, 1983
10. Crandall BF, Matsumoto M: Routine amniotic fluid alphafetoprotein assay: experience with 40,000 pregnancies. **Am J Med Genet 24**:143-149, 1986
11. Crandall BF, Robinson L, Grau P: Risks associated with an elevated maternal serum α-fetoprotein level. **Am J Obstet Gynecol 165**:581-586, 1991
12. Emery AEH: Antenatal diagnosis of genetic disease. **Mod Trends Hum Genet 1**:267, 1970
13. Epley SL, Hanson JW, Cruikshank DP: Fetal injury with midtrimester diagnostic amniocentesis. **Obstet Gynecol 53**:77-80, 1979
14. Fadel HE: Antenatal diagnosis of fetal intracranial anomalies. **J Child Neurol 4 (Suppl)**:107-102, 1989
15. Fraser FC: Genetic counseling. **Am J Hum Genet 26**:636-661, 1974 (Review)
16. Frigoletto FD, Birnholz JC, Driscoll SG, et al: Ultrasound diagnosis of cystic hygroma. **Am J Obstet Gynecol 136**:962-964, 1980
17. Furness ME: Choroid plexus cysts and trisomy 18. **Lancet 2**:693, 1987 (Letter)
18. Gabrielli S, Reece EA, Pilu G, et al: The clinical significance of prenatally diagnosed choroid plexus cysts. **Am J Obstet Gynecol 160**:1207-1210, 1989
19. Jeanty P, Kepple D, Roussis P, et al: *In utero* detection of cardiac failure from an aneurysm of the vein of Galen. **Am J Obstet Gynecol 163**:50-51, 1990
20. Jorde LB, Fineman RM, Martin RA: Epidemiology and genetics of neural tube defects: an application of the Utah Genealogical Data Base. **Am J Phys Anthropol 62**:23-31, 1983
21. Karp LE, Hayden PW: Fetal puncture during midtrimester amniocentesis. **Obstet Gynecol 49**: 115-117, 1977
22. Kennedy KA, Flick KJ, Thurmond AS: First-trimester diagnosis of exencephaly. **Am J Obstet Gynecol 162**: 461-463, 1990
23. Manning FA, Harrison MR, Rodeck C: Catheter shunts for fetal hydronephrosis and hydrocephalus. Report of the International Fetal Surgery Registry. **N Engl J Med 315**:336-340, 1986
24. McCullough DC, Balzer-Martin LA: Current prognosis in overt neonatal hydrocephalus. **J Neurosurg 57**:378-383, 1982
25. Milunsky A, Alpert E, Kitzmiller JL, et al: Prenatal diagnosis of neural tube defects. VIII: The importance of serum alpha-fetoprotein-screening in diabetic pregnant women. **Am J Obstet Gynecol 142**: 1030-1032, 1982
26. Nakahara T, Uozumi T, Monden S, et al: Prenatal diagnosis of open spina bifida by MRI and ultrasonography. **Brain Dev 15**:75-78, 1993
27. NICHD National Registry of Amniocentesis Study Group: Midtrimester amniocentesis for prenatal diagnosis. Safety and accuracy. **JAMA 236**: 1471-1476, 1976
28. Pilu G, De Palma L, Romero R, et al: The fetal subarachnoid cisterns: an ultrasound study with report of a case of congenital communicating hydrocephaly. **J Ultrasound Med 5**:365-372, 1986
29. Pretorius DH, Drose LA, Manco-Johnson ML: Fetal lateral ventricular ratio determination during the second trimester. **J Ultrasound Med 5**:121-124, 1986
30. Revel MP, Pons JC, Lelaidier C, et al: Magnetic resonance imaging of the fetus: a study of 20 cases performed without curarization. **Prenat Diagn 13**: 775-799, 1993
31. Rodríguez JI, García M, Morales C, et al: Trisomy 13 syndrome and neural tube defects. **Am J Med Genet 36**:513-516, 1990
32. Romero R, Pilu GL, Jeanty P, et al: **Prenatal Diagnosis of Congenital Anomalies.** Norwalk, CT: Appleton-Lange, 1987, pp 77-79
33. Sabbagha RE, Sheikh Z, Tamura RK et al: Predictive value, sensitivity, and specificity of ultrasonic targeted imaging for fetal anomalies in gravid women at high risk for birth defects. **Am J Obstet Gynecol 152**: 822-827, 1985
34. Sabbagha RE, Tamura RK, Dal Compo S, et al: Fetal cranial and craniocervical masses: ultrasound characteristics and differential diagnosis. **Am J Obstet Gynecol 138**:511-517, 1980
35. Sakala EP, Andree I: Optimal route of delivery for meningomyelocele. **Obstet Gynecol Surg 4**:209-212, 1990
36. Simpson JL, Elias S: **Essentials of Prenatal Diagnosis.** New York, NY: Churchill Livingstone, 1993

37. Smith AD, Wald NJ, Cuckle HS, et al: AF AChE as a possible diagnostic test for NTDs in early pregnancy. **Lancet 1:**685-688, 1976
38. Thurmond AS, Nelson DW, Lowensohn RI, et al: Enlarged cisterna magna in trisomy 18: prenatal ultrasonographic diagnosis. **Am J Obstet Gynecol 161:**83-85, 1989
39. Wald N, Cuckle H, Boreham J, et al: The effect of maternal weight on maternal serum alpha-fetoprotein levels. **Br J Obstet Gynecol 88:**1094-1096, 1981
40. Wald N, Cuckle H, Nanchahal K: Amniotic fluid acetylcholinesterase measurement in the prenatal diagnosis of open neural tube defects. Second report of the Collaborative Acetylcholinesterase Study. **Prenat Diagn 9:**813-829, 1989
41. Wald NJ, Cuckle H, Brock DJH, et al: Maternal serum-alpha-fetoprotein measurement in antenatal screening for anencephaly and spina bifida in early pregnancy. Report of U.K. collaborative study on alpha-fetoprotein in relation to neural-tube defects. **Lancet 1:**1323-1332, 1977
42. Weinstein P, Weinstein L, Dotters D, et al: Prenatal diagnosis of occipital encephalocele by ultrasound scanning. **Neurosurgery 12:**680-683, 1983
43. Weiss RR, Chatterjee S, Verma U, et al: Early prenatal diagnosis of unusual gestational abnormalities. Department of Obstetrics-Gynecology, Nassau County Medical Center, East Meadow, NY. Presented to the American College of Obstetrics-Gynecology, 1979

CHAPTER 17

THE CURRENT STATUS OF INTRAUTERINE NEUROSURGERY

MICHAEL D. MEDLOCK, MD, AND WILLIAM C. HANIGAN, MD, PHD

INVASIVE FETAL PROCEDURES

Invasive procedures for the diagnosis and treatment of fetal disease have been used for over 40 years. In 1954 Westin[69] was the first to use endoscopy for fetal diagnosis, while in 1963 Liley[43] of New Zealand was the first to use an invasive technique for fetal treatment. The latter procedure involved x-rays and fetal intraperitoneal urographin to perform fetal transfusions for rhesus hemolytic disease. Unfortunately, the first three fetuses died after the procedure, probably from pre-existing hydrops. Over two decades ago, Valenti[65] was the first to use endoscopy for fetal blood sampling and skin biopsy. The fetal tissue samples were used to perform hemoglobin electrophoresis and to diagnose hexosaminidase A and B deficiency, respectively.

Precise, ultrasound-guided intrahepatic transfusions are currently performed in preference to the intraperitoneal approach used by Liley.[4,32] Daffos et al[15] reported no morbidity following 66 successful umbilical vein phlebotomies. Access to the intrahepatic vein requires transgression of the fetal liver with a 20-gauge needle, but with acceptable morbidity. Nicolini et al[52] reported only two deaths in 244 procedures to sample fetal blood from the intrahepatic vein. These techniques appear to improve fetal prognosis. Stewart et al[62] showed that patients in whom anemia was severe enough to require prenatal transfusion did as well on postnatal developmental testing as patients with less severe disease who did not require prenatal transfusion. Muscle biopsy and transplantation of hematopoietic stem cells for bare lymphocyte syndrome have been reported.[4,64]

DIAGNOSTIC IMAGING OF THE FETAL CENTRAL NERVOUS SYSTEM

X-rays, ultrasound, computed tomography (CT), and magnetic resonance imaging (MRI) have been used in prenatal imaging. Conventional x-rays are unable to adequately image fetal soft tissues, and both x-rays and CT expose the fetus to ionizing radiation. Consequently, they are used infrequently in the diagnosis of fetal disease.

MRI yields more soft tissue detail than ultrasound. However, technical difficulties with fetal movement and the cost involved limit its use to a small number of cases, usually as an adjunct to ultrasound.[17,31,73] MRI is probably safe in field strengths of 1 tesla. No increase in chromosomal aberrations or chromatid exchanges in human lymphocytes have been shown following prolonged exposure to 2.3 tesla in a 100-MHz radiofrequency emission.[72] Both CT and MRI are valuable for distinguishing hydranencephaly from maximum hydrocephalus in the neonate, and their superior soft tissue resolution may be helpful with these diagnoses in utero.[63]

Ultrasound remains the gold standard in fetal imaging. Static ultrasound images are sensitive for the diagnosis of fixed anatomical variants of the central nervous system (CNS) and their changes over time. The prenatal diagnoses of microcephaly, Chiari malformation, ventriculomegaly, ventriculitis, anencephaly, spinal dysraphism, Dandy-Walker syndrome, schizencephaly, subdural hemorrhage, intraventricular hemorrhage, and porencephaly can all be made with varying degrees of sensitivity and specificity.[1,26,30,40,42,48,50] Real-time ultrasound can detect indicators of fetal well-being such as respirations, heart rate, and limb movements, and provides accurate landmarks for invasive fetal procedures.

Despite these advances, there are limitations to ultrasound. Madeira et al[45] reported that the ultrasound diagnosis was modified by autopsy in 91 (42%) of 215 aborted mid-trimester fetuses. The false-negative rate in diagnosing extracranial anomalies associated with fetal ventriculomegaly has ranged from 15% to 72%. Nyberg et al[53] correctly identified only 28% of all associated anomalies (Table 1). The sensitivity of ultrasound in diagnosing myelomeningocele approximates 86%.[53] Several factors contribute to its insensitivity in spinal dysraphism. Widening of the fetal lumbar pedicles may be used as an indicator of an open spinal defect, but there is no recognizable ossification of fetal laminae or pedicles in the normal fetus until after the 25th week of gestation in the sacrum and after the 19th week of gestation in the lumbar spine.[22] When fetal and maternal spines are apposed by a supine position of the fetus, the diagnosis of an open neural tube defect may be missed at any gestational age.[22] Even anencephaly may be missed if ultrasound examination is performed before 14 weeks' gestation or if the fetal head is deep in the maternal pelvis.[26,27]

Diagnosis and Prognosis of Fetal Ventriculomegaly

In medical literature, the important distinction between static ventriculomegaly and the physiological state of hydrocephalus is not always made.[23,53,61] Hydrocephalus may be inferred by the presence of progressive ventriculomegaly and elevated intraventricular pressure. While progressive ventriculomegaly can be imaged by consecutive scans, there is no accurate noninvasive measure of intracranial pressure in the fetus.

The diagnosis of fetal ventriculomegaly was initially established by measurements of the biparietal diameter and discrepancies between body and head diameter.[23,57] Since that time, the lateral ventricular ratio (LVR = lateral ventricular width ÷ hemispheric width) has been found to be a more accurate indicator of ventriculomegaly.[39] The LVR decreases to 30% from the 15th to the 24th week of gestation, and remains constant from the 24th week until term.[54] If the LVR remains unchanged during the 15th through 20th weeks of gestation, progressive ventriculomegaly is unlikely.[55] The diagnosis of ventriculomegaly before the 26th week can be unreliable due to the large range of values for the normal LVR.[37,54,55] Finally, ventriculomegaly may not appear until the third trimester of pregnancy.[41]

Other problems include erroneous diagnosis and spontaneous resolution of ventriculomegaly. Rosseau et al[58] reported that 10 of 37 patients with fetal ventriculomegaly had normal-sized ventricles on postnatal imaging. Serial sonograms may show mild ventriculomegaly which resolves before delivery. Although isolated progressive ventriculomegaly is frequently caused by aqueductal stenosis, accurate diagnosis of this condition in utero remains elusive.

Choroid plexus cysts are found in approximately 1% of fetuses and may mimic ventricu-

TABLE 1

OUTCOME OF FETAL VENTRICULOMEGALY

Clinical Series & Year	No. of Fetuses	No. with Other Anomalies	Missed Anomalies	Elective Abortion	Perinatal Death	Total Alive	Alive Poor/Good	Shunted
Cochrane & Myles,[13] 1982	41	30	–	–	26	14	11/3	14
Chervenak et al,[11] 1984	53	44 (26%)	14/53	14	24	15	–	8
Williamson et al,[71]* 1984	30	21	–	–	25	5	–	–
Pretorius et al,[54] 1985	40	28	–	9	25	6	3/3	6
Serlo et al,[61] 1986	38	32	–	5	21	10	6/4	9
Nyberg et al,[53] 1987	61	51 (72%)	96/133	22	19	21	–	–
Vintzileos et al,[67] 1987	20	14 (60%)	12/20	4	7	9	5/4	9
Drugan et al,[18] 1989	43	31 (45%)	10/22	17	7	19	16/3	13
Goldstein et al,[28]+ 1990	55	42 (37%)	11/30	30	10	15	6/9	–
Hanigan,[29] 1991	15	14	–	1	7	7	6/1	3
Rosseau et al,[58]‡ 1992	40	26 (67%)	22/33	3	9	28	12/16	26
Hudgins & Edwards,[35] 1994	47	30 (15%)	7/47	19	7	21	12/9	11
Totals	483	363		124	187	170	77/52	99

*Elective abortions were excluded.
+Included only fetuses with mild ventriculomegaly (10-15 mm diameter).
‡Of 51 consults lost to follow-up, the authors believe 11 probably had terminations.

lomegaly.[3] They may regress during the second and third trimesters or be the harbinger of a lethal genetic trait. Walkinshaw et al[68] studied 15,565 fetuses with ultrasound at 19 weeks' gestation and found 152 (0.98%) fetuses with choroid plexus cysts that were either solitary and >5 mm in diameter or multiple. Of these 152 fetuses, 12 (8%) had other sonographic abnormalities and four (3%) had no other sonographic abnormality, but on amniocentesis or chorionic villi sampling had lethal karyotypes (e.g., trisomies 18 and 21). As the sensitivity of ultrasound diagnosis improves, other such early indicators of genetic anomalies are likely to be clarified.

At least 12 groups have reported their experience with the ultrasound diagnosis of fetal ventriculomegaly and the developmental outcome (Table 1).[10,11,13,14,18,28,29,35,53,54,58,61,67,71] Multiple abnormalities were reported in 75% of the 483 patients in the composite series. The outlook for the fetus with ventriculomegaly is poor: 124 fetuses (26%) were electively aborted and 187 (39%) died in the perinatal period, leaving approximately 170 (35%) alive beyond the neonatal period. Only 129 of the 170 patients had their developmental outcome reported. This outcome was abnormal in 77 (60%) and normal in 52 (40%) during a follow-up of 2 to 3 years.

Among the 129 survivors in the composite series in which the need for postpartum shunting was recorded, only 99 (77%) required shunting. In some, shunts were placed to facilitate custodial care in children with multiple abnormalities. The incidence of isolated progressive ventriculomegaly varied considerably. In Rosseau's series of 27 fetuses and Goldstein's series of 55, no neonate with isolated progressive ventriculomegaly was identified.[28,58] Hudgins et al[36] reported only two (4%) of 47 infants with isolated progressive ventriculomegaly who required shunting. As these studies suggest, a reliable method to predict the need for shunting in the fetus with ventriculomegaly has not been delineated.

Animal Experimentation

Fetal surgery has been used in animal models to study transplantation and regeneration.[7,9] Exceptional wound healing and immunological tolerance make the prenatal environment well-suited for surgical attempts to correct major malformations.[60]

Regeneration experiments with open spinal cord transection in fetal rats have been performed with acceptable morbidity, while craniotomies on healthy fetal rhesus monkeys have shown no increase in fetal wastage.[2,8,16] An animal model of kaolin-induced hydrocephalus was developed in the sheep and the rhesus monkey by Edwards et al.[20,21,25]

Other recent technical advances include a system for fetal endoscopic surgery in sheep developed by Luks et al.[44] This method prevented decompression of the amniotic sac and allowed bipolar cautery in this electrolyte-rich environment. Jennings et al[38] developed an implantable radiotelemetric fetal monitoring device for postoperative fetal monitoring of temperature and electrocardiogram. These represent less invasive means of manipulation that may decrease fetal loss following in utero surgery.

Human Experience

In the early 1980s, advances in ultrasound provided anatomical diagnoses specific enough to allow surgical treatment plans directed at isolated human congenital abnormalities. As the resolution and diagnostic precision of ultrasound improved, many fetal diseases (e.g., supraventricular tachycardia, diaphragmatic hernia, pulmonary cystic adenomatoid malformation, sacrococcygeal teratoma, and obstructive uropathy) were approached with invasive techniques. Some of these treatments have shown limited success in humans. Harrison et al[33] have reported 14 patients on whom they attempted open in utero repair of severe isolated left congenital diaphragmatic hernia. Nine of these patients were successfully repaired. Their technique includes endoscopic catheterization of placental vessels for chronic fetal vascular access.[34] Tocolysis remains a difficult problem that is sometimes uncontrollable, even with toxic doses of tocolytic agents.

Surgical intervention of fetal ventriculomegaly was first performed by Birnholz and Frigoletto.[6,24] Unfortunately, this initial attempt at in utero control of hydrocephalus was undertaken in a patient with undiagnosed Becker's muscular dystrophy. Nevertheless, the novelty of the attempt prompted a widespread interest in the expansion of these techniques for cerebrospinal fluid (CSF) diversion.[47] Subsequent attempts at in utero control of hydrocephalus focused on ventriculo-amniotic shunting.[12,49] This effort was met with difficulties in catheter stabilization, resulting in both intra- and extracranial migration.[12] The procedure-related mortality rate for ventriculo-amniotic shunt placement was 9.8%, compared to 2.3% for transhepatic fetal transfusion.[32,46] Because of difficulties in the identification of an appropriate treatment group and the technical difficulties of in utero shunt placement, a voluntary moratorium on the surgical treatment of fetal hydrocephalus was established in 1983.[13,66] No cases of attempted CSF diversion for fetal hydrocephalus have been reported to the International Fetal Surgery Registry following this moratorium.[46] In a 1994 survey of German-speaking perinatal centers, four of 18 centers had experience in the placement of thoracic, peritoneal, and bladder catheters for amniotic shunting while no catheters were placed for hydrocephalus.[5] The Denver shunt (Denver Biomaterials, Evergreen, CO), used for most ventriculo-amniotic shunts, has been withdrawn from the market.[56]

Ethical and Legal Considerations

There is a substantial body of literature devoted to the ethics of treatment of infants with CNS abnormalities. In the early 1980s several well-publicized cases involved parental refusal of accepted medical interventions. The political debate was defined by antiabortion and disabilities groups advocating access to care, while professional medical organizations advocated physician-patient autonomy. These controversies led to government intervention in the form of amendments to the Child Abuse Prevention and Treatment Act. The Federal Government requested that states prohibit withholding of treatment for life-threatening conditions. The interpretation by the Department of Health and Human Services under the Reagan Administration suggested that a child suffering from Tay-Sachs disease plus a life-threatening intestinal blockage must undergo intestinal surgery (49 Fed Reg 48,164 (1984)).[51] These amendments have been challenged as directives which usurp parents' historical role as agents who act in the best interests of their child.

In the case of therapeutic abortion, the distinction between a condition which is incompatible with life versus a condition which precludes a good quality of life is as difficult in utero as it is postpartum. *Roe v Wade* was decided in 1973 when there were limited options for fetal therapy. As more fetal therapeutic techniques become available, the same arguments to treat may be advanced on the fetus' behalf. Despite the moratorium placed on ventriculo-amniotic shunting over 10 years ago, ongoing progress in neonatal therapy will inevitably lead to further attempts to improve fetal therapy. For the time being, however, our ability to diagnose has far surpassed our ability to treat.

Assuming that parents are desirous of continued attempts at prolongation of fetal life, several conditions must be fulfilled before surgical treatment of fetal disease may be considered a reasonable option:

1. Fetal maturity must be inadequate for ex utero survival. The risks posed to the fetus by continuing the pregnancy must be less than the risks of delivery and neonatal care. If the child is near term with adequate lung maturity, delivery is desirable, since all treatments can be given with greater ease and safety following birth.
2. The natural history of the disease must be of progressive organ damage that compromises fetal health or would compromise the chances for postnatal survival. Nonprogressive disease or static developmental malformations would be excluded from treatment.
3. The treatment must improve on the natural history of the disease. This condition excludes patients with mild disease that would not result in irreparable organ dysfunction prior to delivery and those with severe disease who have already suffered damage from which they cannot recover. While the risks associated with a new procedure may be high due to a "learning curve" effect, techniques can be refined in animal experiments or similar models prior to human use. This reduction in the risk/benefit ratio is a focal point of clinical research.
4. The treatment must pose no more than a limited risk to maternal health. The mother must have adequate counseling to give informed consent and demonstrate an understanding of the risks posed to her health and fertility.

The Road Ahead

Although accurate fetal diagnosis and surgical therapy are improving, there is no well-defined group of fetuses that would benefit from in utero neurosurgery. Diagnostic techniques such as hand-held magnets for real-time MRI and small-bore endoscopy for first trimester fetal visualization have been developed.[19,59] Fetal intracranial tumors may be approached if the natural history warrants therapy. However, it is not known whether children with intracranial malignancies are more likely to achieve long-term survival following earlier in utero surgery. Hemostasis is formidable in such procedures and the frequent necessity of transfusions makes in utero surgery impractical.[70] Other areas for potential surgical therapy such as neural grafting of the dysraphic spinal cord require additional laboratory experience. Since the group of potential patients for in utero neurosurgery is small, the cost of the procedure will undoubtedly be part of the debate over appropriate implementation. Finally, ethical considerations will continue to influence research in human fetal therapy.

REFERENCES

1. Achiron R, Pinhas-Hamiel, Lipitz S, et al: Prenatal ultrasonographic diagnosis of fetal cerebral ventriculitis associated with asymptomatic maternal cytomegalovirus infection. **Prenat Diagn 14**:523-526, 1994
2. Albright L: Techniques of spinal cord surgery in fetal rats. **Neurosurgery 20**:240-242, 1987
3. Benacerraf BR: Asymptomatic cysts of the fetal choroid plexus in the second trimester. **J Ultrasound Med 6**:475-478, 1987
4. Benzie RJ, Ray P, Thompson D, et al: Prenatal exclusion of duchenne muscular dystrophy by fetal muscle biopsy. **Prenat Diagn 14**:235-238, 1994
5. Bernaschek G, Deutinger J, Hansmann M, et al: Feto-amniotic shunting—report of the experience of four European centres. **Prenat Diagn 14**:821-833, 1994
6. Birnholz JC, Frigoletto FD: Antenatal treatment of hydrocephalus. **N Engl J Med 304**:1021-1023, 1981
7. Bleacher JC, Adolph VR, Dillon PW, et al: Isolated fetal mouse limbs: gestational effects on tissue repair in an unperfused system. **J Pediatr Surg 28**: 1312-1315, 1993
8. Brodner RA, Markowitz RS, Lantner HJ: Feasibility of intracranial surgery in the primate fetus. Model and surgical principles. **J Neurosurg 66**:276-282, 1987
9. Chapman SA, Bannister CM: Effect of excision of occipital lobe tissue on about the 70th day of gestation on the growth and development of the sheep's brain. **Surg Neurol 32**:98-104, 1989
10. Chervenak FA, Berkowitz RL, Totora M, et al: The management of fetal hydrocephalus. **Am J Obstet Gynecol 151**:933-942, 1985
11. Chervenak FA, Duncan C, Ment LR, et al: Outcome of fetal ventriculomegaly. **Lancet 2**:179-181, 1984
12. Clewell WH, Johnson ML, Meier PR, et al: A surgical approach to the treatment of fetal hydrocephalus. **N Engl J Med 306**:1320-1325, 1982
13. Cochrane DD, Myles ST: Management of intrauterine hydrocephalus. **J Neurosurg 57**:590-596, 1982
14. Cochrane DD, Myles ST, Nimrod C, et al: Intrauterine hydrocephalus and ventriculomegaly: associated anomalies and fetal outcome. **Can J Neurol Sci 12**: 51-59, 1985
15. Daffos F, Capella-Pavlovsky M, Foresteir F: Fetal blood sampling via the umbilical cord using a needle guided by ultrasound. Report of 66 cases. **Prenat Diagn 3**:271-277, 1983
16. De Beer FC, Thomeer RTWM, Lakke E, et al: Spinal cord transections in fetal rats. Open intrauterine surgery with low morbidity. **Brain Res 454**:397-399, 1988
17. Dinh DH, Wright RM, Hanigan WC: The use of magnetic resonance imaging for the diagnosis of fetal intracranial anomalies. **Childs Nerv Syst 6**:212-215, 1990
18. Drugan A, Krause B, Canady A, et al: The natural history of prenatally diagnosed cerebral ventriculomegaly. **JAMA 261**:1785-1788, 1989
19. Dumez Y, Dommergues M, Gubler MC, et al: Meckel-Gruber syndrome: prenatal diagnosis at 10 menstrual weeks using embryoscopy. **Prenat Diagn 14**: 141-144, 1994
20. Edwards MSB: An evaluation of the in utero neurosurgical treatment of ventriculomegaly. **Clin Neurosurg 33**:347-357, 1986
21. Edwards MSB, Harrison MR, Halks-Miller M, et al: Kaolin-induced congenital hydrocephalus in utero in fetal lambs and rhesus monkeys. **J Neurosurg 60**: 115-122, 1984
22. Filly RA, Simpson GF, Linkowski G: Fetal spine morphology and maturation during the second trimester. Sonographic evaluation. **J Ultrasound Med 6**: 631-636, 1987
23. Freeman RK, McQuown DS, Secrist LJ, et al: The diagnosis of fetal hydrocephalus before viability. **Obstet Gynecol 49**:109, 1977
24. Frigoletto FD, Birnholz JC, Greene MF: Antenatal treatment of hydrocephalus by ventriculoamniotic shunting. **JAMA 248**:2496-2497, 1982
25. Glick PL, Harrison MR, Halks-Miller M, et al: Correction of congenital hydrocephalus in utero II: efficacy of in utero shunting. **J Pediatr Surg 19**: 870-881, 1984
26. Goldstein RB, Filly RA: Prenatal diagnosis of anencephaly: spectrum of sonographic appearances and distinction from the amniotic band syndrome. **AJR 151**:547-550, 1988
27. Goldstein RB, Filly RA, Callen PW: Sonography of anencephaly: pitfalls in early diagnosis. **J Clin Ultrasound 17**:397-402, 1989
28. Goldstein RB, La Pidus AS, Filly RA, et al: Mild lateral cerebral ventricular dilatation in utero: clinical significance and prognosis. **Radiology 176**:237-242, 1990
29. Hanigan WC: The dilemma of fetal ventriculomegaly: research and therapy during the past decade. **Perspect Neurol Surg 2**:111-123, 1991
30. Hanigan WC, Ali MB, Cusack TJ, et al: Diagnosis of subdural hemorrhage in utero. Case report. **J Neurosurg 63**:977-979, 1985
31. Hanigan WC, Gibson J, Kleopoulos NJ, et al: Medical imaging of fetal ventriculomegaly. **J Neurosurg 64**: 575-580, 1986
32. Harman CR, Bowman JM, Manning FA, et al: Intrauterine transfusion—intraperitoneal versus intravascular approach: a case-control comparison. **Am J Obstet Gynecol 162**:1053-1059, 1990
33. Harrison MR, Adzick NS, Flake AW, et al: Correction of congenital diaphragmatic hernia in utero: VI. Hard-earned lessons. **J Pediatr Surg 28**:1411-1418, 1993
34. Hedrick MH, Jennings RW, MacGillivray TE, et al: Endoscopic catheterization of placental vessels for chronic fetal vascular access. **Surg Forum 48**:504-505, 1992
35. Hudgins RJ, Edwards MSB: The fetus with a CNS malformation: natural history and management, in Harrison MR, Golbus MS, Filly RA (eds): **The Unborn Patient, 2nd ed.** Philadelphia, PA: WB Saunders, 1994, pp 437-443
36. Hudgins RJ, Edwards MSB, Goldstein R, et al: Nat-

ural history of fetal ventriculomegaly. **Pediatrics 82:** 692-697, 1988
37. Jeanty P, Dramaix-Wilmet M, Delbeke D, et al: Ultrasonic evaluation of fetal ventricular growth. **Neuroradiology 21:**127-131, 1980
38. Jennings RW, Adzick NS, Longaker MT, et al: Radiotelemetric fetal monitoring during and after open fetal operation. **Surg Gynecol Obstet 176:**59-64, 1993
39. Johnson ML, Dunne MG, Mack LA, et al: Evaluation of fetal intracranial anatomy by static and real-time ultrasound. **J Clin Ultrasound 8:**311-318, 1980
40. Klingensmith WC, Cioffi-Ragan DT: Schizencephaly diagnosis and progression in utero. **Radiology 159:** 617-618, 1986
41. Ko TM, Hwa HL, Tseng LH, et al: Prenatal diagnosis of X-linked hydrocephalus in a Chinese family with four successive affected pregnancies. **Prenat Diagn 14:** 57-60, 1994
42. Kurtz AB, Wapner RJ, Rubin CS, et al: Ultrasound criteria for in utero diagnosis of microcephaly. **J Clin Ultrasound 8:**11-16, 1980
43. Liley AW: Intrauterine transfusion of foetus in haemolytic disease. **Br Med J 2:**1107, 1963
44. Luks Fl, Deprest JA, Vandenberghe K, et al: A model for fetal surgery through intrauterine endoscopy. **J Pediatr Surg 29:**1007-1009, 1994
45. Madeira A, Norman A, Hasiam J, et al: Examination of fetuses after induced abortion for fetal abnormality—a follow-up study. **Prenat Diagn 14:**381-385, 1994
46. Manning FA: The fetus with ventriculomegaly: the Fetal Surgery Registry, in Harrison MR, Golbus MS, Filly RA (eds): **The Unborn Patient, 2nd ed.** Philadelphia, PA: WB Saunders, 1994, pp 448-452
47. Manning FA, Harrison MR, Rodeck C, et al: Catheter shunts for fetal hydronephrosis and hydrocephalus. Report of the International Fetal Surgery Registry. **N Engl J Med 315:**336-340, 1986
48. Mateos F, Esteban J, Ramos JT, et al: Fetal subdural hematoma: diagnosis in utero. Case report. **Pediat Neurosci 13:**125-128, 1987
49. Michejda M, Patronas N, Di Chiro G, et al: Fetal hydrocephalus. II. Amelioration of fetal porencephaly by in utero therapy in nonhuman primates. **JAMA 251:**2548-2552, 1984
50. Newman GC, Buschi AI, Sugg NK, et al: Dandy-Walker syndrome diagnosed in utero by ultrasonography. **Neurology 32:**180-184, 1982
51. Newman SA: Baby Doe, Congress and the States: challenging the Federal treatment standard for impaired infants. **Am J Law Med 15:**1-60, 1989
52. Nicolini U, Nicolaidis P, Fisk NM, et al: Fetal blood sampling from the intrahepatic vein: analysis of safety and clinical experience with 214 procedures. **Obstet Gynecol 76:**47-53, 1990
53. Nyberg DA, Mack LA, Hirsch J, et al: Fetal hydrocephalus: sonographic detection and clinical significance of associated anomalies. **Radiology 163:** 187-191, 1987
54. Pretorius DH, Davis K, Manco-Johnson ML, et al: Clinical course of fetal hydrocephalus: 40 cases. **AJR 144:**827-831, 1985
55. Pretorius DH, Drose JA, Manco-Johnson ML: Fetal lateral ventricular ratio determination during the second trimester. **J Ultrasound Med 5:**121-124, 1986
56. Pringle KC: Fetal diagnosis and fetal surgery. **Clin Perinatol 16:**13-22, 1989
57. Rose J: Fetal abnormalities diagnosed by ultrasound in the second and third trimesters, in Sanders RC, James AE (eds): **Ultrasonography in Obstetrics and Gynecology.** New York, NY: Appleton-Century-Crofts, 1977, p 153
58. Rosseau GL, McCullough DC, Joseph AL: Current prognosis in fetal ventriculomegaly. **J Neurosurg 77:** 551-555, 1992
59. Schenck JF, Jolenz FA, Roemer PB, et al: Superconducting open configuration MRI system for image guided therapy. **Radiology** (In press)
60. Schwartz RH: Acquisition of immunologic self-tolerance: review. **Cell 57:**1073-1081, 1989
61. Serlo W, Kirkinen P, Jouppila P, et al: Prognostic signs in fetal hydrocephalus. **Childs Nerv Syst 2:**93-97, 1986
62. Stewart G, Day RE, Del Priore C, et al: Developmental outcome after intravascular intrauterine transfusion for rhesus haemolytic disease. **Arch Dis Child 70:**F52-F53, 1994
63. Sutton LN, Bruce DA, Schut L: Hydranencephaly versus maximal hydrocephalus: an important clinical distinction. **Neurosurgery 6:**35-38, 1980
64. Touraine JL, Raudrant D, Royo C, et al: In-utero transplantation of stem cells in bare lymphocyte syndrome. **Lancet 1:**1382, 1989 (Letter)
65. Valenti C: Antenatal detection of hemoglobinopathies. A preliminary report. **Am J Obstet Gynecol 115:**851-853, 1973
66. Venes JL: Management of intrauterine hydrocephalus. **J Neurosurg 58:**793-794, 1983 (Letter)
67. Vintzileos AM, Campbell WA, Weinbaum PJ, et al: Perinatal management and outcome of fetal ventriculomegaly. **Obstet Gynecol 69:**5-11, 1987
68. Walkinshaw S, Pilling D, Spriggs A: Isolated choroid plexus cysts—the need for routine offer of karyotyping. **Prenat Diagn 14:**663-667, 1994
69. Westin B: Hysteroscopy in early pregnancy. **Lancet 2:** 872-875, 1954 (Letter)
70. Whittle IR, Simpson DA: Surgical treatment of neonatal intracranial teratoma. **Surg Neurol 15:** 268-273, 1981
71. Williamson RA, Schauberger CW, Varner MW, et al: Heterogeneity of prenatal onset of hydrocephalus: management and counseling implications. **Am J Med Genet 17:**497-508, 1984
72. Wolff S, James TL, Young GB, et al: Magnetic resonance imaging: absence of in vitro cytogenetic damage. **Radiology 155:**163-175, 1985
73. Yun WTC, Nguyen HD, Fisher DJ, et al: MR of fetal central nervous system abnormalities. **AJNR 15:** 459-464, 1994

CHAPTER 18

TREATMENT OF THE PREGNANT PATIENT WHO IS BRAIN DEAD OR IN A PERMANENT VEGETATIVE STATE

HOWARD H. KAUFMAN, MD, JOHN BODENSTEINER, MD, MARK GIBSON, MD, AND ROBERT HOELDTKE, MD

On rare occasions a pregnant woman may suffer brain death or enter the permanent vegetative state. These states can be diagnosed with confidence, and such patients can be supported for prolonged periods. There then arises the question of whether to utilize such support in order for the fetus to mature sufficiently to be able to be born. The following is a discussion of these subjects.

BRAIN DEATH

> . . . the death of persons–of human persons–is of profound moral importance and . . . therefore people generally are very concerned that the criteria of death reflect this importance and provide reliably accurate methods for determining the death of persons.[37]

The question of what is life and when it is lost will be considered first in philosophical and then in physiological terms. In philosophical terms, there is perceived to be something unique about a human being separate from organic or somatic functioning. This is embodied in the dualist concept of body and soul which dates from the teachings of Plato and Aristotle. It is therefore necessary to define what is essential to humanity or personhood and to determine what must be lost in order to define death.

From ancient times it was believed that the locus of this unique quality resided in the brain.[23,76] The mind is identified more specifically with the neocortex, where self-awareness and reasoning are thought to be located. Following this concept, it is not until neocortical functioning occurs that a true human being exists, and once this is lost, human life is over.

However, as mentioned before, it is now possible to support cardiovascular and respiratory functions in patients whose brains have irreversibly ceased all function (and even more easily in those who have lost only neocortical function).[12,34,70,74] This situation has resulted in a need "to define death by criteria that did not depend primarily on the cardiorespiratory function that life support systems artificially preserved."[23] This has been done by "clarifying the definition of death, or by revising the criteria for terminating treatment of the living."[76]

There are several excellent recent reviews about the clinical determination of brain death.[13,26,72] A group of consultants to the President's Commission for the Study of Ethical Problems in Medicine and Biomedical Research and Behavioral Research refined previous criteria.[61,63,80] The consultants advocated that laws should define brain death as "irreversible cessation of all functions of the entire brain."[53,63,80] Their criteria involve clinical evidence of loss of brain function and a period of observation which can be shortened by confirmatory tests, particularly cerebral blood flow (CBF) studies. The difference between these criteria and earlier criteria lies mainly in the rapidity with which brain death can be declared. They provide the current standard, although there are some theoretical problems.[21,61,93] These criteria have proved to be reliable and are further supported since they fulfill the requirement stated by Shewmon, that is, that they are "self-evident on a priori grounds."[93] Since no patient has been reported to have survived when the diagnosis of brain death was made using the criteria, they can be employed with confidence. In cases that fall outside these guidelines, consultation with physicians with particular expertise may be helpful, and other criteria and tests can be used. The evolution of criteria for the declaration of brain death in children less than 5 years old has been considered problematic. But in the last few years, work has begun in this area.[52]

The following procedure for assessment is consistent with the criteria agreed upon by the advisors to the President's Commission.

Clinical Evidence

To be declared brain dead, a patient must first meet accepted *clinical criteria* based on cerebral unresponsivity. The patient should be on a respirator and show no signs of respiratory effort. There should be no sign of eye opening, no spontaneous movement, and no movement elicited by noise or painful stimuli to the face or trunk other than spinal cord reflex movements. The pupils should be midposition.[14] There should be absence of brain stem reflexes (pupillary, oculocephalic [doll's eyes], oculovestibular [iced water irrigation], corneal, gag, and cough reflexes). These reflexes may be difficult to test when there are massive facial injuries. However, it has been pointed out that even when these criteria are met, there may be electroencephalographic (EEG), evoked potential, or neurohumoral function.[42]

The spinal cord reflexes seen after brain death may be quite disconcerting and caregivers as well as friends and family need to be warned about them. Initially after brain death, a state of spinal shock develops, after which there is a stepwise restoration of spinal reflexes.[22,101] Both visceral and somatic reflexes have been observed.[6,20,31,45,49,58,75,101,103,108] They do not preclude the diagnosis of brain death.

Determining the *cause* of apparent brain death can be helpful in establishing that loss of function is not reversible. The most common causes of brain death are trauma, stroke, or ischemia/hypoxia. If the cause is not apparent, studies such as computed tomography, magnetic resonance imaging, or angiography will often clarify the etiology.

Significant levels of a variety of *exogenous substances* (such as alcohol, barbiturates and other depressant drugs, and neuromuscular blocking agents [which may be given for intubation]) and *metabolic abnormalities* (such as those seen in hepatic or renal failure) can reversibly impair neurological functions and might mimic the clinical picture of brain death. If there is any question as to the etiology of apparent brain death, CBF studies can be used to confirm the diagnosis of brain death.

Both *hypothermia* (≤90°F, 32°C) and *hypotension* (≤90 mm Hg systolic blood pressure) might reversibly suppress neurological activity. The diagnosis of brain death should be delayed until body temperature and blood pressure are above these thresholds.

Part of the clinical examination of brain stem function involves evaluation for *apnea*, at least at the end of the period of observation (Table 1). There must be a formal apnea test to prove that brain stem function has been lost. A few patients have been reported who met all other criteria of brain death but did show respiratory efforts.[30] On the other hand, in one series 20% of patients had nonspecific reflex movements during apnea testing that were of no significance.[87] Preoxygenation of 30 minutes has been suggested.[6] Oxygenation must be continued during the test and can be accomplished by using positive end-expiratory pressure, a T-piece, or a tracheal

TABLE 1

APNEA TEST

1. Preoxygenate for at least 10 minutes with 100% O_2 and at the same time adjust the respirator so that pCO_2 is about 40 mm Hg.
2. Disconnect the respirator and give O_2 at 8-12 L/min by tracheal cannula.
3. If hypotension and/or arrhythmias develop at any time, stop the test and place the patient immediately back on the respirator. If this happens, EEG or CBF tests or consultation should be obtained.
4. During disconnection from a respirator, the patient should be observed continuously for spontaneous respirations. If there are none in 10 minutes, draw blood gases and place the patient back on the respirator. The pCO_2 must be >60 torr to be sure of maximally stimulating the medullary respiratory centers. If the pCO_2 is >60 torr and there is no respiratory effort, the patient is apneic.
5. Obviously, if there is any respiratory effort, the patient is not apneic and not brain dead.

catheter.[6] Monitoring should be employed to detect desaturation. Determining apnea requires a specific protocol that insures that the pCO_2 reaches a level which provides a maximal respiratory stimulus, at least 60 mm Hg.[77,88,91] By adjusting the pretest pCO_2 to well above 40 mm Hg, it may be possible to shorten the test to 5 minutes.[8] Since testing will lead to increased pCO_2 and therefore possible elevation of intracranial pressure, it should be reserved until the rest of the initial evaluation makes the diagnosis of brain death reasonably certain or might even be deferred if sufficient observation and testing is done (vide infra). A variety of cardiovascular changes have been noted during testing, including rises and falls in heart rate and blood pressure, and arrythmias, occasionally requiring reconnecting the ventilator.[6-8]

One aspect of brain death which is being better appreciated involves the *hormonal changes* that occur. There can be an initial stress reaction (including a spinal mediated sympathoadrenal response[31]) which may occur due to the original insult, followed by diminished function due to damage to the hypothalamic-pituitary axis (vide infra).

Period of Observation/ Confirmatory Tests

Periods of observation may be needed to confirm the irreversibility of loss of neurological functions. These are not supported by careful study but were designed to be quite cautious. Without confirmatory tests, and if the diagnosis is uncertain or there exist confusing secondary problems (i.e., hypoxia after head injury), it is advisable to wait 12 to 24 hours after the patient first meets the clinical criteria of brain death to make the final declaration. If the cause of coma is hypoxia, the period of observation from the time of loss of brain functions should be 24 hours before the declaration of death. On the other hand, in some situations (such as in patients who have suffered extensive gunshot injuries to the head or who have large intracerebral hematoma) it is reasonable to shorten the period of observation.

Use of certain *confirmatory tests* makes it possible to shorten periods of observation. One family of tests evaluates CBF. Inadequate blood flow to the brain results in irreversible brain damage within minutes. Demonstration of inadequate blood flow confirms the diagnosis of brain death even in cases with drug intoxication, altered metabolic status, shock, or hypothermia. Furthermore, the test is easy for families to understand. *Conventional contrast angiography* has been used to diagnose brain death and has been accepted as the standard of intracranial blood flow evaluation against which to measure other tests. This test can be used to confirm brain death at any time after loss of clinical neurological functions. However, it is complex, costly, potentially damaging to a patient who is in fact alive, and sometimes injures the kidneys of a brain dead donor; it is therefore no longer regularly used for this purpose in the United States. *Radionuclide cerebral angiography* is noninvasive, safe, and can be rapidly performed in a radiology suite or at the bedside with equipment that is likely to be available in many hospitals.[39] Many now view the bedside radionuclide angiogram with radiotracers utilizing technetium as the confirmatory test of choice. It has never been demonstrated to be in error in diagnosing brain death. This test is recommended as a confirmatory study, linked with 6 hours of observed absence of clinical neurological functions. Some experts use this technique immediately after neurological examination has revealed no response or to declare death without a further period of observation, particularly in situations where the etiology is clear, the brain damage is overwhelming (i.e., a large spontaneous intracerebral hematoma), and there are no complicating features. It has also been used to confirm brain death in young children.[92]

An EEG can be done at the bedside, is without risk, and may be helpful when performed by an experienced electroencephalographer. An EEG for brain death should be carried out utilizing the guidelines of the American Electroencephalographic Society.[41] One weakness of the EEG is that it does not directly measure brain stem function. On the other hand, the EEG may still show activity when patients meet the clinical criteria of brain death.[40] Although electrocerebral activity precludes the diagnosis of brain death, electrocerebral silence does not exclude reversible coma (e.g., from intoxication or hypothermia). The patient with electrocerebral inactivity should still have at least 6 hours of observation showing complete loss of brain functions.

Several *newer tests* have been investigated with regard to confirming the diagnosis of brain death, including a new type of brain scan, transcranial Doppler ultrasonography, and evoked potentials. None has been considered in a consensus conference or by a task force, so none yet carries the imprimatur of widespread acceptance.

Apparent contradictions between tests[67] are explainable. For example, EEG activity after clinical brain death may indicate survival of a few cells, and the presence of evoked potentials may indicate survival of a few axons. Blood flow may restart after it has ceased if intracranial pressure drops. Conversely, there may be clinical activity when the EEG is flat or when a radionuclide flow study is negative because of minimal residual brain stem activity, but such patients are not brain dead because they do not meet the clinical criteria.

Documentation and Declaration of Death

There should be careful *documentation* in the hospital record to support a determination of brain death. Date and time of observations should be recorded, as well as details of all clinical evaluation (including apnea testing), pertinent laboratory tests, and results of confirmatory tests. A hospital-approved form may be helpful.

These guidelines are useful:

> This societal resolution has relied upon the perceived clarity of medical criteria for neurological death (as opposed to the obvious uncertainties and delays with most forms of higher brain death), the pressure to achieve permission to save other lives with transplantation, and the political acceptability of incremental change.[61]

Any trained physician should be able to declare brain death. General medical curricula and testing of physician qualifications should encompass brain death. Some criteria (and state laws) suggest that two physicians agree on the diagnosis of brain death, particularly when organ retrieval is being considered. However, if the diagnosis is straightforward and clear, and if the physician involved is well-trained and experienced, it would seem reasonable for a single physician to certify brain death.

Current Judeo-Christian thinking generally supports the concept of brain death.[18,73,99]

The concept that brain death is equivalent to death as diagnosed by the criteria of loss of respiratory and cardiac function is generally accepted by the law. A model brain death law, the Uniform Determination of Death Act, was approved in 1980 by the President's Commission, the American Medical Association (AMA), the American Bar Association, and the National Conference of Commissioners on Uniform State Laws. This law states that brain death is equivalent to death recognized by cardiopulmonary standards. However, it reserves actual criteria and determination for the medical profession. At least 39 states now have brain death laws, and a few others have formally accepted brain death as death in rulings of the state supreme court. Precedents are now so overwhelming that brain death standards probably can be applied anywhere in the United States, although practitioners should know the status of their local laws. Still, there can be problems:

> ... brain death criteria, used in cases where a human being is maintained on artificial ventilation, are far less detectable or even understandable by the ordinary non-medical person, and therefore subject to far greater suspicion.[23]

Cardiovascular and respiratory support was developed particularly in this century (and since the 1950s localized in intensive care units[84]) so that the vegetative activities of the body could be supported after brain death. There are excellent guidelines available for the immediate care of brain dead patients.[24,78,79,85,86] Prolonged support of brain dead patients was first reported in the early 1980s.[33,56] In such patients, physiological derangements, namely lack of respiratory drive, cardiovascular instability, thermovariability, anterior and posterior pituitary insufficiency, and altered nutritional needs, can be corrected. In general such treatment is inappropriate. Exceptions have been made in rare circumstances, usually in an attempt to salvage a viable fetus, the record now being 107 days.[12,27,34,44,56,70]

One aspect of brain death that is being better appreciated and which is important to understand in order to successfully maintain somatic function for long periods is the *hormonal changes* that occur. There can be an initial stress reaction due to the original insult, followed by diminished function caused by damage to the hypothalamic-pituitary axis. The stress reaction has been reviewed in detail, as has herniation with bradycardia and hypertension, the Cushing response.[24,54,89]

Hypothalamic damage of variable severity is almost always present in brain dead patients; evidence of widespread necrotic changes extending to the posterior pituitary and midbrain is occasionally present.[98] Despite this, pituitary function remains intact in the majority of brain dead patients.[57,69,110] However, assessment of pituitary function is problematic in this patient population. Serum cortisol concentrations, an index of adrenocorticotropic hormone secretion, are difficult to interpret in critically ill patients because it is hard to assess the extent of stress in any given individual. A normal serum cortisol, for example, might be inappropriately low in a patient recovering from a subarachnoid hemorrhage. Serum thyroxine and thyroid-stimulating hormone (TSH) concentrations are frequently suppressed in critically ill patients, a physiologically adaptive response to stress (the euthyroid sick syndrome). Thus, low concentrations of thyroxine and TSH in brain dead patients cannot be taken as evidence for true hypopituitarism. Given the difficulties inherent in assessing pituitary function in critically ill patients, it is not surprising that the literature currently available provides conflicting information on the frequency of hypopituitarism in brain dead patients.[57,69,98,110] Although hypothalamic damage would be expected to disrupt pituitary function in this patient population, the occurrence of this has not yet been demonstrated and further studies of this question are needed.

Chronic Support for Brain Dead Patients

There are several helpful reviews that discuss chronic support for brain dead patients in detail, many of which note specific problems of pregnant women:[12,34]

1. Respiratory drive and protective respiratory reflexes are lost with destruction of the brain stem respiratory centers. Other specific problems include neurogenic pulmonary edema and adult respiratory distress syndrome. Since ordinarily a pregnant woman has respiratory alkylosis, pCO_2 should probably be kept above 30 mm Hg to prevent impaired placental perfusion.

2. There is loss of both sympathetic and parasympathetic tone, the result being hypotension. Pressors, specifically dopamine (inotropic, peripheral vasoconstriction) and dobutamine (inotropic), are suggested. Diabetes insipidus with hypovolemia may contribute to hypotension, and a Swan-Ganz catheter should be used to help monitor and treat this. Bradycardia may also be a problem.[12]
3. Hypopituitarism is expected. Postmortem examinations of brain dead patients have revealed progressive changes in the hypothalamus with better preservation of both the anterior and posterior pituitary.[98] This may be explained by the extracranial blood supply to the pituitary and by the fact that it can be protected from increased intracranial pressure by the diaphragma sella. Some hypothalamic hormones may also be produced in extracranial sites such as the pancreas.[98] This explains why after brain death there is initial preservation of endocrine function, at least in part, followed by progressive decline.[98] It is advisable to anticipate hormonal alterations early so that replacement can be utilized to keep the patient stable. Desmopressin is recommended to treat the diabetes insipidus caused by lack of antidiuretic hormone because it has a long duration of action and a low pressor:antidiuretic ratio.[24,25] It has been suggested that triiodothyronine, cortisol, and insulin may be helpful for maintaining somatic function and optimizing activity of organs to be transplanted.[55,67,110] There has been some discussion of the euthyroid sick syndrome in these circumstances.[47,69,78,79]
4. Nutrition and metabolic monitoring is required. Enteral feeding has been used,[12,70] but intravenous hyperalimentation has also been required because of decreased intestinal motility.[34]
5. The patient loses thermoregulation and becomes poikilothermic (thus, hypothermic). Heating blankets or other types of warming devices are indicated.
6. Because of the problem of aortocaval compression, positioning on the sides or use of a tilting bed is indicated.
7. Low-dose heparin has been suggested to prevent deep vein thrombosis and pulmonary emboli. Pulsating boots might also be utilized.
8. Prophylaxis against, monitoring for, and treatment of infections are very important, as infections have been a problem in such patients.[12,34]
9. Endocrine function needs to be monitored frequently in brain dead patients. Patients with hypopituitarism may develop hyponatremia or hypoglycemia. Cortisol therapy should be initiated if serum cortisol levels are consistently low (<8 μg/dL). Thyroid hormone should be given if there is evidence of primary hypothyroidism (low serum thyroxine and high TSH). If thyroxine and TSH are both low, thyroxine therapy should not be given since this profile is most likely the result of the euthyroid sick syndrome. If there are other features of hypopituitarism (a low serum cortisol) or known trauma to the pituitary, thyroxine therapy might be appropriate. Blood sugar should be monitored, and hyperglycemia treated with insulin as necessary. Urine volume and serum sodium should be monitored; if there are indications of diabetes insipidis, serum osmolarity should be measured and arginine vasopressin administered as needed.

The fetus should have fetal heart rate monitoring and frequent ultrasound examinations to follow growth. Betamethasone has been given to promote fetal lung maturation.[12,34]

Permanent Vegetative State

Descartes stated the concept of higher brain function with elegant simplicity, "Cogito ergo sum." Consciousness has been defined as "our immediate sense of the present and what amounts to memory (the source of the revisions of reality . . .)."[82] As to the exact location of consciousness in the brain:

> . . . on the basis of modern evidence for the massive parallel processing of information within the brain, . . . consciousness is not a unitary phenomenon but rather a continually changing, updated and edited version of the world that derives from many neurological sources.[82]

The problem is that there is no consensus about exactly what constitutes consciousness, how to determine whether it is lost, or how to know that loss is irreversible.[111]

The concept of a higher brain or neocortical standard of personhood based on consciousness is already being utilized implicitly if not always explicitly. The problem is that the "key functions" or "higher brain function" must be defined and agreed upon and then subjected to measurement.[106] In recent years it has become widely accepted that it is not ethically required to give any support to breathing patients, not even water, if the patient is not sentient or will not suffer discomfort.[21] Although this approach alters the way we deal with the living, we have not treated such patients as dead, which would mean they could be buried or have their organs harvested.[23,76]

A task force including representatives from the American Academy of Neurology, the American Academy of Pediatrics, the American Neurological Association, the American Association of Neurological Surgeons, and the Child Neurology Society have considered this subject in depth. Their report begins with the definition:

> The vegetative state is a condition of complete unawareness of the self and the environment accompanied by sleep-wake cycles with either complete or partial preservation of brain stem and hypothalamic autonomic functions.[66]

The report includes an extensive literature review of the various causes of the permanent vegetative state, including traumatic and nontraumatic brain injury, degenerative and metabolic disorders, and developmental malformations; times at which it can be known to be permanent; and epidemiology. It notes that there are estimated to be 10,000 to 25,000 adults and 4,000 to 10,000 children in the permanent vegetative state and that their care costs between 1 and 7 billion dollars a year. More research needs to be done to facilitate diagnosis and prognosis of this state. Indeed, a recent survey of ethicists has demonstrated tremendous variations in thoughts about such patients,[35] and there is also the need for explicit discussion to develop standards for dealing with them.[38] It has also been proposed that people should be allowed to choose their own definition of death and to include the option of a higher brain definition as one option.[106]

There is a report of a pregnant woman in the permanent vegetative state who was successfully supported until the birth of her baby.[90] In the circumstance of a pregnant woman who is brain dead or in the permanent vegetative state, the question arises as to when it is appropriate to maintain somatic functions so that the fetus can mature sufficiently to be viable. To try to decide this question requires consideration of philosophical and legal principles.

PHILOSOPHICAL CONSIDERATIONS

Philosophy means literally love of wisdom and is most generally used today to mean "that department of knowledge which deals with ultimate reality, or with the most general causes and principles of things."[94] It encompasses many disciplines. For the purposes of this discussion, bioethics and the law will be considered particularly since the concepts of these disciplines and their interplay are what primarily guide decisions in such matters.

Bioethics is a "form of moral philosophy practiced within medicine."[50] In modern status bioethics may have begun in Seattle during the 1960s in applied ethics utilized when deciding who would be given dialysis. Bioethics expanded in response to the technological developments which extended the natural lifespan of human beings, but at the same time led to many conundrums in initiating and withdrawing care. The discipline is called "bioethics," a term coined by Van Rensselear Potter: "I chose 'bio-' to represent biological knowledge, the science of living systems, and I chose 'ethics' to represent knowledge of human value systems."[50] Landmarks in this movement include founding of the Hastings Center in 1969 and the Kennedy Institute of Ethics in 1970 as well as the establishment of several governmental bodies to consider ethical issues.[105] It has involved philosophers, theologians, social scientists, and lawyers. The importance of this movement has been emphasized:

> By facilitating open discussion and examination of the ethical premises underlying life and death decisions, bioethics has expanded medicine's reflective horizons. In fact, encouraging health practitioners to become self-reflective is the major contribution of bioethics to American health care.[3]

Heifetz[43] has discussed the origin and nature of moral behavior. He describes ethics as a philosophical discipline that develops principles by which to judge right and wrong, and morality as the application of these principles. He feels that these principles should be universal, should be in harmony with human nature, and should benefit the individual and society. He cites three sources of ethics—religion, biological data, and pure reason. Religion gives rise to dogma and religious philosophy, the latter being more flexible. The concepts of religion cannot be verified and therefore should not be forced on others; however, they should be heard and considered. Biological data from lower animals are discounted as being too restricted to use for analyzing human behavior. Pure reason is problematic because it depends on the validity of primary assumptions and is based on the quality of reasoning. Heifetz suggests that ethics must be based on two assumptions: the need to avoid harm to ourselves, our families, and our community, and the need to live in social groups. As the primary moral principles, he cites (in order) nonmaleficence and freedom, qualified by the absence of harm (which is required for a free society), followed by action for the common good (which could cause risks to freedom if given too high a priority), and beneficence. As secondary principles, he includes justice (or the equal treatment of all) and privacy (or the freedom to make a choice of what is not wanted). He recommends using these primary and secondary principles to decide how to resolve moral issues. He states:

> Moral behavior is the product of human reason and emotion, modified by our physical and cultural environment and possibly by our genetic imprint. The degree of importance each factor is given in the final pattern is variable.[43]

Decision-making requires balancing and flexibility. In the case of an incompetent person, consideration of best interests requires intelligence and rational thinking.

An excellent overview of bioethics can be found in the classic text of Beauchamp and Childress,[5] who also utilize a hierarchical system of organization. They describe the two theories which govern choices in cases of conflict: utilitarian and deontological. The utilitarian theory seeks to determine which choice maximizes benefits and minimizes evil. The deontological theory uses criteria of right and wrong based on particular political, religious, and other beliefs. The beliefs of the major cultures and religions of the world relative to the issues discussed here have been reviewed in detail in several publications.[9,11,46,65] Next in the hierarchy are four general and fundamental principles which are listed in order of importance: autonomy; nonmaleficence; beneficence; and justice. Next are rules specific to contexts and restricted in scope; these include veracity, privacy, confidentiality, and fidelity. Lastly are specific decisions and actions. In addition they note that all decisions and actions should be founded in moral ideals (which are to be desired even if not required) and virtuous character traits (which are morally valued). The major problem arises at the level of theory, where a deontological theory may prevent the compromise required to resolve conflicts. But again, this is where respect for the freedom of others and tolerance must be invoked.

The decision-making process requires gathering facts, developing options, and making decisions based on ranking values and principles.[28] Physicians should guide patients or their surrogates through these issues but not decide for them. Patients or their surrogates have a right to be told the truth and to be made aware of the prognosis in order to make spiritual and temporal preparations.[10] Physicians must be trustworthy, and patients or their surrogates must believe that physicians are advocates of their best interests.[10] It is appropriate for such decisions to be difficult and hard fought. It would be best if they were kept from the political arena and freed from the spectre of malpractice.

Callahan put the current status of bioethics in perspective:

> How was the acceptance of bioethics in fact gained? I would say that the first thing those in bioethics had to do . . . was to push religion aside. It was clear that the physician as sole decision maker

> would have to give way to a more complex picture of what moral life is all about. What we began to see was the movement . . . toward a different kind of moral language in the mainstream of public policy, toward a language of rights, worries about questions of pluralism, efforts to find moral consensus and moral strategies in the face of a diverse cultural situation . . . bioethics chose a kind of middle course. That middle course is regulation, regulation being the way we in the United States typically deal with controversial issues. On the one hand you avoid the extreme of simple prohibition of things, while on the other hand you show you are serious and willing to be cautious. What we began to see increasingly was the creation of oversight bodies.... The final factor of great importance I would mention was the emergence ideologically of a form of bioethics that dovetailed very nicely with the reigning political liberalism of the educated classes in America.[50]

In recognition of the current absence of a national forum for analyzing ethical issues in medicine, in 1993 the Congressional Office of Technology Assessment, at the request of United States Senators Mark Hatfield, Edward Kennedy, and Dennis DeConcini, prepared a background paper, entitled "Biomedical Ethics in U.S. Public Policy." They noted the helpfulness of prior Federal bodies and the advantages of a well-funded centralized national forum, and made specific suggestions about the factors to be considered in developing one.[105] If properly established, such a forum could be useful in facilitating accommodations on the controversies in dying and death.[2]

Legal Considerations

It is important to keep in mind that the United States is a heterogeneous culture in which different philosophical systems may be in conflict. However, its unique history with an emphasis on freedom and tolerance provides the political processes and its tradition of the rule of law provides a framework for resolving controversial issues.

The intellectual climate in the United States involves a liberal political philosophy in which personal freedom and privacy are honored and protected, at least if these do not harm others. This concept leads to a way to resolve conflicts:

> Does a state protect a contestable value best by encouraging people to accept it as contestable, understanding that they are responsible for deciding for themselves what it means? Or does the state protect a contestable value best by itself deciding, through the political process, which interpretation is the right one, and then forcing everyone to conform? The goal of responsibility justifies the first choice, the goal of conformity the second. A state cannot pursue both goals at the same time.[29]

Obviously, the proper goal is the former one. For a pluralistic society to function, it is necessary to recognize individuals' rights to make decisions for and about themselves above all other principles, and this tolerance is the price required for our "adventure in liberty."

The political embodiment of the social contract of the United States is the Constitution, including its amendments, specifically the First, Third, Fourth, Fifth, and Fourteenth Amendments.[43] In a superb treatment of the Constitution as it relates to life-and-death decisions, Dworkin[29] pointed out that the Constitution should be interpreted in terms of its broad principles, which is what its framers intended to achieve in terms of liberty and equal concern for its citizens, even if they seem to conflict with apparent details.

Our society is regulated by the rule of law. In the words of Joseph Campbell, "lawyers and law are what hold us together. There is no ethos."[2] It is the Supreme Court's interpretation of the intent of the Constitution which ultimately determines how an issue will be resolved. Consideration of end-of-life decisions in the public arena and government activity involving the judicial, legislative, and executive branches began with the Quinlan case (1976), and there have been many important court cases since.[2,10,11,38,104] Growing legal interest and action, particularly at the state level, has been detailed.[38]

It has been argued that court and legislative action is too easily swayed by political pressure, that the participants are often not well-versed on the issues, that the process is slow and costly, that the venue is too far removed from the actual situation, and that family privacy is violated. In addition, actions may vary from state to state, and cases and laws need to be reconsidered as innovations occur.[38] Some have also argued that in the case of moral choices it is better to keep discussions private, but present court involvement indicates the current failure of private decision-making.[11]

Thus by today's ethical and legal standards, patients or their surrogates have a right to determine what will happen to them based on their own values while physicians must educate them and act as their advocate.[15] This is embodied in the concept of informed consent, which requires that patients be informed of diagnosis, prognosis, and options, but also requires competence, the ability to understand and make reasonable judgments, and that decisions be voluntary. Informed consent can extend into the future in terms of advance directives, including living wills and the appointment of surrogates, or substituted judgment, in which the known wishes of the patient are considered. In the absence of direction by a patient, decisions should be made on best interests, namely what most reasonable people would want.

Direction of Care

A patient or surrogate has a right to treatment, particularly if it is reasonable, and also a right to refuse treatment. Problems may arise when there is a demand for care that a physician feels is inappropriate or a refusal of care that is suggested. If a patient or surrogate demands futile care, in principle a physician need not accede to such a demand. But the physician has no legal protection if care is refused, as indicated in the recent Waglie case in Minnesota in which the court ruled that a husband had the right to demand care for his wife who was in a vegetative state.

That a patient or surrogate can legally refuse treatment has long been established in the United States.[10,64] Indeed, in a 1914 Supreme Court decision, Justice Cardoza declared, "Every human being of adult years and sound mind has the right to determine what shall be done with his own body."[65] This statement is the embodiment of the Constitutional right of liberty and privacy and the common law right of self determination. Another landmark came in 1957 when Pope Pius XII, in response to the development of technologies which at times only prolong dying, proclaimed that extraordinary care is not obligatory.[10] The right to refuse treatment has led to the endorsement by the Hastings Center (1981), the AMA (1982), and the President's Commission (1983) of withholding and withdrawing unwanted care. This principle was accepted in California in 1986 in the Bouvia case, in which the patient was given the right to refuse food and water.[10] Its effect can be seen in such situations as the right of a Jehovah's Witness to refuse blood even if this leads to death, although this right may be limited when it adversely impacts others (i.e., where a mother's refusal of a transfusion will lead to her death and abandonment of a child). There are many cases in which this right has been affirmed.[2,11,29,43,105]

On the other hand, there are religious considerations that obligate a person or surrogate to care for the body, the gift of God. This is true in Catholicism and perhaps even more so in Judaism.[105] There is also historical precedent, at least in terms of cesarean section to save the life of a fetus after the death of the mother, which goes back to Greek mythology and early Roman law.[34,51]

If the wishes of the mother are not known, the decisions should be made by the father and with consideration of the fetus' best interests based on quality of life. Presumably the father would have the right to request or refuse support, but there is no case in which a conflict between a physician and a husband has occurred and been tested in court. There have been cases in which an unmarried father's wishes have been honored ahead of those of a next of kin.[34]

Expensive Care and Scarce Resources

In response to rising costs, health care in the United States is undergoing a revolution, with a focus on cost containment and rationing. Allocation of resources requires consideration of how much money society wants to devote to medical care and, of the total amount, who is to get what portion. Clearly many societies have limited the funds for medicine, which in the United States has been done only in a fragmented, ad hoc fashion. Similarly, determination of who gets what portions of health care dollars has not been discussed comprehensively. Attempts to do so, such as that in Oregon, have been unsuccessful. On the other hand, many parties, including payers, hospital administrators and lawyers, and governmental watchdogs are intruding into patient-physician decision-making and influencing that decision-making based on considerations of cost as well as perceived benefits and risks. Ethics committees can act as patient advocates and counterbalance inappropriate rulings.[28,62] Recent work of interest involves how to determine the dollar worth of medical interventions in terms of years of functional life and satisfaction, how much different members of society are owed and should request, and what they are willing to pay for themselves and for others.[2,15]

The Fetus

Humanism, the dominant secular philosophy of our time, emphasizes the value of the life of each individual.[23] However, the absolute sanctity of life is a contestable value. If human life is inherently sacred, the fetus would need to be protected except to save the life of the mother. If, on the other hand, its rights had to be balanced against the rights of the mother, other relatives, and society, its rights might be altered, especially depending on its age. It has been argued that a mother has rights of privacy and self-determination, that she should not be forced to assume risk for another person, that her rights supersede the rights of a fetus even to the point of aborting it, and that she is in the best position to choose when abortion is appropriate.[2] In this discussion, only the last condition might be relevant.

A middle-of-the-road approach involves trying to determine a point at which the fetus does have rights–the point at which the potential to become a human being is realized sufficiently to warrant protection. Several stages in development might be considered significant besides the conceptus (which is a new genotype with the potential for life). These include: implantation (6-14 days' gestation); sufficient development of the nervous system so there is limited (reflex) response to stimuli and the possibility of a personal identity (8 weeks' gestation); recognizability as a human (12-16 weeks' gestation); development of a neocortex and an integrated nervous system, a patterned EEG, the presumed ability to react to painful stimuli, the possibility of self-consciousness, and viability (the ability to survive ex utero), all of which occur at about 23 to 24 weeks' gestation; and, finally, birth with breathing. Some even feel what is important is the development of such characteristics as consciousness, language, abstract reasoning, and self-awareness,[1,48,55,97] which occur well after birth; in many cultures even a young infant does not have human status.

Different parties have different interests. The child has an interest in living only if it is healthy and may expect a socially satisfying life, the mother has an interest in controlling her life as she feels is most appropriate, the father has a similar interest, and society has a need to protect the rights of the father and mother and to avoid the burden of an impaired child or one without parental support. On the other hand, the child has an interest in existing, the mother and father may need to be protected from making a poor decision, and society needs to protect the vulnerable. Resolution of these interests is at times difficult and must be individualized to some extent. Shaw developed a formula to help evaluate the potential quality of life of an infant: Quality of life = natural endowment × (home and societal support).[3,104] This reflects the problem that, in many cases, children who are saved may have inadequate support. Decision-making should be done by informed and wise parents in the child's best interest.

When management of the patient and her pregnancy on behalf of the fetus is elected, the chief considerations are: monitoring of fetal well-being (growth, adequacy of placental function); determination of fetal lung maturity (the chief predictor of newborn well-being); and timing and mode of delivery.

Determination of fetal well-being involves regular assessment of maternal and fetal physiology as in routine prenatal care, including screening for maternal glucose intolerance, hypertension, and isoimmunization. Specific deviations from normal (e.g., the development of diabetes mellitus or the emergence of pre-eclampsia) should be managed as in a normal pregnancy. In addition, monitoring of fetal well-being by nonstressed assessment of the fetal heart, by sonographic determinants for adequate fetal growth, and by biophysical profile (which includes fetal heart rate variability, amniotic fluid volume, fine and gross motor activity of the fetus, and total breathing movements) should be conducted at regular intervals to determine if they are appropriate for gestational age, as well as to determine any other additional complicating factors. Deterioration of fetal status with or without observable contributing maternal factors may precipitate need for delivery.[12,33] Since the primary aim is delivery of a viable newborn, prolongation of maternal life to assure healthy postnatal newborn adaptation is paramount and complications injurious to the mother should be treated rather than predisposing to early delivery, as there is no concern about long-term consequences to the mother.

Fetal pulmonary maturity, the most important consideration, can be assessed by weekly amniotic fluid analysis of the lecithin/sphingomyelin ratio (L/S ratio). Because there may be unanticipated maternal or fetal circumstances that would require preterm delivery, prophylactic administration of glucocorticoids to hasten fetal lung maturity is advisable beginning at 28 weeks' gestation (when such treatment is known to become effective).[19] When maternal functions are stable, the administration of glucoids might allow earlier delivery without respiratory compromise in the newborn course, but at the cost of other morbidities of newborn adaptation of the premature system (nutritional, metabolic) that would be contrary to the underlying goal of optimal newborn outcome. This can be accomplished with occasional success as early as 23 weeks' gestation, although with much higher rates of success at 28 weeks' gestation.[1,27,60] With effort and use of expensive resources, much longer support is possible and leads to even better outcome. Therefore, in the absence of maternal or fetal complications, delivery at or about the 36th week of gestation, contingent on a favorable L/S ratio, would constitute a reasonable aim.

As to delivery, labor in any instance entails small but measurable fetal risks, which under normal circumstances are counterbalanced by maternal considerations. As the latter do not prevail here, cesarean section has been the mode of delivery selected in most case reports.[12,27,34] There are also the possibilities for research on and use of an aborted fetus even if it is not viable.[102] It should always be remembered that the fetus is a symbol of human life and should be treated with respect. However, living human beings have vital interest in use of the fetus in research and treatment. Transplantation of fetal tissue has received great interest. There is growing evidence that fetal tissue transplantation may be helpful for Parkinson's disease as well as other diseases.[97,100] More research in these and other applications is needed, but must be done thoughtfully and with sufficient oversight to avoid any suggestion of impropriety. Research of the fetus in utero has been useful, but here protection similar to that in any living human must be observed. Research on the living fetus ex utero is useful, but must be done with sensitivity.[55,97] The moratorium on federal funding for fetal research established during the administration of President George Bush was eliminated by President Bill Clinton when he took office.[48] New guidelines for the use of fetal tissue have been issued (National Institutes of Health (NIH) Revitalization Act of 1993 [PL 103-43]), and the first new NIH grant for human implantation of fetal tissue has been awarded. Thus, even if the fetus will not be carried to viability, it could still be desirable to support the mother so it can be employed in research and treatment of others.

Transplantation

Recent advances in transplantation provide the opportunity of using the organs of a brain dead person to improve or even to save the lives of others and even conserve money because of diminished medical costs and increased productivity.[71,81,85,86] The advances currently being made are reflected in the rising numbers of transplants (now about 20,000/year)[32] and rising rates of organ and donor survival. However, between 1988 and 1991, when candidates increased 55%, donors only increased by 16%. By March 1993, 30,000 patients were on waiting lists, and six people awaiting a transplanted heart or a liver died every day. Cadaver donors remain at about 4,000/year even though more potential donors exist.[24]

The causes for this problem are numerous. Currently, organ donation is based on voluntarism and altruism.[17] Although surveys have suggested the public largely understands brain death and generally looks favorably on donation, this is not a universal attitude, particularly among a number of minorities.[16,36,59,83,85,86] Also, many people who would wish to donate do not tell their families, while families who have not been told are more reluctant to donate organs.[36] In addition, organs are lost when patients were not vigorously resuscitated or supported.

The Uniform Anatomical Gift Act (1968), now adopted in all states, permits the patient to make a directive in advance. Forty-nine states have rules to encourage this statement on the driver's license. Thirty-eight states have Routine Inquiry/Required Request laws (1987) mandating inquiry of next of kin, but these have not had much effect.[16,17] National laws to promote transplantation include the National Organ Transplantation Act of 1984 (PL 98-507) and Amendments in 1988 (PL 100-607) and 1990 (PL 101-616). They established a national organ procurement network and a scientific registry as well as a Task Force and have led to ongoing activities.[32,85,86] The Surgeon General sponsored a workshop in July 1991; recommendations from this workshop include strategies to increase donations.[68,81] There have been many proposals including improvement in donor identification and care, more effective contact with donor families, universal checking for donor cards, and public education. Other solutions suggested include presumed consent, mandated decision-making, and rewarded gifting.[16,17,85,86,96,107] In several countries, organs are harvested based on "presumed consent" if the deceased had not previously objected. However, it has been suggested that "mandated choice" is a better solution.[95] A recent Gallup poll suggested financial rewards would not be helpful.[36]

Because facilitating transplantation has many benefits and in many cases may save a life, it is permissible, virtuous, and believed by many to be obligatory.[55] Professional obligations as well as the ethical and religious imperatives of beneficence, charity, and honesty compel physicians to be proactive and facilitate transplantation by informing the family about this possibility when it exists. The AMA Code of Medical Ethics (1992) declares, "The voluntary donation of organs in appropriate circumstances is to be encouraged," and organized neurosurgery has supported this approach.

Other solutions are being considered: xenographs are being attempted, creating their own ethical issues; artificial organs are being investigated; the use of life donors is being expanded; and the use of non-heart-beating cadaver donors is again being explored. The University of Pittsburgh has developed a protocol in which terminal patients who have elected to have life-sustaining treatment stopped and who have expressed a wish to donate organs are taken into an operating room, treatment is stopped, and their organs harvested if they do not breathe and their heart stops in a short period. This may increase the donor pool by 20% to 25%. A review of the evolution of this controversial protocol, its status, the experience with it, and critiques about it have been published.[4,109]

Conclusion

The conditions of brain death and the permanent vegetative state can be diagnosed with certainty. It is possible to support somatic functions of a pregnant woman in these states until a viable baby can be delivered, although this can be a complicated and expensive undertaking, especially if the mother's incapacitation comes early in her pregnancy and support must be continued for a long period.[12,34] Current bioethical priniciples and legal rules can be applied to such situations. The prior wishes of the mother and the wishes of the father/husband or other surrogate should be considered, as well as the possibilities for a healthy and acceptable social life for the child. More discussion is needed at a societal level to decide if and what limits should be placed on this undertaking.

REFERENCES

1. Allen MC, Donohue PK, Dusman AE: The limit of viability: neonatal outcome of infants born at 22 to 25 weeks' gestation. **N Engl J Med 329:**1597-1601, 1993
2. Annas GJ: **Standard of Care: The Law of American Bioethics.** New York, NY: Oxford University Press, 1993
3. Anspach RR: **Deciding Who Lives: Fateful Choices in the Intensive-Care Nursery.** Berkeley, CA: University of California Press, 1993
4. Arnold RM, Youngner SJ: Back to the future: obtaining organs from non-heart-beating cadavers. **Kennedy Instit Ethics J 3:**103-111, 1993
5. Beauchamp TL, Childress JF: **Principles of Biomedical Ethics, 3rd ed.** New York, NY: Oxford University Press, 1989
6. Belsh JM, Blatt R, Schiffman PL: Apnea testing in brain death. **Arch Intern Med** 146:2385-2388, 1986
7. Benzel EC, Gross CD, Hadden TA, et al: The apnea test for the determination of brain death. **J Neurosurg 71:**191-194, 1989
8. Benzel EC, Mashburn JP, Conrad S, et al: Apnea testing for the determination of brain death: a modified protocol. Technical note. **J Neurosurg 76:**1029-1031, 1992
9. Berger A, Badham RP, Kutscher AH, et al: **Perspectives on Death and Dying: Cross-Cultural and Multi-Disciplinary Views.** Philadelphia, PA: Charles Press, 1989
10. Berger AS: **Dying & Death in Law & Medicine: A Forensic Primer for Health and Legal Professionals.** Westport, CT: Praeger, 1993
11. Berger AS, Berger J (eds): **To Die or Not to Die? Cross-Disciplinary, Cultural, and Legal Perspectives on the Right to Choose Death.** New York, NY: Praeger, 1990
12. Bernstein IM, Watson M, Simmons GM, et al: Maternal brain death and prolonged fetal survival. **Obstet Gynecol 74:**434-437, 1989
13. Black PM: Conceptual and practical issues in the declaration of death by brain criteria. **Neurosurg Clin North Am 2:**493-501, 1991
14. Bleck TP: Dilated pupils and brain death. **Ann Intern Med 112:**632, 1990 (Letter)
15. Brock DW: **Life and Death.** Cambridge, England: Cambridge University Press, 1993
16. Caplan A, Siminoff L, Arnold R, et al: Increasing organ and tissue donation: what are the obstacles, what are our options?, in: **The Surgeon General's Workshop on Increasing Organ Donation. Background Papers.** Washington, DC: US Department of Health and Human Services, 1991, pp 199-232
17. Caplan AL, Virnig B: Is altruism enough? Required request and the donation of cadaver organs and tissues in the United States. **Crit Care Clin 6:** 1007-1018, 1990
18. Childress JF: Protestant perspectives on organ donation, in Kaufman HH (ed): **Pediatric Brain Death and Organ/Tissue Retrieval. Medical, Ethical, and Legal Aspects.** New York, NY: Plenum Press, 1989, pp 45-53
19. Collaborative Group on Antenatal Steroid Therapy: Effects of antenatal dexamethasone administration on the prevention of respiratory distress syndrome. **Am J Obstet Gynecol 141:**276-286, 1981
20. Conci F, Procaccio F, Arosio M, et al: Viscera-somatic and viscero-visceral reflexes in brain death. **J Neurol Neurosurg Psychiatry 49:**695-698, 1986
21. Council on Scientific Affairs and Council on Ethical and Judicial Affairs: Persistent vegetative state and the decision to withdraw or withhold life support. **JAMA 263:**426-430, 1990
22. Crenna P, Conci F, Boselli L: Changes in spinal reflex excitability in brain-dead humans. **Electroencephalogr Clin Neurophysiol 73:**206-214, 1989
23. Dagi TF: Death-defining acts: historical and cultural observations on the end of life, in Kaufman HH (ed): **Pediatric Brain Death and Organ/Tissue Retrieval. Medical, Ethical and Legal Aspects.** New York, NY: Plenum Press, 1989, pp 1-30
24. Darby JM, Stein K, Grenvik A, et al: Approach to management of the heartbeating "brain dead" organ donor. **JAMA 261:**2222-2228, 1989
25. Debelak L, Pollak R, Reckard C: Arginine vasopressin versus desmopressin for the treatment of diabetes insipidus in the brain dead organ donor. **Transplant Proc 22:**351-352, 1990
26. de Villiers JC: Pitfalls and problems in the diagnosis of cerebral death. **Prog Neurol Surg 13:**180-202, 1990
27. Dillon WP, Lee RV, Tronolone MJ, et al: Life support and maternal brain death during pregnancy. **JAMA 248:**1089-1091, 1982
28. Dubler N, Nimmons D: **Ethics on Call. Taking Charge of Life-and-Death Choices in Today's Health Care System.** New York, NY: Vintage Books, 1993
29. Dworkin R: **Life's Dominion. An Argument About Abortion, Euthanasia, and Individual Freedom.** New York, NY: Alfred A Knopf, 1993
30. Earnest MP, Beresford HR, McIntyre HB: Testing for apnea in suspected brain death: Methods used by 129 clinicians. **Neurology 36:**542-544, 1986
31. Ebata T, Watanabe Y, Amaha K, et al: Haemodynamic changes during the apnoea test for diagnosis of brain death. **Can J Anaesth 38:**436-440, 1991
32. Evans RW, Orians CE, Ascher NL: The potential supply of organ donors. An assessment of the efficiency of organ procurement efforts in the United States. **JAMA 267:**239-246, 1992
33. Fabro F: Brain death with prolonged somatic survival. **N Engl J Med 306:**1361, 1982 (Letter)
34. Field DR, Gates EA, Creasy RK, et al: Maternal brain death during pregnancy. Medical and ethical issues. **JAMA 260:**816-822, 1988
35. Fox E, Stocking C: Ethics consultants' recommendations for life-prolonging treatment of patients in a persistent vegetative state. **JAMA 270:**2578-2582, 1993
36. Gallup Organization: **The American Public's Attitudes Toward Organ Donation and Transplantation.** Boston, MA: The Partnership for Organ Donation, February 1993
37. Gillon R: Death. **J Med Ethics 16:**3-4, 1990 (Editorial)
38. Glick HR: **The Right to Die. Policy Innovation and Its Consequences.** New York, NY: Columbia University Press, 1992
39. Goodman JM, Heck LL, Moore BD: Confirmation of brain death with portable isotope angiography: a review of 204 consecutive cases. **Neurosurgery 16:**492-497, 1985

40. Grigg MM, Kelly MA, Celesia GG, et al: Electroencephalographic activity after brain death. **Arch Neurol 44:**948-954, 1987
41. Guideline Three: minimum technical standards for EEG recording in suspected cerebral death. American Electroencephalographic Society. **J Clin Neurophysiol 11:**10-3, 1994
42. Halevy A, Brody B: Brain death: reconciling definitions, criteria, and tests. **Ann Intern Med 119:** 519-525, 1983
43. Heifetz MD: **Easier Said Than Done. Moral Decisions in Medical Uncertainty.** Buffalo, NY: Prometheus Books, 1992
44. Heikkinen JE, Rinne RI, Alahuhta SM, et al: Life support for 10 weeks with successful fetal outcome after fatal maternal brain damage. **Br Med J 290:**1237-1238, 1985
45. Heytens L, Verlooy J, Gheuens J, et al: Lazarus sign and extensor posturing in a brain-dead patient. Case report. **J Neurosurg 71:**449-451, 1989
46. Hill TP, Shirley D: **A Good Death. Taking More Control at the End of Your Life.** Reading, MA: Addison-Wesley, 1992
47. Howlett TA, Keogh AM, Perry L, et al: Anterior and posterior pituitary function in brain-stem-dead donors. A possible role for hormonal replacement therapy. **Transplantation 47:**828-834, 1989
48. Humber JM, Almeder RF (eds): **Bioethics and the Fetus. Medical, Moral and Legal Issues.** Clifton, NJ: Humana Press, 1991
49. Jastremski MS, Powner D, Snyder J, et al: Spontaneous decerebrate movement after declaration of brain death. **Neurosurgery 29:**479-480, 1991 (Letter)
50. Jonsen AR (ed): The birth of bioethics. Report of a conference. **Hastings Cent Rep 23 (Special Suppl):** 1-16, November/December 1993
51. Katz VL, Dotters DJ, Droegemueller W: Perimortem cesarean delivery. **Obstet Gynecol 68:**571-576, 1986
52. Kaufman HH (ed): **Pediatric Brain Death and Organ/Tissue Retrieval. Medical, Ethical and Legal Aspects.** New York, NY: Plenum Press, 1989
53. Kaufman HH, Lynn J: Brain death. **Neurosurgery 19:**850-856, 1986
54. Kaufman HH, Timberlake G, Voelker J, et al: Medical complications of head injury. **Med Clin North Am 77:**43-60, 1993
55. Keyes CD, Wiest WE (eds): **New Harvest. Transplanting Body Parts and Reaping the Benefits.** Clifton, NJ: Humana Press, 1991
56. Klein RC: Brain death with prolonged somatic survival. **N Engl J Med 306:**1362, 1982 (Letter)
57. Koller J, Wieser C, Gottardis M, et al: Thyroid hormones and their impact on the hemodynamic and metabolic stability of organ donors and on kidney graft function after transplantation. **Transplant Proc 22:**355-357, 1990
58. Kuwagata Y, Sugimoto H, Yoshioka T, et al: Hemodynamic response with passive neck flexion in brain death. **Neurosurgery 29:**239-241, 1991
59. Lange SS: Psychosocial, legal, ethical, and cultural aspects of organ donation and transplantation. **Crit Care Nurs Clin North Am 4:**25-42, 1992
60. Loewy EH: The pregnant brain dead and the fetus: must we always try to wrest life from death? **Am J Obstet Gynecol 157:**1097-1101, 1987
61. Lynn J: Brain death: historical perspectives and current concerns, in Kaufman HH (ed): **Pediatric Brain Death and Organ/Tissue Retrieval. Medical, Ethical and Legal Aspects.** New York, NY: Plenum Press, 1989, pp 65-72
62. Macklin R: **Enemies of Patients.** New York, NY: Oxford University Press, 1993
63. Medical Consultants on the Diagnosis of Death: Guidelines for the determination of death: report of the Medical Consultants on the Diagnosis of Death to the President's Commission for the Study of Ethical Problems in Medicine and Biomedical and Behavioral Research. **JAMA 246:**2184-2186, 1981
64. Meisel A: The legal consensus about foregoing life-sustaining treatment: its status and its prospects. **Kennedy Instit Ethics J 2:**309-345, 1993
65. Misbin R: **Euthanasia: The Good of the Patient—The Good of Society.** Frederick, MD: University Publishing Group, 1992
66. Multi-Society Task Force on PVS: Medical aspects of the persistent vegetative state. Parts 1 and 2. **N Engl J Med 330:**1499-1508, 1572-1579, 1994
67. Nau R, Prange HW, Klingelhöfer J, et al: Results of four technical investigations in fifty clinically brain dead patients. **Intensive Care Med 18:**82-88, 1992
68. Novello AC: From the surgeon general, US Public Health Service: increasing organ donation. **JAMA 267:**213, 1992
69. Novitzky D: Triiodothyronine replacement, the euthyroid sick syndrome, and organ transplantation. **Transplant Proc 23:**2460-2462, 1991
70. Nuutinen LS, Alahuhta SM, Heikkinen JE: Nutrition during ten-week life support with successful fetal outcome in a case with fatal maternal brain damage. **JPEN J Parenter Enteral Nutr 13:**432-435, 1989
71. Olson CM (ed): Diagnostic and therapeutic technology assessment (DATTA): lung transplantation. **JAMA 269:**931-936, 1993
72. Pallis C: Brainstem death: the evolution of a concept. **Semin Thorac Cardiovasc Surg 2:**135-152, 1990
73. Paris JJ: Catholic considerations of brain death and organ retrieval, in Kaufman HH (ed): **Pediatric Brain Death and Organ/Tissue Retrieval. Medical, Ethical and Legal Aspects.** New York, NY: Plenum Press, 1989, pp 35-43
74. Parisi JE, Kim RC, Collins GH, et al: Brain death with prolonged somatic survival. **N Engl J Med 306:**14-16, 1982
75. Patterson KW, McShane A: Reflex spinal cord activity as a cause of a delay in the diagnosis of brain death. **Ir Med J 84:**27-28, 1991
76. Pernick MS: Back from the grave: recurring controversies over defining and diagnosing death in history, in Zaner RM (ed): **Death: Beyond Whole-Brain Criteria.** Boston, MA: Kluwer Academic, 1988, pp 17-74
77. Posner JB: Coma and other states of consciousness: the differential diagnosis of brain death. **Ann NY Acad Sci 315:**215-227, 1978
78. Powner DJ, Darby JM, Stein KL: Organ donor management in the intensive care unit, in Grande CM (ed): **Textbook of Trauma, Anesthesia and Critical Care.** St Louis, MO: CV Mosby, 1993, pp 1007-1012
79. Prager MC: Care of organ donors. **Int Anesthesiol Clin 29:**1-16, 1991
80. President's Commission for the Study of Ethical Problems in Medicine and Biomedical and Behavioral Research (ed): **Defining Death: A Report on the**

Medical, Legal, and Ethical Issues in the Determination of Death. Washington, DC: US Government Printing Office, 1981
81. Public Health Service: **The Surgeon General's Workshop on Increasing Organ Donation: Proceedings.** Washington, DC: US Department of Health and Human Services, 1991
82. Purves D: Book review of Dennett DC: *Consciousness Explained, 1991.* **Science 257:**1291-1292, 1992
83. Randall T: Too few human organs for transplantation, too many in need . . . and the gap widens. **JAMA 265:**1223, 1227, 1991
84. Reiser SJ: The intensive care unit: the unfolding and ambiguities of survival therapy. **Int J Technol Assess Health Care 8:**382-394, 1992
85. Rivers EP, Buse SM, Bivins BA, et al: Organ and tissue procurement in the acute care setting: principles and practice, I. **Ann Emerg Med 19:**78-85, 1990
86. Rivers EP, Buse SM, Bivins BA, et al: Organ and tissue procurement in the acute care setting: principles and practice, II. **Ann Emerg Med 19:**193-200, 1990
87. Ropper AH: Unusual spontaneous movements in brain-dead patients. **Neurology 34:**1089-1092, 1984
88. Ropper AH, Kennedy SK, Russell L: Apnea testing in the diagnosis of brain death. Clinical and physiological observations. **J Neurosurg 55:**942-946, 1981
89. Rowlands BJ, Kaufman HH: Metabolic physiology, pathophysiology, and management, in Wirth FP, Ratcheson RA (eds): **Neurosurgical Critical Care.** Baltimore, MD: Williams & Wilkins, 1987, pp 81-107
90. Sampson MB, Petersen LP: Post-traumatic coma during pregnancy. **Obstet Gynecol (Suppl) 53:**2-3, 1979
91. Schafer JA, Caronna JJ: Duration of apnea needed to confirm brain death. **Neurology 28:**661-666, 1978
92. Schwartz JA, Brill D, Baxter J: Detection of blood flow to the brain by radionuclide cerebral imaging, in Kaufman HH (ed): **Pediatric Brain Death and Organ/Tissue Retrieval. Medical, Ethical and Legal Aspects.** New York, NY: Plenum Press, 1989, pp 149-156
93. Shewmon DA: The probability of inevitability: the inherent impossibility of validating criteria for brain death or "irreversibility" through clinical studies. **Stat Med 6:**535-553, 1987
94. Simpson JA, Weiner ESC (eds): **The Oxford English Dictionary, 2nd ed, Vol XI.** Oxford, England: Clarendon Press, 1989
95. Spital A: Mandated choice. The preferred solution to the organ shortage? **Arch Intern Med 152:** 2421-2424, 1992
96. Spital A: The shortage of organs for transplantation: where do we go from here? **N Engl J Med 325:** 1243-1246, 1991 (Sounding Board)
97. Steinbock B: **Life Before Birth. The Moral and Legal Status of Embryos and Fetuses.** New York, NY: Oxford University Press, 1992
98. Sugimoto T, Sakano T, Kinoshita Y, et al: Morphological and functional alterations of the hypothalamic-pituitary system in brain death with long term bodily living. **Acta Neurochir 115:**31-36, 1992
99. Tendler RM: A Jewish approach to ethical issues in brain death and organ transplantation, in Kaufman HH (ed): **Pediatric Brain Death and Organ/Tissue Retrieval. Medical, Ethical and Legal Aspects.** New York, NY: Plenum Press, 1989, pp 31-34
100. Truog RD: Do-not-resuscitate orders during anesthesia and surgery. **Anesthesiology 74:**606-608, 1991
101. Turmel A, Roux A, Bojanowski MW: Spinal man after declaration of brain death. **Neurosurgery 28:**298-302, 1991
102. Turner DA, Kearney W: Scientific and ethical concerns in neural fetal tissue transplantation. **Neurosurgery 33:**1031-1037, 1993
103. Urasaki E, Tokimura T, Kumai J, et al: Preserved spinal dorsal horn potentials in a brain-dead patient with Lazarus' sign. Case report. **J Neurosurg 76:** 710-713, 1992
104. Urofsky MI: **Letting Go; Death, Dying & the Law.** New York, NY: Macmillan, 1993
105. US Congress, Office of Technology Assessment: **Biomedical Ethics in U.S. Public Policy—Background Paper.** Washington, DC: US Government Printing Office, 1993, OTA-BP-BBS-105
106. Veatch RM: The impending collapse of the whole-brain definition of death. **Hastings Cent Rep 23:** 18-24, July/August, 1993
107. Veatch RM: Routine inquiry about organ donation: an alternative to presumed consent. **N Engl J Med 325:**1246-1249, 1991 (Sounding Board)
108. Wetzel RC, Setzer N, Stiff JL, et al: Hemodynamic responses in brain dead organ donor patients. **Anesth Analg 64:**125-128, 1985
109. Youngner SJ, Arnold RM: Ethical, psychosocial, and public policy implications of procuring organs from non-heart-beating cadaver donors. **JAMA 269:** 2769-2774, 1993
110. Zaloga GP: Endocrine function after brain death. **Crit Care Med 18:**785-786, 1990 (Editorial)
111. Zaner RM: Introduction, in Zaner RM (ed): **Death: Beyond Whole-Brain Criteria.** Boston, MA: Kluwer Academic, 1988, pp 1-14

QUESTIONS FOR *Neurosurgical Aspects of Pregnancy*

The following questions have been provided to give physicians the option of testing their comprehension of the material provided in *Neurosurgical Aspects of Pregnancy.* The test is to be self-scored. Answers may be found in the back of this book. A Continuing Medical Education (CME) certificate will be mailed upon the return of the enclosed test evaluation/feedback card along with a $25 administrative fee. Telephone 708-692-9500 (after 1/20/96 847-692-9500) to order additional evaluation/feedback cards or information about other CME products from the American Association of Neurological Surgeons.

After reading this book, a physician should be able to:

- understand specific neurosurgical disorders that arise exclusively during pregnancy
- comprehend the basic physiological changes associated with pregnancy
- understand the toxicity of common neurosurgical drugs and radiation exposure to mother and fetus
- understand the cardinal principles of positioning and fetal monitoring in neurosurgery of pregnancy patients
- tailor specific neurosurgical procedures to the needs of the pregnant woman.

CHAPTER 1

Fetal Toxicity of Common Neurosurgical Drugs

1. During which trimester(s) of pregnancy is the fetus most susceptible to the teratogenic effects of medications?
   (A) first trimester
   (B) second trimester
   (C) third trimester
   (D) second and third trimesters
   (E) all trimesters equally

2. Which of the following factors is involved in the teratogenicity of medications?
   (A) the type of drug
   (B) the drug dose
   (C) changes in pharmacokinetics during pregnancy
   (D) placental metabolism
   (E) all of the above

3. Anticonvulsant medications can increase:
   (A) maternal complications.
   (B) fetal complications.
   (C) both
   (D) neither

4. Which of the following is a potential etiological factor in the teratogenicity of anticonvulsants?
   (A) genetic makeup
   (B) epoxide metabolites
   (C) folic acid deficiency
   (D) all of the above
   (E) A and B

5. Which of the following factors is known to increase the safety of various anticonvulsant medications during pregnancy?
   (A) adherence to monotherapy when possible
   (B) close monitoring of anticonvulsant levels
   (C) folic acid supplementation
   (D) maternal vitamin K prophylaxis prior to delivery with certain anticonvulsants
   (E) all of the above

6. Bromocriptine:
   (A) should be continued throughout the duration of pregnancy.
   (B) should never be given during pregnancy due to its teratogenic effects.
   (C) should be stopped during pregnancy and restarted only if signs and symptoms of tumor recurrence develop.
   (D) does not interfere with breast-feeding.

7. Fetal warfarin syndrome occurs from exposure to coumarin derivatives during the:
   (A) first trimester.
   (B) second trimester.
   (C) third trimester.
   (D) second and third trimesters.
   (E) first and third trimesters.

8. When used during pregnancy, heparin:
   (A) crosses the placenta but is safe.
   (B) crosses the placenta and produces severe teratogenic effects.
   (C) does not cross the placenta and therefore causes no adverse effects.
   (D) does not cross the placenta but still produces adverse effects.
   (E) none of the above

9. Glucocorticoid therapy during pregnancy:
   (A) is always contraindicated.
   (B) may be associated with adverse effects but typically at higher doses.
   (C) precipitates spontaneous abortions.
   (D) delays fetal lung maturation.
   (E) none of the above

10. Nimodipine:
    (A) has been thoroughly studied and has no known adverse effects when used during pregnancy.
    (B) is associated with severe teratogenic effects in human beings but has no adverse effects in animal studies.
    (C) produces folic acid deficiency.
    (D) should be used with caution since few studies are available which address the safety of this drug in pregnancy.
    (E) is compatible with breast-feeding.

CHAPTER 2

Neuroradiological Diagnosis During Pregnancy: Risks and Guidelines

1. Ionizing radiation reacts with biological tissues to form:
   (A) ion pairs.
   (B) free radicals.
   (C) both
   (D) neither

2. What is the major difference between ionizing waves and ionizing particles?
   (A) Waves exhibit low energy and particles exhibit high energy.
   (B) Waves exhibit low penetrance and particles exhibit low energy.
   (C) Waves exhibit high energy and particles exhibit low energy.
   (D) Waves exhibit high penetrance and particles exhibit low penetrance.

3. One "rad" (radiation absorbed dose) is equal to:
   (A) 100 Gy.
   (B) approximately 100 roentgen.
   (C) 10 cGy.
   (D) approximately 1 roentgen.

4. Which of the following is true?
   (A) 1 rad equals 1 rem equals 1 roentgen
   (B) 1 sievert equals 100 rem equals 100 rad
   (C) both
   (D) neither

5. Which of the following is *not* true regarding the data concerning radiation effects on the fetus?
   (A) There is little reliable human data.
   (B) Animal data can be readily extrapolated to humans.
   (C) Data from atomic bomb survivors have been a major source of information.
   (D) Therapeutic irradiation during the early part of the century has been a source of data.

6. Which of the following is a true radiation effect of the fetus?
   (A) During implantation (Days 1-15), the most likely effect is growth retardation.
   (B) During organogenesis (Days 15-50), the most likely effect is death.
   (C) both
   (D) neither

7. Which of the following statement is *true*?
   (A) During preimplantation, the major effect of radiation on the fetus is death.
   (B) The effect of radiation to the fetus prior to implantation is usually an "all or none" phenomenon.
   (C) During organogenesis, the central nervous system is highly sensitive to radiation.
   (D) all of the above

8. Which statement is most accurate regarding diagnostic imaging during pregnancy?
   (A) Most studies show no statistical correlation between diagnostic x-rays and congenital malformation.
   (B) Diagnostic x-rays should never be performed during pregnancy.
   (C) For most routine diagnostic studies, the maximum radiation dose to the fetus is considerably higher than the threshold at which malformations are thought to occur.
   (D) Computed tomography scans of the brain expose the fetus to high levels of radiation through scatter.

9. Which statement is most accurate regarding occupational exposure during pregnancy?
   (A) Pregnant radiologists should refrain completely from performing angiography.
   (B) Pregnant radiologists may have unlimited exposure as long as a lead shield is worn to protect the fetus.
   (C) By following strict guideline for radiation protection and quality assurance, the radiation exposure to the fetus of a pregnant radiologist should

fall well below the guidelines set by the National Council on Radiation Protection and Measurements and the International Commission on Radiological Protection.
(D) The primary concern for occupational exposure is during the second trimester of pregnancy.

10. Which of the following most accurately reflects the use of magnetic resonance imaging (MRI) during pregnancy?
(A) MRI should not be used during pregnancy for any reason.
(B) The Food and Drug Administration prohibits the use of MRI during pregnancy.
(C) MRI should be used during the first trimester only if clear medical indications exist and there is a definite advantage over other tests.
(D) MRI can be used safely during the entire period of gestation without concern.

CHAPTER 3

FETAL EFFECTS OF ANESTHESIA

1. Important physiological changes of pregnancy that impact on anesthetic practice include which of the following?
(A) soft tissue swelling of the airway
(B) an increase in cardiac output
(C) an increased sensitivity to anesthetic drugs
(D) despite fasting, the parturient is at risk for aspiration of gastric contents
(E) all of the above

2. Uterine blood flow:
(A) is autoregulated.
(B) arises from the inferior epigastric artery.
(C) is unaffected by maternal position.
(D) increases by 700% near term.
(E) all of the above

3. Fetal monitoring during surgery:
(A) is rarely possible.
(B) is not reliable until 34 weeks' gestational age.
(C) may be possible at 18 weeks' gestational age.
(D) is unaffected by anesthetic agents.
(E) should not be continued into the postoperative period.

4. Raised intracranial pressure in parturients has been safely treated by:
(A) barbiturates.
(B) mannitol.
(C) maternal hyperventilation.
(D) furosemide.
(E) all of the above.

5. Concerning the effects of hyperventilation in pregnancy,
(A) hyperventilation is associated with increased uterine blood flow.
(B) the change in blood flow is likely due to the effects of positive pressure ventilation on venous return and cardiac output.
(C) the safe lower limit of maternal hypocapnia is 35 mm Hg.
(D) the normal maternal $PaCO_2$ at term is 40 mm Hg.
(E) all of the above

6. Concerning induced hypotension during pregnancy:
(A) one minimum alveolar concentration isoflurane is not associated with significant decreases in uterine blood flow.
(B) sodium nitroprusside use may be associated with fetal cyanide toxicity.
(C) trimethaphan may impair neurological examination.
(D) nitroglycerin has been used safely as a hypotensive agent in pregnancy.
(E) all of the above

7. Mannitol:
(A) is probably safe in moderate doses (<1.0 gm/kg maternal weight).
(B) will not lead to fetal dehydration.
(C) is contraindicated in pregnancy.
(D) does not cross the placenta.

8. Patient positioning may be complicated in pregnancy since:
   (A) there is little experience on the sitting position in parturients.
   (B) position and site of surgery may make fetal monitoring difficult.
   (C) aortocaval compression by the gravid uterus may produce fetal hypoxemia without maternal symptoms.
   (D) all of the above

9. General comments on the effects of anesthesia during pregnancy include which one of the following?
   (A) Anesthesia has been associated with human fetal anomalies.
   (B) The relative risk of anesthesia or surgery alone is not known.
   (C) Neurosurgery should never occur during the first trimester.
   (D) It is pointless to perform fetal monitoring in pre-viable (i.e., <24 weeks' gestational age) fetuses.
   (E) Regional anesthesia is associated with lower fetal morbidity and mortality than general anesthesia.

10. Regarding specific anesthetic agents:
   (A) muscle relaxants cross the placenta in clinically significant amounts.
   (B) the normally useful induction drug thiopental should not be used in pregnancy.
   (C) most intravenous and inhalational anesthetic agents cross the placenta readily and may sedate or anesthetize the fetus.
   (D) small doses of benzodiazepines have little effect on fetal heart rate beat-to-beat variability.
   (E) all of the above

CHAPTER 4

CHANGES IN CARDIOVASCULAR AND CEREBROVASCULAR FUNCTION DURING PREGNANCY

1. Which of the following hemodynamic measurements decreases during the course of normal pregnancy?
   (A) heart rate
   (B) blood pressure
   (C) blood volume
   (D) cardiac output
   (E) all of the above

2. The anemia observed in normal pregnancy:
   (A) is due to increased iron metabolism by the fetus.
   (B) occurs in spite of increases in the total red blood cell mass.
   (C) is refractory to iron supplementation.
   (D) is due to impaired gastrointestinal absorption of iron.
   (E) all of the above

3. During normal pregnancy, the supine position:
   (A) may result in compression of the vena cava.
   (B) may result in compression of the aorta.
   (C) both
   (D) neither

4. Cardiac failure is most likely during:
   (A) the first trimester of normal pregnancy.
   (B) the second trimester of normal pregnancy.
   (C) the third trimester of normal pregnancy.
   (D) labor.
   (E) none of the above

5. Hypertension observed during pregnancy:
   (A) may be transient.
   (B) is often associated with renal artery stenosis.

(C) occurs only during first pregnancies.
(D) occurs only in women with pre-existing or latent hypertension.
(E) all of the above

6. Categories of hypertension associated with pregnancy include:
(A) pre-eclampsia/eclampsia.
(B) chronic hypertension.
(C) pre-eclampsia superimposed on chronic hypertension.
(D) transient hypertension.
(E) all of the above

7. Cardiac output:
(A) increases only during active labor.
(B) returns to normal immediately after delivery.
(C) increases during the first trimester and then remains stable.
(D) remains elevated through the second day after delivery.
(E) none of the above

8. The decrease in peripheral vascular resistance seen during normal pregnancy may:
(A) stimulate increases in plasma volume.
(B) be due to the presence of the utero-placental circulation.
(C) be due to direct vasodilatory effects of circulating hormones.
(D) all of the above
(E) none of the above

9. Blood loss during delivery:
(A) corrects the increased blood volume which occurs during pregnancy.
(B) increases with delivery of twins.
(C) is less with cesarean than with vaginal delivery.
(D) all of the above
(E) none of the above

10. Cerebral blood flow during pregnancy:
(A) is known definitively to increase.
(B) is known definitively to decrease.
(C) probably increases but is insufficiently studied.
(D) probably decreases but is insufficiently studied.

CHAPTER 5

Hemostasis and Thrombosis Considerations in Pregnancy

1. Pregnant patients with Type I von Willebrand's disease are at greatest risk of hemorrhage in the:
(A) first trimester.
(B) second trimester.
(C) third trimester.
(D) peripartum period.
(E) first and second week postpartum.

2. All of the following are true concerning DDAVP (desmopressin acetate) *except*:
(A) DDAVP is an effective treatment of mild factor VIII deficiency.
(B) DDAVP treatment shortens the bleeding time in uremia.
(C) DDAVP is an effective treatment of thrombotic thrombocytopenia purpura.
(D) DDAVP can cause hyponatremia in the fetus.
(E) DDAVP is an effective treatment of Type I von Willebrand's disease.

3. The most frequent naturally occurring coagulation factor inhibitor is directed at:
(A) factor X.
(B) factor VIII.
(C) fibrinogen.
(D) the von Willebrand factor.
(E) factor VII.

4. Which of the following complications of pregnancy is associated with disseminated intravascular coagulation (DIC)?
(A) abruptio placenta
(B) amniotic fluid embolism
(C) retained dead fetus
(D) tubal pregnancy
(E) all are correct

5. The most important treatment of DIC is:
   (A) anticoagulation with heparin.
   (B) inhibition of fibrinolysis with Amicar.
   (C) coagulation factor replacement.
   (D) treatment of the underlying cause.
   (E) platelet infusion.

6. How frequently does deep venous thrombosis complicate pregnancy?
   (A) less than one in 10,000 persons
   (B) one to four in 10,000 persons
   (C) one to four in 1,000 persons
   (D) one to three in 100 persons
   (E) three to five in 100 persons

7. What percent of maternal deaths are due to pulmonary embolus?
   (A) 21%
   (B) 11%
   (C) 1%
   (D) 0.5%
   (E) 0.11%

8. Severe deficiency of factor XII is associated with all of the following *except*:
   (A) reduced activation of the fibrinolytic system.
   (B) moderately severe bleeding disorder.
   (C) markedly prolonged APTT.
   (D) increased risk of thrombosis.
   (E) reduced activation of factor XI in vitro.

9. Coumadin therapy reduces the functional levels of all of the following factors *except*:
   (A) factor X.
   (B) prothrombin.
   (C) protein S.
   (D) factor V.
   (E) factor VII.

10. In pregnant patients with idiopathic thrombocytopenic purpura, the mortality rate is approximately:
   (A) 0.1 %
   (B) 0.5%
   (C) 1%
   (D) 5%
   (E) 10%

CHAPTER 6

Back Pain in Pregnancy

1. What percentage of pregnant women experience some degree of back pain during pregnancy?
   (A) 10%
   (B) 30%
   (C) 50%
   (D) 90%

2. What factor has been clearly associated with an increased incidence of back pain during pregnancy?
   (A) patient age
   (B) parity
   (C) antenatal history of pain
   (D) strenuous activity
   (C) all of the above

3. Which of the following modalities would be most effective in reducing the incidence of back pain in the perinatal period?
   (A) antenatal counseling
   (B) posture training
   (C) regular exercise
   (D) limiting weight gain

4. During pregnancy, the hormone relaxin exerts its effects by:
   (A) causing proliferation of connective tissue.
   (B) causing proliferation and increasing the vascularity of connective tissue.
   (C) resulting in vascularization and softening of the proliferative connective tissue.
   (D) relaxing the tension on ligamentous structures allowing for adaptive changes to occur during growth of the fetus and delivery.

5. The tendency to herniate an intervertebral disc during pregnancy:
   (A) approximates that of the general population.
   (B) occurs at a frequency of about one in 10,000.

(C) does not change during the pregnancy; however, the greater the number of pregnancies resulting in a live birth that the woman has, the greater the tendency for a herniated intervertebral disc.
(D) all of the above

6. Scoliosis, spondylytic disease, and pain related to rheumatoid arthritis of the spine have been shown to exacerbate with pregnancy.
A) true B) false

7. Night pain during pregnancy most likely results from fatigue.
A) true B) false

8. Most back pain during pregnancy is self-limited and as such requires conservative care and usually no diagnostic evaluation.
A) true B) false

9. The risk associated with magnetic resonance imaging appears to be acceptable during pregnancy; however, the results of imaging should be interpreted carefully as findings may not correlate with the clinical history or examination.
A) true B) false

10. Antenatal counseling will reduce a significant portion of back pain during pregnancy and may be the most effective treatment modality.
A) true B) false

CHAPTER 7

Carpal Tunnel Syndrome in Pregnancy

1. The author(s) credited with the first description of the carpal tunnel syndrome (CTS) is/are:
(A) Soferman et al
(B) Putnam
(C) Tobin
(D) Wallace and Cook

2. The author(s) credited with being the first to recognize the possible relationship between CTS and pregnancy is/are?
(A) Soferman et al
(B) Putnam
(C) Tobin
(D) Wallace and Cook

3. The incidence of CTS in pregnancy is:
(A) 1%-10%.
(B) 2%-15%.
(C) 2%-35%.
(D) 5%-20%.

4. What is considered to be the best conservative treatment for CTS in pregnancy?
(A) hydrocortisone injection
(B) estrogen therapy
(C) nonsteroidal anti-inflammatory medications
(D) splinting

5. CTS in pregnancy is usually:
(A) bilateral.
(B) left-sided.
(C) right-sided.

6. When is the onset of CTS most prevalent?
(A) first trimester
(B) second trimester
(C) third trimester

7. What is the most common natural history of CTS in pregnancy?
(A) spontaneous relief with parturition
(B) relief in the postpartum period only after surgical decompression of the median nerve
(C) relief only after high-dose estrogen therapy
(D) no relief obtainable

8. Is there a correlation between weight gain and the onset of CTS in pregnancy?
(A) yes
(B) no

9. What is the calculated morbidity ratio for women to develop CTS in pregnancy?
(A) 1
(B) 2.5
(C) 3
(D) 3.5

10. In most studies discussed in this review did parity correlate with the development of CTS in pregnancy?
    (A) yes
    (B) no
    (C) unknown

CHAPTER 8

Pituitary Tumors and Sheehan's Syndrome in Pregnant Women

1. The pituitary gland enlarges during pregnancy by approximately:
    (A) 10%-20%.
    (B) 25%-30%.
    (C) 30%-50%.
    (D) 50%-70%.
    (E) 70%-100%.

2. During pregnancy, physiological changes of endocrinological importance include:
    (A) lower gonadotropin concentrations and a diminished response to gonadotropin-releasing hormone.
    (B) attenuated growth hormone response to insulin and arginine.
    (C) elevated adrenocorticotropic hormone concentrations, despite a rise in plasma cortisol.
    (D) no significant change in thyrotropin, free thyroxine, or tri-iodothyronine concentrations.
    (E) all of the above

3. Regarding the natural history of pituitary tumors during pregnancy, all are true *except:*
    (A) headaches usually manifest during the first trimester.
    (B) visual disturbances occur equally during all trimesters of pregnancy.
    (C) prolactinomas usually decrease in size but all other tumors increase in size.
    (D) most patients with microadenoms do not require treatment during pregnancy.

4. A patient harboring a prolactinoma should:
    (A) not lactate since suckling would significantly increase prolactin levels.
    (B) be given estrogen to inhibit lactation.
    (C) be treated prior to pregnancy if the tumor is a macroprolactinoma.
    (D) not be given bromocriptine during pregnancy because of the significant risk of teratogenicity associated with this drug.

5. In pregnant patients with a growth hormone-secreting pituitary tumor and acromegaly, the following are true *except:*
    (A) somatomedin-C concentrations may be spuriously decreased during pregnancy, therefore results should be interpreted cautiously.
    (B) pregnancy may result in significant tumor expansion.
    (C) bromocriptine can be given during pregnancy and can be effective in limiting tumor expansion.
    (D) all of the above

6. In pregnant patients with Cushing's disease:
    (A) plasma cortisol is reduced because of increased metabolic turnover.
    (B) the usual diurnal variation of plasma cortisol is maintained during pregnancy.
    (C) urinary-free cortisol is reduced secondary to the reduction in plasma cortisol during pregnancy.
    (D) there may be an increase in the incidence of miscarriage.

7. Concerning Sheehan's syndrome, which of the following is *true?*
    (A) Clinical presentation includes altered menstrual pattern, diminished or absent lactation, fatigue, altered level of consciousness, heat intolerance, hyperthyroidism, and genital hypertrophy.
    (B) Hormone therapy may result in successful pregnancy. An established pregnancy is incontrovertible evidence against the diagnosis of Sheehan's syndrome.

(C) An established pregnancy is incontrovertible evidence against the diagnosis of Sheehan's syndrome.
(D) none of the above

8. Most cases of lymphocytic hypophysitis are:
(A) associated with a co-existing pituitary adenoma.
(B) in males aged over 65 years.
(C) associated with a hyperfunctioning anterior pituitary gland.
(D) usually diagnosed at or before conception.
(E) none of the above

9. Diabetes insipidus:
(A) may significantly reduce a woman's fertility.
(B) may retard the progress of labor.
(C) usually worsens during pregnancy.
(D) all of the above

10. During pregnancy:
(A) prolactinomas are the most common pituitary tumor encountered.
(B) a patient presenting with acute visual loss from an expanding macroprolactinoma should only be treated by medical therapy.
(C) hypopituitarism may result in abortion.
(D) A and C
(E) all of the above

CHAPTER 9

Spontaneous SAH in Pregnancy and the Puerperium

1. The most common cause of subarachnoid hemorrhage (SAH) in pregnancy is:
(A) saccular (berry) aneurysm.
(B) arteriovenous malformation (AVM).
(C) venous angioma.
(D) trauma.

2. Which of the following may be found in association with both aneurysmal rupture and eclampsia?
(A) proteinuria
(B) hypertension
(C) intraparenchymal hemorrhage
(D) SAH
(E) all of the above

3. Which of the following is not a normal (physiological) hemodynamic change associated with pregnancy?
(A) increased cardiac output
(B) increased blood volume
(C) decreased central venous pressure
(D) decreased mean arterial pressure
(E) decreased hematocrit

4. Aneurysmal rupture is most likely to occur initially during:
(A) the first trimester.
(B) the second trimester.
(C) the third trimester.
(D) labor and delivery.

5. Women suffering aneurysmal SAH:
(A) rarely have had a previous uncomplicated pregnancy.
(B) frequently have had a previous uncomplicated pregnancy.
(C) are less likely than those with AVM to have had a previous uncomplicated pregnancy.
(D) rarely rehemorrhage.

6. Which of the following pharmacological agents is absolutely contraindicated for use in the pregnant patient with SAH?
(A) phenytoin
(B) nimodipine
(C) mannitol
(D) aminocaproic acid
(E) none of the above

7. A 25-year-old gravida 3 para 2 woman presents at 20 weeks of gestation with the acute onset of severe headache and nuchal rigidity, but demonstrates no focal neurological deficit or depression of consciousness. Diffuse SAH is identified on a computed tomography scan of the brain. Cerebral angiography demonstrates a 15-mm right posterior communicating artery aneurysm. The most appropriate management would consist of:
   (A) craniotomy, then clip ligation of the aneurysm within 24°.
   (B) endovascular balloon embolization.
   (C) expectant (nonoperative) management.
   (D) medical management until the third trimester, then surgical clip ligation of the aneurysm.

8. Which of the following statements regarding cerebral angiography is *true?*
   (A) The positive yield of cerebral angiography is lower in pregnant patients than in the general population.
   (B) Iodinated intravascular contrast agents are teratogenic.
   (C) Angiography may be performed safely in the third trimester, but should be avoided prior to this time.
   (D) Angiography may cause fetal dehydration.
   (E) Vertebrobasilar angiography is not essential because posterior circulation aneurysms rarely rupture during pregnancy.

9. Which of the following statements regarding AVM in the pregnant patient is false?
   (A) The parietal lobe is involved in one-third to one-half of cases.
   (B) Rehemorrhage is more common than in the general population.
   (C) The initial manifestation of an AVM is usually SAH.
   (D) Angiomatous SAH occurs most frequently in the first trimester of pregnancy.
   (E) Vasospasm following angiomatous hemorrhage is rare.

10. Which of the following statements regarding anesthetic management of the pregnant patient with SAH is *false*?
   (A) Hypothermia is well-tolerated by both mother and fetus.
   (B) The requirement for volatile anesthetic agents is reduced.
   (C) Mechanical hyperventilation may precipitate fetal hypoxia and acidosis.
   (D) The supine position is well-tolerated for craniotomy during the third trimester.
   (E) The use of sodium nitroprusside may induce fetal cyanide toxicity.

CHAPTER 10

VENOUS THROMBOTIC DISORDERS IN PREGNANCY

1. Pregnancy increases the risk of thromboembolic disease:
   (A) two-fold.
   (B) three- to four-fold.
   (C) five- to six-fold.
   (D) seven- to eight-fold.

2. Thromboembolic complications:
   (A) present at any time during pregnancy or the puerperium.
   (B) occur more frequently during the puerperium.
   (C) originate from deep vein thrombosis (DVT) occurring more frequently in the right leg during pregnancy.
   (D) originate from DVT occurring more frequently in the pelvic veins.

3. The clinical diagnosis of DVT is correct:
   (A) 20% of the time.
   (B) 50% of the time.
   (C) 75% of the time.
   (D) 85% of the time.

4. Identify the laboratory test not yet confirmed effective for diagnosis of DVT with Level I evidence.
   (A) impedance plethysmography
   (B) venography
   (C) B-mode imaging/Doppler ultrasonography
   (D) nuclear venogram

5. Diagnosis of pulmonary embolism can be established with any of the following *except*:
   (A) pulmonary angiogram
   (B) ventilation-perfusion scan
   (C) arterial blood gas measurement
   (D) venogram or impedance plethysmography

6. Which of the following statements is *false*?
   (A) Radiation exposure to the fetus during venography is about 500 mrad.
   (B) Radiation exposure to the fetus during pulmonary angiography is about 405 mrad.
   (C) Radiation exposure to the fetus during pulmonary angiography performed through a brachial artery is about 250 mrad.
   (D) Radiation exposure to the fetus for ventilation-perfusion scanning is about 55 mrad.

7. The risk for developing DVT is:
   (A) as high as 50% in patients with spinal cord injury.
   (B) up to 53% in the nonparalyzed leg of stroke patients.
   (C) lowest in brain tumor patients.
   (D) higher in patients with meningioma compared with glioma.

8. Which of the following drugs or mechanisms is contraindicated for prophylaxis of thromboembolic events (DVT or pulmonary embolism) during pregnancy?
   (A) heparin
   (B) intermittent pneumatic compression
   (C) low molecular weight heparin (LMWH)
   (D) warfarin

9. Which of the following statements is *false*?
   (A) Heparin requirements can fluctuate tremendously during pregnancy.
   (B) Osteoporosis occurs in 20% of patients treated for more than 4 weeks with heparin.
   (C) LMWH is administered subcutaneously in a fixed-dose based on body weight and does not require monitoring of the activated partial thromboplastin time.
   (D) LMWH requirements do not appear to fluctuate during pregnancy.

10. Which of the following statements is *true*?
   (A) The diagnosis of intracranial venous thrombosis can be established with either magnetic resonance imaging or angiography.
   (B) Intracranial venous thrombosis occurs with a frequency of one in 1,000 deliveries.
   (C) Intracranial venous thrombosis occurs with equal frequency during pregnancy and during the puerperium.
   (D) Standard treatment of intracranial venous thrombosis includes administration of thrombolytic agents such as tissue-type plasminogen activator or streptokinase.

CHAPTER 11

Cerebral Embolism in Pregnant Women

1. Pathognomonic signs exist for diagnosis of:
   (A) air embolism.
   (B) fat embolism.
   (C) amniotic fluid embolism.
   (D) none of the above.

2. All of the following are true *except:*
   (A) Liebermeister's sign and a "mill-wheel" murmur may suggest a diagnosis of air embolism.
   (B) Dyspnea, stupor, and conjunctival petechia suggest a diagnosis of fat embolism.
   (C) Neurological sequelae are usually helpful in diagnosing amniotic fluid embolism.
   (D) A history of a molar pregnancy in a patient with sudden hemiparesis is suggestive of metastatic choriocarcinoma.

3. Which of the following is *false?*
   (A) Fetal debris in the buffy coat may be found with amniotic fluid embolism.
   (B) The pregnant patient is probably at increased risk of air embolism through vaginal air insufflation.
   (C) Cocaine causes ischemic stroke primarily through vasospasm of small intracerebral vessels.
   (D) Arterial dissection occurs more commonly during labor or delivery.

4. All of the following are false *except:*
   (A) Pregnant patients with mechanical prosthetic valves should be treated with aspirin alone.
   (B) Cocaine use increases the risk of stroke.
   (C) Delayed hyperbaric oxygen treatment is the treatment of choice for stroke due to air embolism.
   (D) The investigation of the etiology of embolic stroke should be delayed until the pregnancy has been completed.

5. Which of the following is *false?*
   (A) Only amniotic fluid embolism and metastatic choriocarcinoma are unique to pregnancy.
   (B) Pregnancy may place a patient at increased risk of stroke due to air embolism.
   (C) There is no effective therapy for air embolism.
   (D) It is unclear if pregnancy increases the risk of dissection.

6. Warfarin use during pregnancy is:
   (A) completely safe.
   (B) associated with an embryopathy if used between 6 and 12 weeks of gestation.
   (C) not associated with central nervous system malformations.
   (D) is associated with high rates of thromboembolism.

7. Patients with all of the following conditions should be given antibiotic prophylaxis prior to labor and delivery *except*:
   (A) patent foramen ovale.
   (B) prosthetic heart valves.
   (C) rheumatic valvular disease.
   (D) mitral valve prolapse.

8. Heparin use in pregnancy:
   (A) may be associated with Dandy-Walker syndrome in the fetus.
   (B) can cause osteoporosis with long-term use.
   (C) should always be via an intravenous route.
   (D) is contraindicated in the weeks preceding delivery.

9. Peripartum cardiomyopathy:
   (A) is due to poorly controlled hypertension.
   (B) is more common in Caucasians.
   (C) usually occurs in the first trimester.
   (D) can present with cerebral embolism.

10. Paradoxical embolism can occur in the following conditions *except* when:
   (A) there is a left-to-right shunting.
   (B) right atrial pressure is elevated due to a Valsalva manuver.
   (C) there is venous thrombophlebitis.
   (D) a patent foramen ovale is present.

CHAPTER 12

CHORIOCARCINOMA IN PREGNANCY

1. Each of the following is a true statement *except*:
   (A) Choriocarcinoma is the most malignant tumor associated with pregnancy.
   (B) It involves the nervous system in 1% of cases.
   (C) It is preceded by hydatidiform mole in half the cases.
   (D) It is a leading cause of post-partum stroke.
   (E) It is a leading cause of oncotic aneurysms.

2. The pathology of choriocarcinoma includes all of the following *except*:
   (A) syncytotrophoblastic elements.
   (B) immunoreactivity for human chorionic gonadotropin (hCG).
   (C) well-differentiated cytotrophoblasts.
   (D) immunoreactivity for human placental lactogen.
   (E) pleomorphism, hemorrhage, and vascular invasion.

3. The following are true about cerebral metastases from choriocarcinoma *except*:
   (A) the majority of lesions are hemorrhagic.
   (B) the majority of cases are solitary lesions.
   (C) the majority are in the middle cerebral artery distribution.
   (D) the majority spread by the cerebrospinal fluid pathway.
   (E) the majority are preceded by pulmonary lesions.

4. The typical patient with central nervous system (CNS) choriocarcinoma is:
   (A) young, female, Asian, post-partum.
   (B) middle-aged, female, Asian, with hydatidiform mole.
   (C) young, male, Asian, with testicular tumor.
   (D) young, female, Caucasian, with pineal lesion.
   (E) young, female, Asian, with no history of pregnancy.

5. The classic clinical triad for CNS choriocarcinoma includes each of the following *except*:
   (A) childbearing age and menstrual abnormalities.
   (B) recent or remote pregnancy or abortion.
   (C) acute cerebrovascular event with evidence of mass lesion.
   (D) undiagnosed primary tumor.

6. Prognosis in patients with systemic choriocarcinoma is adversely affected by each of the following *except*:
   (A) metastases to the brain.
   (B) presence of hydatidiform mole rather than pregnancy event.
   (C) delay in diagnosis >4 months.
   (D) high plasma beta-hCG titers.
   (E) term pregnancy rather than spontaneous abortion.

7. Treatment options in metastatic choriocarcinoma include each of the following *except*:
   (A) chemotherapy in patients with or without CNS disease.
   (B) chemotherapy without cranial radiation for a single brain lesion.
   (C) chemotherapy and cranial radiation for multiple CNS lesions.
   (D) craniotomy, chemotherapy, and radiation for solitary hemorrhagic CNS lesion.
   (E) multiagent chemotherapy up-front in high-risk patients.

8. The following statements about multi-agent chemotherapy for choriocarcinoma are true *except*:
   (A) the response rate is lower for patients with extrapulmonary metastatic lesions.
   (B) the response rate is lower after a term pregnancy.
   (C) the response rate is lower when used up-front.
   (D) methotrexate, cytoxan, and actinomycin-D are often used.
   (E) normalization of hCG is one criterion of response.

CHAPTER 13

Nerve Injuries Related to Childbirth

1. Obstetrical factors known to cause birth-related brachial plexus injury include all but one of the following:
   (A) shoulder dystocia.
   (B) high infant birth weight.
   (C) primigravida.
   (D) multiparous mother.

2. The incidence of birth-related brachial plexus injury is:
   (A) one in 100.
   (B) one in 1000.
   (C) 10 in 100.
   (D) 10 in 1000.

3. Improvement from a birth-related brachial plexus injury should begin by:
   (A) 1 month of age.
   (B) 2 months of age.
   (C) 3 months of age.
   (D) 4 months of age.

4. Neurological improvement from a birth-related brachial plexus injury can be predicted by:
   (A) electromyography (EMG).
   (B) neurological examination.
   (C) computed tomography-myelogram.
   (D) nerve conduction.

5. Avulsions are:
   (A) nerve root breakage.
   (B) nerve rootlet breakage.
   (C) nerve trunk breakage.
   (D) peripheral nerve breakage.

6. Ruptures are breakages of all but which one of the following?
   (A) nerve root
   (B) nerve rootlet
   (C) nerve trunk
   (D) peripheral nerve

7. Avulsions occur primarily at which one or more nerve root levels?
   (A) C5
   (B) C6
   (C) C7
   (D) C8

8. Ruptures occur primarily at which one or more nerve root levels?
   (A) C5
   (B) C6
   (C) C7
   (D) C8

9. Intraoperative electrodiagnostic testing (EMG, evoked responses) is used to determine:
   (A) nerve rootlet transmission to spinal cord.
   (B) avulsions.
   (C) distal muscle responses.
   (D) ruptures.
   (E) all of the above

10. Major structures to consider when exploring the upper brachial plexus via the supraclavicular approach include the:
    (A) pleura.
    (B) vertebral artery.
    (C) phrenic nerve.
    (D) thoracic duct.
    (E) all of the above

CHAPTER 14

Idiopathic Intracranial Hypertension (Pseudotumor Cerebri), Hydrocephalus, and Ventriculoperitoneal Shunts in Pregnancy

1. Common signs of pseudotumor cerebri include all of the following *except*:
   (A) headache.
   (B) seizures.

(C) dizziness.
(D) diplopia.

2. According to Durcan's review, the average annual incidence of idiopathic intracranial hypertension (IIH) in the normal population is approximately:
   (A) one in 10,000.
   (B) one in 100,000.
   (C) four in 1,000,000.
   (D) four in 100,000.

3. In the same survey by Durcan et al, the incidence of IIH in pregnant females is increased by how many in comparison to the normal population?
   (A) two-fold
   (B) four-fold
   (C) 10-fold
   (D) 20-fold

4. In women who are over 20% above their ideal body weight, the incidence of IIH is increased by approximately how many?
   (A) two-fold
   (B) four-fold
   (C) 10-fold
   (D) 20-fold

5. Conditions believed to be associated with IIH include all of the following *except:*
   (A) rapid steroid withdrawal.
   (B) Addison's disease.
   (C) vitamin A intake.
   (D) anorexia.

6. The percentage of IIH patients who present with diplopia is approximately:
   (A) 10%.
   (B) 20%.
   (C) 30%.
   (D) 40%.

7. The most sensitive method of following visual function in pregnant patients with IIH is:
   (A) serial visual field examinations.
   (B) visual evoked responses.
   (C) indirect ophthalmoscopy.
   (D) retinal fluoroscopy.

8. According to the available literature, which of the following statements is *false?*
   (A) Extracranial shunting is generally a contraindication for vaginal delivery.
   (B) Hydrocephalus is not a contraindication for intrauterine pregnancy.
   (C) Exacerbation of hydrocephalus during pregnancy has been managed with shunt pumping.
   (D) Most authors avoid antibiotic prophylaxis for delivery in pregnant women with shunts.

9. The incidence of bacteremia during delivery has been estimated at:
   (A) 0.1%.
   (B) 0.5%.
   (C) 1.0%.
   (D) 5.0%.

10. In the largest available literature series published to date, what percentage of pregnant patients with shunts required cesarean section for delivery?
   (A) 1%
   (B) 5%
   (C) 15%
   (D) 30%

CHAPTER 15

Operative Positioning and Fetal Monitoring Considerations

1. Which of the following maneuvers does *not* threaten fetal physiology during a surgical procedure involving a pregnant patient?
   (A) maternal hyperventilation
   (B) maternal hypothermia
   (C) maternal hypotension
   (D) supine positioning

2. Which of the following hematological changes is *atypical* for a normal pregnancy?
   (A) increased hematocrit
   (B) increased erythrocyte volume
   (C) increased blood volume
   (D) increased platelet count

3. Uterine blood flow is influenced by which of the following?
   (A) cardiac output
   (B) progesterone
   (C) maternal blood pressure
   (D) maternal position
   (E) all of the above

4. The "supine hypotensive syndrome" relates primarily to which of the following?
   (A) dilutional anemia
   (B) extracellular fluid retention
   (C) compression of the aorta and vena cava
   (D) occult hemorrhage

5. A 35-year-old woman in her 33rd week of pregnancy suffers subarachnoid hemorrhage. Admission electrocardiogram demonstrates left axis deviation and paroxysmal supraventricular tachycardia. These findings are suggestive of which of the following?
   (A) subendocardial myocardial infarction
   (B) increased myocardial workload due to catecholamine release
   (C) normal physiology
   (D) increased risk during general anesthesia

6. Which of the following pulmonary changes is not expected in pregnancy?
   (A) reduced functional residual capacity
   (B) increased tidal volume
   (C) increased respiratory rate
   (D) decreased oxygen extraction

7. Maternal hypotension is related to all of the following *except:*
   (A) increased cardiac output.
   (B) failure of the uteroplacental vasculature to vasodilate.
   (C) fetal bradycardia.
   (D) spinal anesthesia.

8. Which of the following is associated with fetal distress?
   (A) light halothane anesthesia
   (B) fetal tachycardia
   (C) maternal pCO_2 of 35 mm Hg
   (D) fetal bradycardia
   (E) all of the above
   (F) B and D
   (G) A and C

9. The most desirable position for a patient in the third trimester undergoing craniotomy for aneurysm is which of the following?
   (A) concorde
   (B) supine with large right hip roll
   (C) supine, neutral
   (D) prone

10. Lumbar laminectomy can be complicated in the pregnant patient by which of the following?
   (A) epidural venous engorgement
   (B) excessive dose of regional anesthetic agent
   (C) maternal hypotension
   (D) fetal bradycardia
   (E) all of the above
   (F) A and C
   (G) B and D
   (H) A, B, and C

CHAPTER 16

INTRAUTERINE DIAGNOSIS OF DEVELOPMENTAL NEUROSURGICAL DISORDERS

1. Which of the following clinical states is not associated with an elevated maternal serum alpha-fetoprotein?
   (A) normal pregnancy
   (B) twin pregnancy
   (C) open neural tube defect
   (D) maternal insulin-dependent diabetes mellitus
   (E) fetal death

2. Which of the following statements is *true* concerning alpha-fetoprotein measurements?
   (A) Maternal serum alpha-fetoprotein levels decline steadily throughout pregnancy.
   (B) Mean amniotic fluid alpha-fetoprotein levels rise sharply during the 12th week of gestation, peak at Week 13, and then decline approximately 12% per week.
   (C) Amniotic fluid alpha-fetoprotein levels rise throughout pregnancy.
   (D) Amniotic fluid alpha-fetoprotein levels decline steadily throughout pregnancy.
   (E) Maternal serum alpha-fetoprotein levels rise through the 20th week of gestation, peak, and then decline approximately 15% per week.

3. The most common cause for an elevated amniotic fluid alpha-fetoprotein level is:
   (A) anencephaly.
   (B) gastroschisis.
   (C) fetal blood contamination of the amniotic fluid.
   (D) hydrocephaly.
   (E) twin pregnancy.

4. Which of the following statements concerning intrauterine fetal ultrasound is *false*?
   (A) The threshold for imaging the lateral ventricles is approximately 12 weeks of gestation.
   (B) At 15 weeks' gestation, the lateral ventricles are mostly filled with choroid plexus.
   (C) Normal ventricular to hemispheric ratio during the second trimester is 50% ± 10%.
   (D) A second trimester fetal ultrasound on which the choroid plexus appears small with reference to the lateral ventricle portends a diagnosis of hydrocephalus.
   (E) Biparietal diameter of the fetal head is a sensitive indicator of early hydrocephalus.

5. With an established diagnosis of fetal hydrocephalus, which the following is *not* indicated for further evaluation?
   (A) complete ultrasound examination of the fetus to rule out other structural abnormalities
   (B) amniocentesis to measure alpha-fetoprotein, karyotype, and sex determination
   (C) amniotic fluid analysis for congenital infections such as toxoplasmosis, rubella, cytomegaloviral encephalus
   (D) cephalocentesis
   (E) serial ultrasonography to monitor for progressive hydrocephalus

6. Which of the following is *false* with reference to neural tube defects?
   (A) Open spina bifida requires surgical repair within 24 to 72 hours postpartum.
   (B) Ultrasound is capable of detecting bony defects as well as mass lesions.
   (C) Maternal serum alpha-fetoprotein levels are abnormally elevated in both open and closed neural tube defects.
   (D) Ultrasound study of the fetus is not useful for detecting integrity of the skin over a neural tube defect.
   (E) The presence of a sibling with spina bifida increases the chance for this anomaly in the fetus approximately 100 times.

7. Which of the following statements is *true* regarding a fetus with an encephalocele?
   (A) An encephalocele sac filled with cerebrospinal fluid predicts a poor outcome.
   (B) The presence of relative microcephaly improves the prognosis.
   (C) Occipital encephaloceles are associated with progressive hydrocephalus.
   (D) The prenatal diagnosis of encephalocele is usually made by elevated amniotic fluid alpha-fetoprotein.
   (E) Interval treatment of hydrocephalus is not acceptable management for encephalocele.

8. Which of the following statements is *false* with reference to intrauterine ultrasonography of the fetus?
   (A) A diagnosis of meningocele cannot be excluded by lack of demonstration of a neural tube defect.
   (B) Fetal edema is similar in appearance to intrauterine fetal death.
   (C) Cystic hygroma cannot be differentiated from a meningocele by ultrasonographic study.
   (D) Stunted twin gestational sac is often difficult to differentiate from meningocele.
   (E) Conjoined twins can have a similar appearance to that of a cephalic mass.

9. Which of the following is not an indication for ultrasound of the fetal central nervous system?
   (A) maternal diabetes mellitus
   (B) history of a neurological deficit in a sibling
   (C) low serum or amniotic fluid alpha-fetoprotein level
   (D) breech presentation
   (E) amniotic fluid volume abnormalities

10. Which of the following modalities of intrauterine evaluation is useful for differentiating aneurysm of the great vein of Galen from other anomalies such as colloid cysts, choroid plexus cysts, porencephalic cysts, and pineal tumors?
   (A) maternal serum alpha-fetoprotein
   (B) Doppler ultrasound examination
   (C) amniotic fluid alpha-fetoprotein level
   (D) intrauterine magnetic resonance imaging
   (E) fetal umbilical blood sampling

CHAPTER 17

THE CURRENT STATUS OF INTRAUTERINE NEUROSURGERY

1. What percent of fetuses with ventriculomegaly will have other associated abnormalities?
   (A) 20%-30%
   (B) 40%-50%
   (C) 60%-70%
   (D) 80%-90%

2. What is the risk of undetected fetal anomalies associated with ventriculomegaly?
   (A) 10%
   (B) 20%
   (C) variable, but probably >50%
   (D) >95%

3. After what point can anencephaly be diagnosed with a high degree of sensitivity?
   (A) 10 weeks' gestation
   (B) 12 weeks' gestation
   (C) 14 weeks' gestation
   (D) 16 weeks' gestation

4. The ultrasound finding most sensitive for ventriculomegaly is:
   (A) head circumference.
   (B) biparietal diameter.
   (C) lateral ventricular width.
   (D) lateral ventricular ratio.

5. At what age is ultrasound of the fetal ventricular system an accurate predictor of the development of hydrocephalus?
   (A) 14 weeks' gestation
   (B) 18 weeks' gestation
   (C) 22 weeks' gestation
   (D) 26 weeks' gestation

6. A single choroid plexus cyst measuring >5 mm in diameter is *not* associated with:
   (A) choroid plexus carcinoma.
   (B) lethal karyotypic abnormalities.
   (C) an inadvertent diagnosis of ventriculomegaly.
   (D) a benign clinical course.

7. The number of attempts at in utero cerebrospinal fluid diversion reported to the International Fetal Surgery Registry in the past 5 years is:
   (A) none.
   (B) five.
   (C) 10.
   (D) 15.

8. Which procedure or imaging study is not commonly used in prenatal diagnosis?
   (A) ultrasound
   (B) umbilical cord blood sampling
   (C) intrahepatic vein blood sampling
   (D) magnetic resonance imaging

9. The lateral ventricular ratio is defined as:
   (A) bicaudate width divided by lateral ventricular distance.
   (B) bicaudate width divided by hemispheric width.
   (C) lateral ventricular width divided by hemispheric width.
   (D) hemispheric width divided by lateral ventricular width.

CHAPTER 18

Treatment of the Pregnant Patient Who is Brain Dead or in a Permanent Vegetative State

1. The human state:
   (A) makes man unique.
   (B) must be defined to determine what is death.
   (C) resides in the brain.
   (D) resides in the neocortex.
   (E) all of the above

2. Death may be defined as:
   (A) permanent loss of brain function.
   (B) permanent loss of neocortical function.
   (C) loss of clinical brain function.
   (D) loss of electroencephalographic (EEG) recordings.
   (E) A and B

3. The most recently widely accepted criteria for brain death:
   (A) are the Harvard criteria.
   (B) are the criteria of the President's Commission.
   (C) are the same for children and adults.
   (D) require a specialist to confirm.
   (E) require laboratory testing.

4. The diagnosis of death requires:
   (A) cerebral unresponsivity.
   (B) an isotope cerebral blood flow study.
   (C) an EEG.
   (D) testing for apnea.
   (E) A and D

5. Brain death:
   (A) is accepted in Judeo-Christian thinking.
   (B) is accepted by law and court precedent.
   (C) may be difficult for a layman to understand.
   (D) precludes long-term support of vegetative functions.
   (E) A, B, and C

6. Consciousness:
   (A) can be easily defined.
   (B) arises from the neocortex.
   (C) does not require awareness of self.
   (D) requires a sleep-wake cycle.
   (E) is not an important subject to study.

7. Philosophy:
   (A) means "love of wisdom."
   (B) deals with ultimate reality.
   (C) deals with causes and principles.
   (D) encompasses bioethics.
   (E) all of the above

8. Bioethics:
   (A) is a form of moral philosophy.
   (B) began in its modern form in 1960.
   (C) arose because of technical developments relating to life support.
   (D) is studied at the Hastings Center and the Kennedy Institute.
   (E) all of the above

9. Bioethics as described by Beanchamp and Childress:
   (A) may be based on two theories: deontologic and utilitarian.
   (B) has four principles: paternalism, non maleficence, beneficence, and justice.
   (C) has several rules which are all encompassing.
   (D) involves ideals and character traits which are required.
   (E) makes it easy to come to conclusions.

10. A pleuralistic nation requires:
   (A) strict rules to ensure conformity.
   (B) everyone to submerge their personal convictions.
   (C) personal freedom and privacy.
   (D) freedom from all laws.
   (E) rapid resolution of conflicting ideas.

11. The patient:
   (A) has the right to any treatment he wants.
   (B) has the right to refuse treatment.
   (C) cannot refuse food and water.
   (D) cannot demand a physician give him specific treatments.
   (E) cannot spell out his wishes in advance.

12. The fetus:
   (A) attains human status at a defined time after conception.
   (B) has rights which supercedes the mother's.
   (C) has no moral obligations from the mother.
   (D) may survive birth as early as 23 weeks' gestation.
   (E) if aborted can be used by anyone as a brain tissue donor.

INDEX

Page numbers for figures and tables are followed by *f* and *t*, respectively.

A

B

C

D

E

F

G

H

K

L

M

N

W

Neurosurgical Aspects of Pregnancy

ANSWERS TO CME QUESTIONS

Chapter 1
1. A 2. E 3. C 4. D 5. E
6. C 7. A 8. D 9. B 10. D

Chapter 2
1. C 2. D 3. D 4. C 5. B
6. D 7. D 8. A 9 C 10. C

Chapter 3
1. E 2. D 3. C 4. E 5. B
6. E 7. A 8. D 9. B 10. C

Chapter 4
1. B 2. B 3. C 4. E 5. A
6. E 7. D 8. D 9. B 10. C

Chapter 5
1. E 2. C 3. B 4. E 5. D
6. C 7. B 8. B 9. D 10. C

Chapter 6
1. C 2. E 3. A 4. C 5. D
6. B 7. B 8. A 9. A 10. A

Chapter 7
1. B 2. B 3. C 4. D 5. A
6. C 7. A 8. B 9. B 10. B

Chapter 8
1. E 2. E 3. C 4. C 5. A
6. D 7. B 8. E 9. C 10. D

Chapter 9
1. D 2. E 3. C 4. C 5. B
6. E 7. A 8. D 9. D 10. D

Chapter 10
1. C 2. A 3. B 4. D 5. C
6. C 7. D 8. D 9. B 10. A

Chapter 11
1. A 2. C 3. C 4. B 5. C
6. B 7. A 8. A 9. C 10. A

Chapter 12
1. B 2. C 3. D 4. A 5. D
6. B 7. B 8. C

Chapter 13
1. C 2. B 3. D 4. B 5. B
6. B 7. C, D 8. A, B 9. E 10. E

Chapter 14
1. B 2. B 3. B 4. D 5. D
6. C 7. A 8. A 9. B 10. C

Chapter 15
1. B 2. A 3. E 4. C 5. C
6. D 7. A 8. F 9. B 10. E

Chapter 16
1. D 2. B 3. C 4. E 5. D
6. C 7. C 8. C 9. D 10. B

Chapter 17
1. C 2. C 3. C 4. D 5. D
6. A 7. A 8. D 9. C

Chapter 18
1. E 2. E 3. B 4. E 5. E
6. B 7. E 8. E 9. A 10. C
11. B 12. D

PREVIOUSLY PUBLISHED BOOKS IN THE *Neurosurgical Topics* SERIES

Endovascular Neurological Intervention
Edited by Robert J. Maciunas, MD

Benign Cerebral Glioma, Volume II
Edited by Michael L. J. Apuzzo, MD

Benign Cerebral Glioma, Volume I
Edited by Michael L. J. Apuzzo, MD

Contemporary Management of Spinal Cord Injury
Edited by Edward C. Benzel, MD, and Charles H. Tator, MD

Philosophy of Neurosurgery
Edited by Issam A. Awad, MD

Neurosurgical Emergencies, Volume II
Edited by Christopher M. Loftus, MD

Neurosurgical Emergencies, Volume I
Edited by Christopher M. Loftus, MD

Interactive Image-Guided Neurosurgery
Edited by Robert J. Maciunas, MD

Spinal Instrumentation
Edited by Edward C. Benzel, MD

Current Management of Cerebral Aneurysms
Edited by Issam A. Awad, MD

Spinal Trauma: Current Evaluation and Management
Edited by Gary L. Rea, MD, and Carole A. Miller, MD

Surgery of the Cranial Nerves of the Posterior Fossa
Edited by Daniel L. Barrow, MD

Degenerative Disease of the Cervical Spine
Edited by Paul R. Cooper, MD

Neurosurgery for the Third Millennium
Edited by Michael L.J. Apuzzo, MD

Cerebrovascular Occlusive Disease and Brain Ischemia
Edited by Issam A. Awad, MD

Practical Approaches to Peripheral Nerve Surgery
Edited by Edward C. Benzel, MD

Complications and Sequelae of Head Injury
Edited by Daniel L. Barrow, MD

Neurosurgical Aspects of Epilepsy
Edited by Michael L.J. Apuzzo, MD

Complications of Spinal Surgery
Edited by Edward C. Tarlov, MD

Contemporary Diagnosis and Management of Pituitary Adenomas
Edited by Paul R. Cooper, MD

Neurosurgical Treatment of Disorders of the Thoracic Spine
Edited by Edward C. Tarlov, MD

Intracranial Vascular Malformations
Edited by Daniel L. Barrow, MD

Malignant Cerebral Glioma
Edited by Michael L.J. Apuzzo, MD

Management of Posttraumatic Spinal Instability
Edited by Paul R. Cooper, MD

For order information before 1/20/96 call (708) 692-9500.
After 1/20/96 call (847) 692-9500.

Dr. Loftus is Professor of Surgery (Neurological Surgery) at the University of Iowa College of Medicine. His clinical and investigative interests are dedicated to cerebrovascular neurosurgery, and he currently serves as Secretary/Treasurer of the AANS/CNS Joint Section of Cerebrovascular Surgery. Dr. Loftus is the Editor-In-Chief of *Clinical Neurosurgery* and *Techniques in Neurosurgery* and serves on the editorial boards of *Neurosurgery* and the *Journal of Stroke and Cerebrovascular Diseases.*

Neurosurgical Aspects of Pregnancy is Dr. Loftus' seventh book and his third contribution to this series.

Publications Office
Gay Palazzo
Joanne B. Needham
Patti Lawson

Lebanon, NH

Compositor
Barbara Homeyer

Indexer
Linda Dorr